FOCUS ON NUTRITION RESEARCH

FOCUS ON NUTRITION RESEARCH

TONY P. STARKS
EDITOR

Nova Biomedical Books
New York

For permission to use material from this book please contact us:
Telephone 631-231-7269; Fax 631-231-8175
Web Site: http://www.novapublishers.com

NOTICE TO THE READER

The Publisher has taken reasonable care in the preparation of this book, but makes no expressed or implied warranty of any kind and assumes no responsibility for any errors or omissions. No liability is assumed for incidental or consequential damages in connection with or arising out of information contained in this book. The Publisher shall not be liable for any special, consequential, or exemplary damages resulting, in whole or in part, from the readers' use of, or reliance upon, this material.

Independent verification should be sought for any data, advice or recommendations contained in this book. In addition, no responsibility is assumed by the publisher for any injury and/or damage to persons or property arising from any methods, products, instructions, ideas or otherwise contained in this publication.

This publication is designed to provide accurate and authoritative information with regard to the subject matter cover herein. It is sold with the clear understanding that the Publisher is not engaged in rendering legal or any other professional services. If legal, medical or any other expert assistance is required, the services of a competent person should be sought. FROM A DECLARATION OF PARTICIPANTS JOINTLY ADOPTED BY A COMMITTEE OF THE AMERICAN BAR ASSOCIATION AND A COMMITTEE OF PUBLISHERS.

Library of Congress Cataloging-in-Publication Data
Focus on nutrition research / Tony P. Starks, editor.
    p. ; cm.
Includes bibliographical references and index.
ISBN 1-59454-768-8
1. Nutrition. 2. Malnutrition.
[DNLM: 1. Nutrition. 2. Malnutrition. QU 145 F652 2006] I. Starks, Tony P.
QP141.F65   2006
612.3--dc22   2005026637

Published by Nova Science Publishers, Inc. ✚New York

Contents

Preface   vii

Chapter I   **Nutraceuticals for Cardiovascular Protection**   1
                   Emily Payne, Louise Potts and Brian Lockwood

Chapter II   **Protective Effect of Vitamin C against Protein Modification in**
                   Brain: Its Importance to Neurodegenerative Conditions   33
                   Concepción Sánchez-Moreno and Antonio Martín

Chapter III   **Food Restriction Effects on Plasma Amino Acids, Myofibrillar**
                   Protein Profiles, Plasma and Muscle Free and Sterified Fatty
                   Acids on Monogastric and Ruminants: A Review   49
                   André Martinho de Almeida, Sofia van Harten and Luís Alfaro Cardoso

Chapter IV   **Food and Weight-Related Behaviours: Do Beliefs Matter More**
                   than Nutrition Knowledge?   71
                   Madeleine Nowak, Petra G. Buettner, David Woodward and Anna Hawkes

Chapter V   **Hypothalamic Serotonin in the Control of Food Intake:**
                   Physiological Interactions and Effect of Obesity   121
                   Eliane B. Ribeiro, Mônica M. Telles, Lila M. Oyama, Vera L.F. Silveira
                   and Cláudia M.O. Nascimento

Chapter VI   **Hypovitaminosis D in Elderly People Living in an Overpopulated**
                   City: Buenos Aires, Argentina   149
                   L. Plantalech, A. Bagur, J. Fassi, H. Salerni, M.J. Pozzo, M. Ercolano,
                   M. Ladizesky, C. Casco, S.N. Zeni, J. Somoza and B. Oliveri

Chapter VII   **The Intestinal Transportation of Zinc Sulfate and Zinc Methionine**
                   and Their Effects on Growth in Mice   165
                   Y.U. Ze-Peng, Shi Yong-Hui, L.E. Guo-Wei and L.I. Lu-Mu

Chapter VIII   **In Vivo and in Vitro Immunomodulatory Effects of Peptidoglycan**
                   Derived from *Lactobacillus*   187
                   Jin Sun, Guowei Le, Yonghui Shi, Xiyi Ma and Guanhong Li

Chapter IX   **Advances in the Diagnosis and Treatment of Feeding Disorders in**
                   Children with Developmental Disabilities   207
                   Steven M. Schwarz, William McCarthy and Mimi N. Ton

Index   223

Preface

Nutrition is the taking in and use of food and other nourishing material by the body. Nutrition is a 3-part process. First, food or drink is consumed. Second, the body breaks down the food or drink into nutrients. Third, the nutrients travel through the bloodstream to different parts of the body where they are used as "fuel" and for many other purposes. To give the body proper nutrition, a person has to eat and drink enough of the foods that contain key nutrients. This new book examines new research in this field which is belatedly receiving the proper attention.

Cardiovascular diseases (CVD) which affect the heart and circulatory system are known to cause millions of deaths each year worldwide, comprising the largest contribution to mortality in Europe and North America. As a result, in recent years high focus has been centred on developing new treatments and methods of prevention of CVD.

In addition to receiving appropriate pharmaceutical medicines to either reduce the risk of developing CVD or slow the rate of progression of CVD, individuals with a predisposition and those with established CVD are given advice relating to their dietary habits. This advice is based upon knowledge of the impact of the fat and cholesterol content of diet on the risk of developing coronary heart disease (CHD) which has been demonstrated in both epidemiology and laboratory-based research.

Over the past two decades the field of nutrition has evolved to consider how diet can be used to prevent and treat chronic disease states including CVD. Whilst classic essential nutrients remain the subject of many studies, there is growing interest in evaluating the biological health effects of a wide range of bioactive compounds.

Nutraceutical supplements which could be used safely to reduce the risk factors and decrease the chances of developing cardiovascular diseases, such as angina, myocardial infarction or heart failure, would be desirable and advantageous both to patients and healthcare providers.

A number of nutraceuticals have been claimed to be beneficial in the prevention or symptom reduction of cardiovascular disease, these include black and green tea and their flavonoids, soy protein and isoflavones, essential fatty acids, coenzyme Q10, lycopene, policosanol and pycogenol. The aim of chapter 1 is to look at this selection of nutraceutical compounds to determine what effects they have on the cardiovascular system and what evidence there is to support their use, both experimentally and clinically.

The debilitating consequences of age-related brain deterioration are extensive and extremely costly in terms of quality of life and longevity. One of the potential causes of age-related destruction of neuronal tissue appears to be caused by the free radicals-mediated toxic damage. Free radicals and other reactive oxygen species are derived either from normal essential metabolic processes in the human body or from external sources such as exposure to X-rays, ozone, cigarette smoking, air pollutants and industrial chemicals. The brain appears to be particularly susceptible to free radical attack because it generates more of these compounds per gram of tissue than any other organ in the body. Protein modification can be induced by several mechanisms including: oxidative cleavage of the peptide chain, oxidation of specific amino acid residues such as lysine, arginine, proline, and threonine, advanced glycation (reaction of reducing sugars with lysine). Protein modification results in cross-linking and aggregation, as well as loss of enzyme activity. Oxidative modification of proteins has been implicated in various neurodegenerative conditions including Alzheimer's disease (AD) and Parkinson's disease (PD). Modified amino acid residues have been detected in brains from Alzheimer's patients.

Chapter 2 explores the fact that recent studies have shown that various vitamin compounds with antioxidant-like properties can slow the progression of AD. In addition, vitamin C is also known to act as a scavenger of free radicals substances that play a role in causing diseases. Because of its redox potential, vitamin C, as an electron donor in biological systems, modulates several metabolic and enzymatic reactions. As a corollary of the "free radical hypothesis, oxidative modification, and cell function impairment", antioxidants that can inhibit protein oxidation may slow the progression of cognitive decline and neurodegenerative disease. In fact, significant reductions in vitamin C have been observed in patients with AD, vascular dementia (VD), and PD. Interestingly, vitamin C is present in brain's tissue at higher concentrations than any other tissue in the body. Therefore, better understanding of the roles of vitamin C in brain is important in the quest to improve its intake and recommendations.

Undernutrition is a major setback of animal production in the tropics. Progressive weight loss is characterized by a mobilization of body depots, especially fat and to a lesser extent protein. Muscle and therefore protein breaks down in order to supply amino acid as an energy source, generating a vast array of responses in serum free amino acid concentrations, myofibrillar protein (with special reference to Myosin Heavy Chains, Actin, Protein C, α Actinin and Tropomyosin + Troponin T) profiles and free fatty acids and fatty acids incorporated in triacylglycerol as a consequence of several factors: animal species and the severity of food restriction. The objective of chapter 3 is to present a review regarding these very important aspects of undernutrition. Several domestic animals species, both ruminant and monogastric will be considered with significance to both laboratory and farm animals. Special relevance will be given to works conducted at our group particularly on two experiments, first with laboratory rats and in a latter point *Boer goat* bucks in an applied prospective.

Western societies are faced with two diametrically opposed weight-related problems. Firstly, the average weight of their populations is rising, together with the health, social and economic problems associated with overweight and obesity. The rise in weight is probably due to a combination of: time constraints; readily available inexpensive prepared foods, beverages and snack foods; and lower activity levels due to energy saving devices and more sedentary leisure activities. Secondly, the slim image, prevalent in these societies, results in weight loss measures even among those who are not overweight. This unnecessary and unrealistic 'striving for slimness' may result in poor eating habits, inadequate dietary intake, needless psychological pressure, and eating disorders. Preoccupation with a slim body image and restrictive eating practices is not solely an issue among adult populations, but is also alarmingly prevalent in adolescents.

In order to better understand some of these issues, the authors of chapter 4 have examined the food, nutrition, weight and shape-related beliefs and behaviours of a group of adolescents in Northern Australia. In this chapter they: report on a study showing that beliefs of adolescents predict their weight loss behaviour; review information from the same population showing that beliefs are a better predictor of food choice than nutrition knowledge; and propose a model for food and weight related behaviour, which incorporates the individual's beliefs into the well established Transtheoretical Model of Change.

The hypothalamic serotonergic system has long been known to have an anorexigenic effect, which is likely to play a role in the control of energy homeostasis. Although the exact nature of the likely serotonergic influence on the pathogenesis of obesity remains unclear, the feeding-inhibition induced by central serotonergic stimulation has been the basis of many appetite suppressant drugs.

A complex network of hypothalamic factors has been shown to participate in the control of energy intake. This system includes anabolic effectors (which stimulate feeding), namely neuropeptide Y, orexins, melanin-concentrating hormone, and agouti-related protein, as well as catabolic effectors (which inhibit feeding), such as melanocyte-stimulating hormone, cocaine-and amphetamine-regulated transcript, corticotropin releasing hormone, and, most likely, serotonin. This system operates under the influence of peripherally borne adiposity/satiety signals, which include the adipocyte hormone leptin, the pancreatic hormone insulin, and the gastric hormone ghrelin. A large number of studies have been dedicated to elucidate the precise relationships among those multiple factors and their relevance to obesity.

Chapter 5 will focus on the available data concerning the interactions of serotonin with the anabolic and catabolic hypothalamic systems as well as its putative participation as a physiological target of the adiposity signals. The authors also consider the status of these interactions in rodent models of hypothalamic and genetic obesity.

Elderly people are susceptible to hypovitaminosis D. Bone loss and fractures have been associated with Vitamin D deficiency. Urban populations are prone to suffering Hypovitaminosis D due to the type of housing (large apartment buildings), lack of green spaces, and indoor lifestyle. In addition, low-income elderly subjects have been reported to be a risk population. The aim of the study in chapter 6 was to determine winter 25OHD serum levels of the non-institutionalized elderly population of a large overpopulated city, and to analyze their determining factors. The conclusion show that Hypovitaminosis D is common in elderly people living in a big city, as is the case of Buenos Aires, during winter; it is related to low sunlight exposure and poor intake of Vitamin D rich foods, which counteract seasonal changes in Vitamin D synthesis. Subjects with low income are most vulnerable.

The objective of chapter 7 was an experiment conducted to investigate the effect of zinc sulfate ($ZnSO_4$) and zinc methionine (Zn-Met) on growth and the expression of growth-related genes in mice; the further purpose was to study the transportation regulation of different zinc forms in the intestine of mice. The conclusion indicates Zn-Met could improve the weight gain efficiently by up-regulating the expression of IGF-I mRNA. It was deduced that there might be different transportation ways in organic and inorganic zinc base on their different effects on the expression of ZnTs, DCT1 and MT-1 gene.

The aim of chapter 8 was to show that the functioning of host immune system, at the systemic as well as local (gastraintestinal tract) level, can be influenced by signals provided by commensal-associated molecular patterns (CAMPs) of probiotics (such as Lactobacilli). Peptidoglycan (PG) is an important CAMP present on the cell surface of *Lactobacillus*. The purpose of this study was to evaluate the immunomodulatory activity of PG. derived from *Lactobacillus*. The conclusion of the study has demonstrated that PG derived from *Lactobacillus* possesses immunostimulating activity on healthy and tumor-inoculated mice. PG is responsible for certain immune responses induced by *Lactobacillus*. Anti-tumor effect of *Lactobacillus* is likely attributable to activation of MФ by PG expressed on the bacterial cell surface.

Feeding difficulties, secondary nutritional deficiencies and growth failure frequently complicate management and heighten morbidity for infants, children and adults with developmental disabilities. Oral-motor dysfunction, poor coordination of swallowing, esophageal motility disorders and aversive feeding behaviors represent common problems that comprise significant obstacles to growth, hinder the achievement of developmental potential and increase dependency upon both acute and chronic healthcare resources. The association between feeding disorders and significant malnutrition has been reported in up to 90% of non-ambulatory children with cerebral palsy. Failure to assess and treat these problems in a timely fashion results in malnutrition and growth failure, maximizes the risk of feeding-related complications, increases hospitalization rates and contributes to impaired quality of life.

In chapter 9, the authors consider the background and significance of feeding disorders in children with disabilities, and review their proposed diagnostic and therapeutic algorithm for managing these problems. The influences of diagnosis-specific management strategies on patient growth and clinical outcomes are evaluated, and newer methods for calculating energy requirements are discussed. Utilizing a diagnosis-specific approach, they recently reported their clinical experiences in a group of 79 children with moderate to severe motor and/or cognitive disabilities, who were referred for feeding problems. Their initial two-year follow-up data demonstrated that interventions directed at increasing energy intake significantly improved overall nutritional status and reduced clinical morbidity. Further clinical, nutritional and growth data were collected over a 5-year period, in 21 developmentally disabled children who required percutaneous endoscopic gastrostomy (PEG) feedings to achieve nutritional rehabilitation. At the conclusion of the monitoring period, 21 patients had undergone 109.3 patient-years of PEG feedings (mean 5.2 years, range 1-11 years). Gastrostomy feedings resulted in significant weight gain and were associated with marked improvements in body mass index (BMI) and BMI *Z*-scores. The data herein also confirm the authors' earlier observations, suggesting that reductions in feeding-associated morbidity and acute care hospitalization rates occurred as a consequence of aggressive nutritional management. The significance of these findings for subsequent treatment of feeding disorders in developmentally disabled children is discussed.

In: Focus on Nutrition Research
Editor: Tony P. Starks, pp. 1-32

ISBN 1-59454-768-8
© 2006 Nova Science Publishers, Inc.

Chapter I

Nutraceuticals for Cardiovascular Protection

Emily Payne, Louise Potts and Brian Lockwood
School of Pharmacy and Pharmaceutical Sciences,
University of Manchester,
Manchester M13 9PL
UK

Abstract

Cardiovascular diseases (CVD) which affect the heart and circulatory system are known to cause millions of deaths each year worldwide, comprising the largest contribution to mortality in Europe and North America [1]. As a result, in recent years high focus has been centred on developing new treatments and methods of prevention of CVD [2].

Nutraceutical supplements which could be used safely to reduce the risk factors and decrease the chances of developing cardiovascular diseases, such as angina, myocardial infarction or heart failure, would be desirable and advantageous both to patients and healthcare providers.

A number of nutraceuticals have been claimed to be beneficial in the prevention or symptom reduction of cardiovascular disease, these include black and green tea and their flavonoids, soy protein and isoflavones, essential fatty acids, coenzyme Q10, lycopene, policosanol and pycogenol. The aim of this review is to look at this selection of nutraceutical compounds to determine what effects they have on the cardiovascular system and what evidence there is to support their use, both experimentally and clinically.

The findings collated from the wide variety of *in vitro* experiments, animal studies and clinical trials previously discussed strongly suggest that supplementation of an individual's diet with certain of these nutraceuticals can have beneficial effects on cardiovascular health. Indeed, substantial evidence has been collected from studies involving soy protein supplementation of subjects' diets that the Food and Drug Administration gave their approval to the manufacturers of soy foods to use the health claim that consumption of at least 25g of soy protein per day is related to a reduced risk of developing CHD [55].

It is clear that there is the potential for benefit to be gained from the use of these nutraceutical supplements. Most are able to reduce various risk factors associated with cardiovascular diseases, such as cholesterol or hypertension, others are antiarrhythmic and therefore can reduce coronary heart disease mortality. However it is difficult to accurately define a recommended dosage, due to the fact that many of these nutraceuticals may be obtained as part of a healthy diet, resulting in some people having higher levels in their body compared to others. For effective cardiovascular protection, monitoring of plasma levels may be required before these products can be safely and effectively used to reduce cardiovascular disease.

Introduction

Cardiovascular diseases (CVD) which affect the heart and circulatory system are known to cause millions of deaths each year worldwide, comprising the largest contribution to mortality in Europe and North America [1]. As a result, in recent years high focus has been centred on developing new treatments and methods of prevention of CVD [2].

In addition to receiving appropriate pharmaceutical medicines to either reduce the risk of developing CVD or slow the rate of progression of CVD, individuals with a predisposition and those with established CVD are given advice relating to their dietary habits. This advice is based upon knowledge of the impact of the fat and cholesterol content of diet on the risk of developing coronary heart disease (CHD) which has been demonstrated in both epidemiology and laboratory-based research [3].

Over the past two decades the field of nutrition has evolved to consider how diet can be used to prevent and treat chronic disease states including CVD. Whilst classic essential nutrients remain the subject of many studies, there is growing interest in evaluating the biological health effects of a wide range of bioactive compounds [4].

Nutraceutical supplements which could be used safely to reduce the risk factors and decrease the chances of developing cardiovascular diseases, such as angina, myocardial infarction or heart failure, would be desirable and advantageous both to patients and healthcare providers.

A number of nutraceuticals have been claimed to be beneficial in the prevention or symptom reduction of cardiovascular disease, these include black and green tea and their flavonoids, soy protein and isoflavones, essential fatty acids, coenzyme Q10, lycopene, policosanol and pycogenol. The aim of this review is to look at this selection of nutraceutical compounds to determine what effects they have on the cardiovascular system and what evidence there is to support their use, both experimentally and clinically.

Black and Green Tea

The prevalence of flavonoids in tea has led to its use for long term prevention of CVD [5]. Being one of the most popular beverages in the world, second in consumption only to water, tea has been the subject of a vast array of biomedical research and clinical trials over the last decade [6]. In particular, discovery of the chemical composition of tea leaves, predominantly their high content of various classes of bioactive polyphenolic compounds known as flavonoids, fuelled intense research into the possible health benefits of drinking tea [7].

Tea is derived from the leaves of the *Camellia sinensis* plant, from which there are three different types of tea manufactured worldwide: black, green and oolong. In the production of green 'unfermented' tea, freshly harvested leaves are rapidly steamed or pan-fried. This procedure results in deactivation of naturally occurring polyphenol oxidase enzymes, thereby preventing fermentation of polyphenols present in the plant material [8]. The resultant product has a similar chemical composition to the fresh leaves, being rich in flavonoids, most notably catechins. It is the presence of these compounds within the prepared tea that is responsible for the characteristic colour and flavour of green tea [9]. Structures of the major constituents are outlined in Figure 1.

In contrast, black 'fermented' tea is produced by storing the harvested leaves at room temperature for several hours prior to rolling, cutting and drying them, a process that promotes the oxidation, and therefore fermentation, of the tea polyphenols [4]. During the fermentation process, simple catechin polyphenols are converted into more complex and condensed polyphenolic compounds including theaflavins and thearubigin polymers, making black tea a rich source of these particular flavonoids [9]. The chemical composition of most black teas varies slightly depending on the extent of fermentation undergone [10]. Partial fermentation following rolling of the plant leaves produces oolong tea, which contains monomeric catechins, theaflavins and thearubigins [10]. Some of the major flavonoids of black tea are outlined in Figure 2.

A number of epidemiological studies have evaluated the effect of tea consumption on the incidence of CVD. Initially centred on green tea, the focus of more recent research has shifted to also include black tea, and the findings of such studies and research are discussed in detail below.

Plasma Lipid-Lowering Activity of Tea

It has been proposed that consumption of both black and green teas is linked to reduced cholesterol and triglyceride plasma concentrations in humans [10]. Hypercholesterolaemia is a well-known risk factor for CVD, which suggests that ingestion of tea could exert a cardioprotective effect via its cholesterol-lowering potential [1, 6].

A recent study was conducted to determine the effects of black tea consumption on the blood lipid profiles of a group of mildly hypercholesterolaemic volunteers. The findings revealed that ingestion of 5 servings of black tea per day for a duration of 3 weeks reduced total cholesterol 6.5%, low-density lipoprotein (LDL) cholesterol 11.1%, apolipoprotein B 5% and lipoprotein(a) 16.4%, compared with a caffeine-containing placebo [11].

In addition, an inverse relationship between green tea consumption and serum cholesterol and triglyceride levels was identified in an earlier epidemiology study conducted in Japan. Whilst green tea did not lower the plasma total cholesterol levels of postmenopausal female subjects, male subjects were found to have decreased serum levels of both total cholesterol and triglycerides [12].

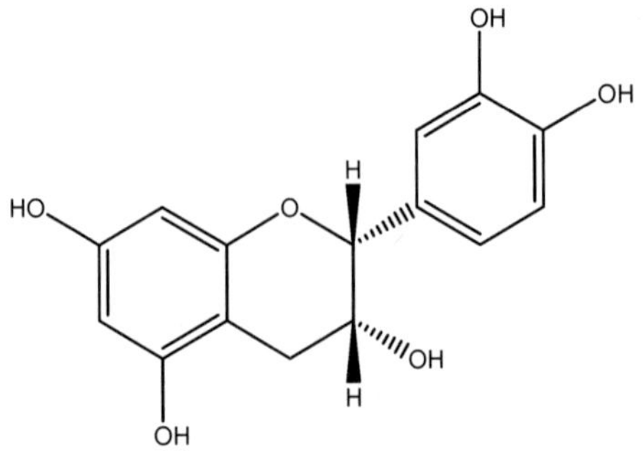

epicatechin

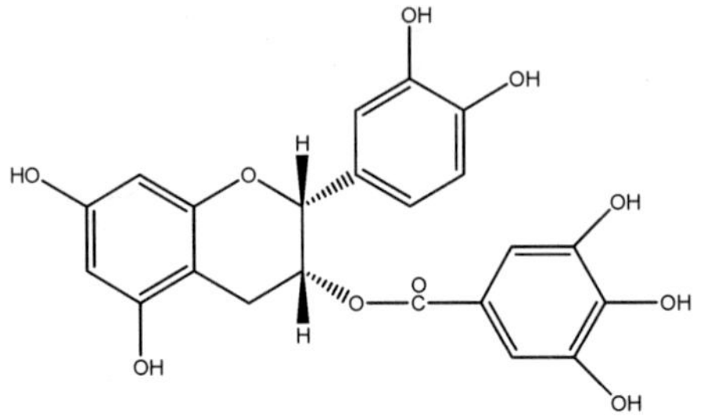

epicatechin gallate

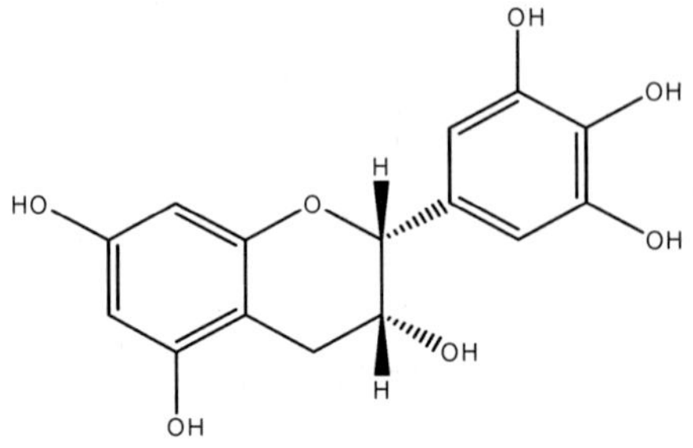

epigallocatechin

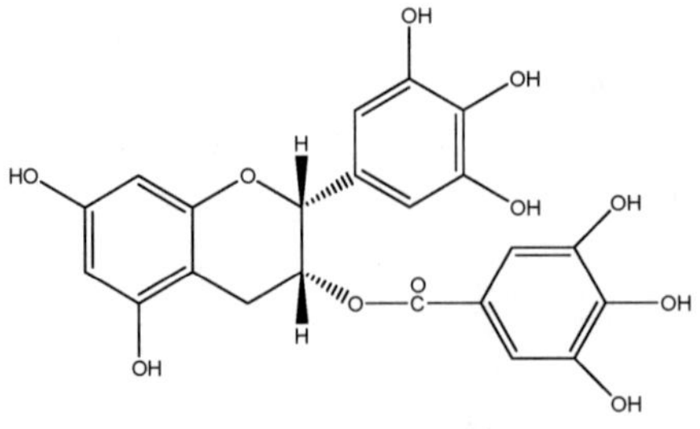

epigallocatechin gallate

Figure 1. The major catechins of green tea.

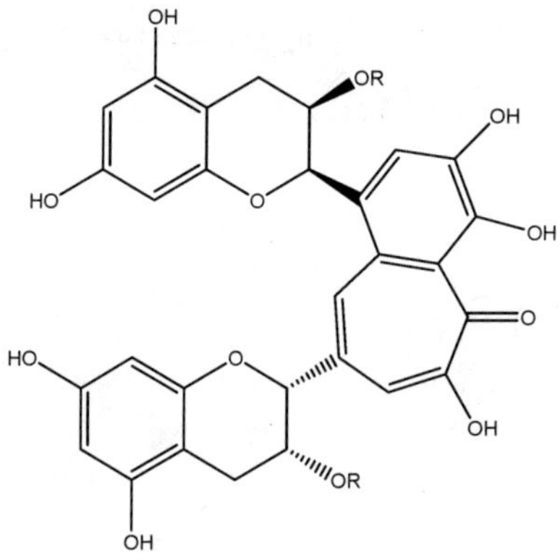

theaflavins

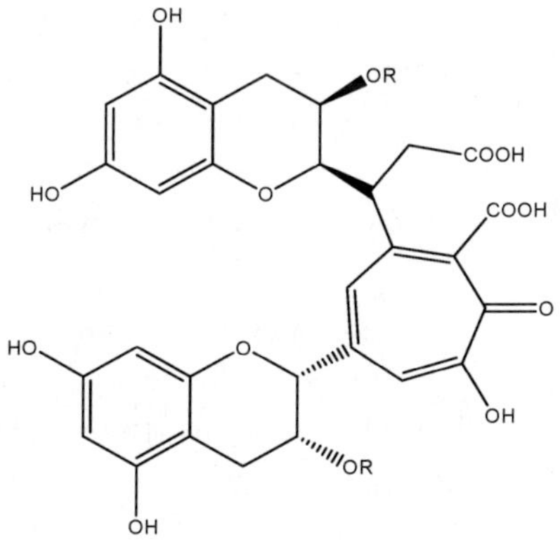

thearubigins

Figure 2. The major catechins of black tea.

Futhermore, a randomised controlled trial completed in China investigated the cholesterol-lowering effect of a theaflavin-enriched green tea extract on adults with mild to moderate hypercholesterolaemia. The results of the study showed that ingestion of the extract resulted in an 11.3% reduction in serum total cholesterol, and a 16.4% reduction in LDL cholesterol, compared to baseline measurements [6].

Animal studies involving rats showed that tea catechins reduced the absorption of cholesterol *in vivo* whilst precipitating cholesterol from micelles *in vitro*, indicating that the hypocholesterolaemic activity of tea could be linked to reduced intestinal absorption of cholesterol [6].

Further studies conducted with rodents have revealed that green tea catechins and black tea polyphenols may exert their hypocholesterolaemic activity via a number of mechanisms, including increased faecal excretion of fat and cholesterol, up-regulated LDL receptors in liver cells, and reduced hepatic cholesterol concentration [6]. However, additional research is necessary in order to determine if such mechanisms are also applicable to humans.

Whilst there is much evidence to suggest that drinking tea can help to lower cholesterol levels, several human-based trials have failed to identify any association between tea consumption and a more favourable lipid profile in subjects [6]. This suggests that more extensive research is needed to consolidate the findings of the trials detailed previously.

Effects of Tea Consumption on Endothelial Function

Endothelial cells that line blood and lymphatic vessels and the heart have an integral role in vascular homeostasis, mediating their effects via the production and release of certain locally acting chemical factors. Probably the most important of such factors, nitric oxide (NO) exerts a wide range of effects, partially due to its contribution to anti-inflammatory and anti-thrombotic processes, but primarily due to its role as a vasodilator [13].

If the normal functioning of endothelial cells is disrupted, a loss of NO is often observed, impairing vasodilator function in conduit arteries and resulting in an increased risk of developing CVD [13].

It is thought that increased antioxidant defences in the body and decreased production of reactive oxygen species may contribute to reduced breakdown and/or enhanced synthesis and release of endothelial-derived NO, thereby improving vascular function. This theory has been the subject of many studies that have considered the possible beneficial effects of tea consumption on endothelial function. In such studies, brachial artery flow-mediated dilation (FMD) was used as a marker of vasodilator function, which in turn reflects endothelial function [14].

One study reported that relative to ingestion of hot water, endothelium-dependent FMD improved approximately 41% in subjects with mildly elevated serum cholesterol or triglyceride concentrations, following black tea consumption [14]. Another study found that ingestion of black tea correlated with improved vascular function in patients with established coronary artery disease (CAD) [14]. In a further study, a 65% improvement in brachial artery FMD was observed following acute consumption of black tea; regular ingestion of black tea over a four week period was found to improve FMD 56%, whilst a 77% acute improvement was reported in those subjects who ingested black tea chronically [14].

As endothelial dysfunction is associated with a state of increased oxidative stress, it follows that ingestion of antioxidants could reverse the associated impaired vascular function [15]. Knowledge of the potent antioxidant properties of tea polyphenols has led to the belief that ingestion of tea may lead to enhanced endothelial function via a polyphenol-mediated reduction in oxidative stress [14].

However, the results of certain studies, considering the effect of tea on endothelium-independent vasodilation, have cast some doubt over the proposed mechanism by which improved vascular function is achieved following ingestion of tea. In some such studies, polyphenol antioxidants have proved to enhance vasodilation in response to glyceryl trinitrate, thereby indicating that the effects of tea polyphenols on vascular function are not solely restricted to improving endothelial function. Other proposed mechanisms include improved smooth muscle cell function and/or enhanced bioavailability of endogenously released NO [14].

Further research is necessary to determine the full range of mechanisms by which vascular function can be improved by black tea polyphenols. However, it is clear that the improvement of endothelial function that is observed following ingestion of tea contributes to this enhanced vascular function, suggesting one possible mechanism by which black tea consumption reduces the risk and/or extent of cardiovascular disease [14]. Future research could be extended to consider the potential effects of green tea extracts on endothelial function.

Tea Consumption and Atherogenesis

Over 6.5 million people worldwide die each year as a result of CHD – the majority of cases being attributable to atherosclerosis of the coronary arteries [1]. Various *ex vivo* epidemiological studies have shown that consumption of approximately two cups of black tea per day correlates with a decreased risk of developing CHD, and it is thought that this observation may be mediated by reduced incidence and degree of progression of atherogenesis in tea-drinking individuals [16].

The evidence collated from several animal studies and human trials supports this hypothesis. One such trial, conducted in Japan, found that consumption of green tea correlated with a reduced extent of atherosclerosis in both male and female subjects [8]. In addition, following consumption of black tea a reduction in early atherosclerosis was observed in hamsters that had been fed a saturated fat diet. In this animal model of atherosclerosis, an inverse association was also identified between green tea consumption and atherogenesis [8]. Furthermore, studies involving rabbits have shown that reduced atherosclerosis results from ingestion of either green or black tea [8].

In order to consider the possible mechanisms by which tea drinking could exert a beneficial effect on atherosclerosis, it is important to understand the trigger factors that are implicated in atherogenesis. It is thought that the oxidation of both LDL cholesterol and very low-density lipoproteins (VLDL) contributes to the development of atherosclerosis [8]. It can therefore be inferred that by preventing the oxidation of these plasma lipids, a corresponding reduction in atherogenesis will be observed.

Following consumption of tea, absorption of flavonoids into the bloodstream has been found to significantly increase the total radical-trapping antioxidant status of the plasma [16]. A range of *in vitro* studies has demonstrated that tea flavonoids are capable of inhibiting the oxidation of LDL cholesterol by virtue of their free-radical scavenging activity [10, 16]. Furthermore, a significant decrease in foam cell formation, the early form of atherosclerosis, was observed in the hamster model of atherosclerosis detailed previously following the independent consumption of green and black teas [8]. It is therefore plausible that consumption of tea can have beneficial effects on atherosclerosis, which could explain the mechanism by which green and black teas exert their protective effects against CHD.

Although there is substantial evidence to suggest that drinking tea can reduce an individual's risk of developing CHD, some trials have failed to provide a conclusive link between tea consumption and increased plasma antioxidant status [13]. This suggests that more research and *in vivo* studies are necessary in order to determine the full range of mechanisms by which tea flavonoids can exert a beneficial effect on atherosclerosis, thereby reducing the risk of CHD.

Anti-Hypertensive Activity of Tea

In many countries throughout the world, approximately 20 per cent of the adult population suffer from hypertension – the most common form of CVD [7]. High blood pressure presents as one of the greatest risk factors associated with cardiovascular-related death, and as such, hypertension has been the subject of many studies that look into the possible health-benefits associated with tea drinking [7].

Conflicting evidence has been yielded from human trials and animal studies that have focussed on the potential short-term effects of tea drinking on blood pressure. Human clinical trials conducted in both Australia and England failed to reveal a correlation between short-term consumption of high quantities of green or black tea and a drop in the subjects' blood pressures. However, animal studies conducted in Japan concluded that a substantial hypotensive effect was observed in rats following short-term supplementation of their diet with green tea extracts. Furthermore, an epidemiological study completed in Norway revealed that subjects experienced a fall in systolic blood pressure with increased consumption of black tea, whilst a further study conducted in Japan showed no relation between green tea intake and blood pressure [7].

The conflicting findings of the afore-mentioned epidemiological studies led to confusion over the real anti-hypertensive effect attributable to green and black teas. In an attempt to consolidate the evidence previously gathered, a further epidemiology-based study was initiated in 1996, involving the participation of the Chinese adult population of Taiwan [7]. The aim of this study was to examine the long-term effects of tea drinking on the risk of developing hypertension, taking into account various lifestyle and dietary factors which could also contribute to fluctuations in blood pressure [7].

The findings of this study contrasted those associated with the short-term clinical trials conducted in Australia and England, detailed previously. Overall, an inverse association was identified between consumption of tea and the subjects' mean blood pressures. Furthermore, it was noted that those participants who had consumed at least 120ml of tea per day for one year had a significantly lower risk of being diagnosed with hypertension than non-habitual tea drinkers. It was therefore concluded from this study that the threshold level of tea consumption that is likely to reduce the risk of developing hypertension would be 120ml or more of either green or oolong tea per day for at least one year [7].

Hypertension is characterised by increased peripheral vascular tone, which could be a result of endothelial dysfunction. A state of oxidative stress is also commonly observed in the hypertensive patient, where there is an abnormally high concentration of reactive oxygen species. It is thought that the presence of superoxide radicals could result in impaired nitric oxide synthesis, or even increased deactivation of NO, a theory that could explain the increased peripheral vascular resistance observed in hypertension [7].

It is well known that tea polyphenols, for example green tea catechins, act as potent antioxidants via free-radical scavenging, chelation of transition metals and inhibition of enzymes [10, 17]. Furthermore, green tea is amongst the top five plant extracts that have demonstrated the greatest ability to induce vascular smooth muscle relaxation [7].

It has therefore been proposed that green and oolong tea extracts exert their anti-hypertensive effects by reversing the endothelial dysfunction associated with hypertension, primarily via their antioxidant activity, and through their capacity to relax vascular smooth muscle [7].

Myocardial Infarction Incidence in Relation to Tea Consumption

Myocardial infarctions (MI) occur in patients who have established CHD where there is severe and/or prolonged impaired supply of oxygenated blood to the cardiac tissue. There are a wide range of risk factors associated with the development of CHD, including family history, hypertension, raised serum cholesterol, diabetes, smoking, poor diet and lack of exercise [1].

As previously discussed, tea consumption is thought to have beneficial effects against hypertension and serum cholesterol levels, as well as exerting anti-atherogenic effects and improving vascular function [7, 10]. In addition, flavonoids are believed to have anti-platelet and anti-thrombotic properties, which suggests that ingestion of tea could minimise the risk of developing CHD and of suffering a MI via a wide range of beneficial effects on the cardiovascular system [18].

The potential benefit of tea consumption against MI has been the subject of many epidemiological studies. The Boston Area Health Study reported that subjects who consumed at least one cup of black tea per day had roughly half the risk of suffering a MI compared with non tea-drinkers [10]. Another study found that ingestion of one or more cups of green tea per day correlated with a significant decrease in MI, despite an apparent lack of effect on CAD [10]. Likewise, the Zutphen Elderly Study claimed an inverse association between age-adjusted catechin intake and MI incidence, and a study involving the general Dutch population found that tea drinkers consuming more than 375ml per day had a lower relative risk of incident MI than non tea-drinkers [17, 18].

In addition, a meta-analysis of tea consumption in relation to MI, based on ten cohort studies and seven case-control studies, reported that an increase in tea consumption of three cups per day was associated with an 11% decrease in the incidence rate of MI [19].

Furthermore a prospective cohort study, involving 1,900 patients who had suffered an acute MI, concluded that post-MI mortality was lower amongst moderate to heavy tea drinkers (consuming more than 14 cups of tea per week) compared with non-drinkers [20].

However, the results of some studies are not consistent with the hypothesis that tea consumption reduces the incidence of MI. Several studies conducted within the US showed very little, if any, association between tea consumption and reduced MI incidence [19]. Furthermore, two studies conducted within the UK actually identified a positive correlation between tea consumption and CHD risk [19]. The lack of consistency in the findings of such studies indicates that further research is necessary in order to consolidate the preliminary evidence suggesting a beneficial effect of tea consumption on MI.

Soy

In 1999, the Food and Drug Administration gave their approval to the manufacturers of soy foods to use the health claim that consumption of at least 25g of soy protein per day is related to a reduced risk of developing CHD [21]. The granting of this approval stemmed from the knowledge that soy beans and the majority of soy protein products provide a rich source of phytoestrogen compounds known as isoflavones [22]. Figure 3 shows some of the major phytoestrogens of soy.

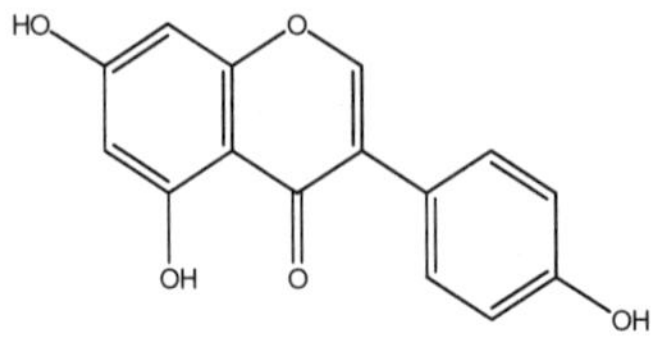

genistein

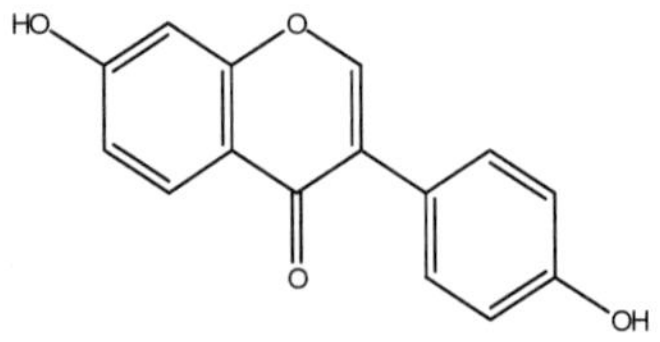

daidzein

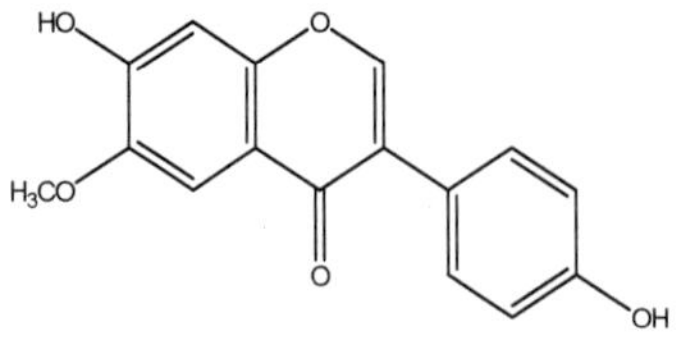

glycitein

Figure 3. The major phytoestrogens of soy.

A substantial number of recent clinical trials have considered the possible health-promoting effects of these isoflavones. One of the prime objectives of a number of these trials was to evaluate the reduction in CVD risk that is attributable to the isoflavone content of the soy protein used to supplement subjects' diets. The findings of such trials and the conclusions of further research are discussed in detail below.

Effects of Soy on Plasma Lipids

It has been claimed that ingestion of moderate quantities of soy protein can lower an individual's plasma cholesterol levels, thereby reducing their risk of developing CVD [23].

Whilst there remains some debate as to which compounds are responsible for the biological effects of soy proteins, the isoflavones are a strong candidate and as such, have been the subject of many animal studies and human trials considering the lipid-lowering effects of soy products [23].

The results of many animal studies have indicated that ingestion of isoflavone-rich soy protein is associated with decreased LDL and increased high-density lipoprotein (HDL) cholesterol plasma concentrations [2, 24]. However, the findings of several clinical trials have proved less conclusive [3].

Analysis of the data collected during a human intervention trial involving hypercholesterolaemic postmenopausal women showed significantly improved blood lipid profiles in those subjects receiving 40g of soy protein per day, which contained either moderate or high concentrations of isoflavones, compared to those receiving 40g of protein per day obtained from casein and nonfat dry milk [25].

In addition, an earlier study revealed that mildly hypercholesterolaemic men consuming 50g of soy protein daily experienced an 11-12% reduction in total and LDL cholesterol concentrations [25]. Another trial involving male subjects showed a 5-6% reduction in total cholesterol concentrations in those subjects consuming 25g of soy protein per day [25].

Several studies have compared the effects of isoflavone-rich soy protein and isoflavone-depleted soy protein on the plasma lipid profiles of subjects [23]. One such study found that consumption of isoflavone-rich soy protein significantly decreased total and LDL cholesterol levels in those subjects with the highest baseline LDL cholesterol concentrations [23]. A study of premenopausal women showed that subjects ingesting isoflavone-rich soy protein had lower LDL cholesterol concentrations and lower ratios of total to HDL cholesterol and of LDL to HDL cholesterol than did those subjects consuming isoflavone-depleted soy protein [23].

The findings of these studies support the hypothesis that the isoflavone content of soy protein is responsible for the cholesterol-lowering capacity of soy products that has been observed in many trials [3].

It has been proposed that isoflavones could exert their hypocholesterolaemic effect by virtue of their oestrogenic properties. Isoflavone compounds, in particular genistein and daidzein, are similar in both chemical structure and biological activity to endogenous oestrogen, possessing both the phenolic ring and the two hydroxyl groups that are essential for binding to oestrogen receptors [26].

Oestrogen replacement therapy in postmenopausal women is known to cause a decrease in their plasma cholesterol concentrations. It is therefore plausible that the oestrogenic activity of isoflavones could contribute to the reduction of cholesterol levels observed in mildly hypercholesterolaemic subjects receiving soy products rich in genistein and daidzein [5].

Other mechanisms implicated in the cholesterol-lowering activity of the isoflavones include altered thyroid status; enhanced bile acid excretion, leading to increased rates of cholesterol excretion; upregulation of LDL receptors; altered liver metabolism; and heightened levels of oestrogen resulting from competition between the endogenous hormone and the soy isoflavones for sex-hormone binding globulin proteins [3, 27-29].

Whilst there is substantial evidence to suggest that consumption of soy protein rich in isoflavones can lead to a more favourable plasma lipid profile in humans, a significant amount of conflicting evidence has been collated from additional clinical trials.

Two separate studies concluded that isoflavone intake had no significant effect on plasma lipid concentrations in normocholesterolaemic and hypercholesterolaemic subjects when compared with a placebo [2]. In addition, an eight-week intervention study, which involved healthy middle-aged subjects receiving dietary supplementation with 55mg of isoflavonoids per day in tablet form, found that the active tablets had no significant influence on serum lipid or lipoprotein concentrations when compared to the effects of the placebo tablets [5]. Furthermore, a trial that involved healthy volunteers receiving a four-week soy milk supplementation failed to identify any significant correlation between soy intake and altered serum cholesterol levels [30].

The inconsistencies in the evidence presented to date suggest that further research and trials are necessary to consolidate the generally accepted view that replacement of animal protein in the diet with soy protein could reduce plasma lipid and lipoprotein concentrations.

Soy Consumption and Vascular Function

It has been hypothesised that phytoestrogens may have a beneficial effect on vascular function by acting directly on vessel walls, perhaps via improved arterial compliance and enhanced FMD [28, 31]. Many animal studies and human trials have been conducted to test this hypothesis, investigating the improvement in vascular function that is attributable to the isoflavone component of soy products.

One trial involving normotensive male and postmenopausal female subjects found that a three-month dietary soy protein supplementation significantly improved distal pulse wave velocity, reflecting a reduction in the extent of vasoconstriction in peripheral resistance vessels. However, the same trial revealed that soy supplementation failed to have any affect on arterial compliance, and even correlated with a reduction in mean brachial artery FMD in male subjects [31].

Trials involving atherosclerotic female macaques have however provided more promising evidence. When assessed for their coronary vascular reactivity, administration of acetylcholine dilated the arteries of those monkeys receiving a diet rich in isoflavones, whereas vessel constriction was observed in those primates that were being fed a low isoflavone diet [3]. Subsequent intravenous administration of genistein to those animals receiving the low isoflavone diet proved to dilate previously constricted vessels, indicating that isoflavones can play an important role in vessel dilation [3].

Furthermore, one clinical trial demonstrated an increase in blood flow within the microcirculation of subjects' forearms following infusion of genistein into the brachial artery [28]. Another trial reported an improvement in brachial artery FMD in women who had been taking genistein for six months, whilst an additional trial observed a significant improvement in the systemic arterial compliance of perimenopausal subjects following administration of 45mg of genistein for a duration of five to ten weeks [3, 28].

The evidence collated from these studies suggests that consumption of soy products rich in isoflavones could lead to improved vascular function via a variety of mechanisms. Due to their similarities in structure to oestrogen, it is thought that soy isoflavones may mediate these effects by binding to beta oestrogen receptors present in the vasculature [28].

Oestrogen therapy is associated with improved large artery function, enhanced brachial artery FMD, and restoration of normal vasomotion in postmenopausal women [27, 31]. As previously discussed, impaired brachial artery FMD correlates with coronary artery endothelial dysfunction and is positively associated with cardiovascular risk factors [31]. It can therefore be concluded that via biological oestrogenic mechanisms, dietary soy could improve vascular function, hence reducing CVD risk [31].

Despite the promising results of some studies, conflicting findings of certain trials have cast some doubt over the true effects of soy isoflavones on vascular function. The observed effects of genistein on vascular reactivity indicate that the compound may be of some use in treating angina, however further trials are necessary to confirm this notion and to determine the true degree of benefit conferred to vascular function through consumption of soy [27].

Anti-Atherogenic Effects of Soy

Atherogenesis of the coronary arteries is one of the major contributing factors implicated in the pathogenesis of CHD [1]. Data collected from a range of experimental animal studies have indicated that diets rich in soy protein may have beneficial effects in preventing the onset and development of atherosclerosis, suggesting that ingestion of soy could result in a reduced risk of developing CHD [27].

One trial involving male and female cynomolgus monkeys reported that those fed a diet containing intact soy protein were found to have the least atherosclerosis whilst those fed protein from casein-lactalbumin had the most [27]. A third group of monkeys received soy protein isolates, from which the majority of isoflavones had been extracted, and were found to have only marginally less atherosclerosis than the casein-lactalbumin group. From the results of this study it was concluded that soy consumption could aid the prevention of atherosclerotic plaque development in monkeys. It was also suggested that this property of soy is likely to be attributable to its isoflavone content [27].

Based on these findings, a number of *in vitro* studies and human-based trials have been conducted with the aim of identifying mechanisms implicated in the anti-atherogenic activity of isoflavones.

As the trigger for a cascade of events including accelerated platelet aggregation, injury to arterial endothelial cells, and stimulation of foam cell and fatty streak development, LDL oxidation has a central role in the pathogenesis of atherosclerosis. It has therefore been suggested that prevention of this oxidation process could result in an improvement in atherosclerosis and interestingly, soy isoflavones are known to have antioxidant properties [32].

Studies in rats have shown that consumption of an isoflavone-rich soy-protein isolate results in significant inhibition of LDL oxidation. In addition, *in vitro* experiments have indicated that both genistein and daidzein cause inhibition of LDL oxidation in the vascular subendothelium [32]. It is thought that this antioxidative activity of the isoflavones can be attributed to their ability to scavenge free radicals, thereby reducing oxidative stress [3].

It has therefore been hypothesised that soy isoflavones may exert an anti-atherogenic effect in humans through inhibition of LDL oxidation – an essential process involved in the development of atherosclerosis – by nature of their antioxidant activity [27, 32]. Proposed alternative mechanisms include agonist activity at oestrogen receptors; reduction in hyperlipidaemia; inhibition of the migration and proliferation of smooth muscle cells by genistein; and inhibition of tyrosine kinase by genistein [27].

Further epidemiological trials are necessary in order to confirm the effect of soy consumption on atherosclerosis before health claims relating to reduced CHD risk can be made. In particular, the possible contribution of the metabolites of genistein and daidzein to the anti-atherogenic activity of soy products could be investigated further, as recent work has suggested that these metabolites in particular, may actually have a more potent inhibiting effect on LDL oxidation than the parent isoflavones themselves [33].

Effects of Soy Products on Blood Pressure

As the most common form of CVD, hypertension has been the focus of several trials that have compared the cardioprotective effects of ingestion of soy protein to those of animal protein consumption [7]. To date, conflicting evidence has been collated from these trials and has thus cast some confusion over the true improvement in blood pressure that can be derived from ingestion of soy protein.

In one study, consumption of a soy-based diet was found to attenuate the development of hypertension in spontaneously hypertensive rats [34]. Furthermore, trials in perimenopausal women have revealed that subjects' diastolic blood pressure was significantly reduced following dietary soy protein supplementation, whilst a three-month trial involving normotensive subjects concluded that soy protein supplementation correlated with a significant reduction in the systolic, diastolic and mean blood pressures of subjects [31, 34].

In an attempt to elucidate the real contribution of soy protein ingestion to a more favourable blood pressure profile in humans, a further trial involving male and female subjects with mild-to-moderate hypertension was conducted [34]. Subjects received 500ml of either soy milk or cow's milk twice daily for a three-month period. At the end of the trial, those subjects who had received soy milk were found to have significantly lower systolic, diastolic and mean blood pressures than their initial baseline values. Furthermore, these reductions proved to be of a greater magnitude than those observed in the subjects who received cow's milk [34].

Further data collected from this trial exposed a negative correlation between the decreases in blood pressure and the daily urinary isoflavonoid excretions that were observed in subjects. In particular, urinary excretion of genistein was found to strongly correlate with reductions in diastolic blood pressure, whilst lower systolic blood pressures tended to be associated with increased levels of urinary excretion of equol (a metabolite of daidzein) [34].

It was concluded from this trial that soy milk consumption successfully reduces blood pressure in subjects with mild-to-moderate hypertension, an effect thought to be mediated by the isoflavonoid component of soy. This theory is supported by the results of other studies that have indicated that both genistein and equol exert vasorelaxant and natriuretic effects in rats [34].

As previously mentioned, a state of oxidative stress is often associated with hypertension, and soy isoflavones are known to possess antioxidant properties [7, 32]. It has therefore been postulated that some of the hypotensive effects induced by soy products could be afforded to the antioxidant nature of their isoflavone content [34].

However, the data collected from one particular human trial, in which patients with essential hypertension received 55mg of isoflavonoids in tablet form per day for eight weeks, showed that ingestion of isoflavonoids failed to exert any significant hypotensive effect in subjects [34].

The findings of this trial contrast those of many other studies that have been conducted with the aim of investigating the potential anti-hypertensive activity of soy products. It is therefore clearly important that further research is undertaken in order to clarify the true degree of blood pressure-lowering activity that can be attributed to soy consumption. Additionally, future trials could focus on identifying the full range of mechanisms implicated in this activity, including the possible hypotensive effects of soy components other than the isoflavones [34].

n-3 and n-6 Essential Fatty Acids

It has been well documented that high levels of serum cholesterol are associated with atherosclerosis and an increased risk of developing cardiovascular complications. A high dietary intake of saturated fat is thought to increase cholesterol levels and increase this risk. Conversely, polyunsaturated fatty acids (PUFAs) of the n-3 and n-6 series are believed to be beneficial against coronary heart disease mortality [35]. Current advice recommends reducing cholesterol, saturated fat and trans fatty acid intake in preference to saturated fat, in order to reduce serum cholesterol levels by consuming a healthy diet [36].

The n-3 and n-6 essential fatty acids are not produced endogenously by the body, and have been established as important for neurodevelopment and vascular health, therefore it is crucial that sufficient amounts are obtained in the diet, or signs of clinical deficiency can be observed, therefore a constant dietary supply of both n-3 and n-6 PUFAS is needed to maintain health [37].

Linoleic acid (LA) is the primary n-6 PUFA, sources comprise vegetable oils including safflower, sunflower and corn oils [37]. It is extensively incorporated into phospholipid membranes and lipoproteins and can be elongated and desaturated *in vivo* to form other fatty acids such as arachidonic acid [35].

The n-3 fatty acid group consists of eicosapentaenoic acid (EPA), docosahexaenoic acid (DHA) and α-linolenic acid (ALA). EPA and DHA are found primarily in fish oils, ALA is found in vegetable oils such as soybean and canola oil. EPA and DHA can also be formed from the desaturation and elongation of ALA in the liver, although only a small percentage will be produced by this method. It is currently recommended to eat at least one portion of oily fish per week to meet the required dietary amount of n-3 PUFAs [38]. The structures of the major n-3 and n-6 PUFAs are shown in Figure 4.

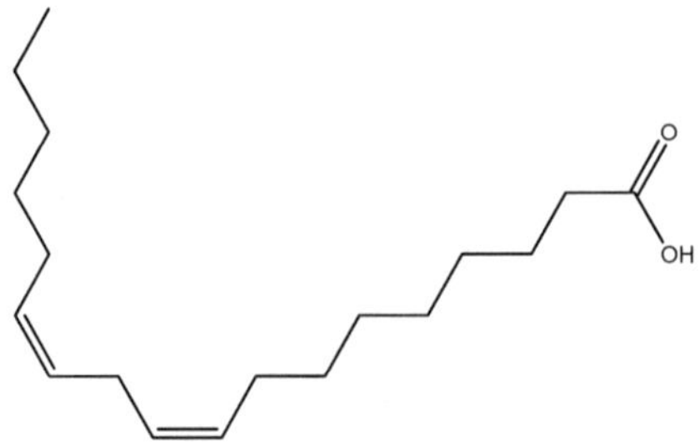

linoleic acid

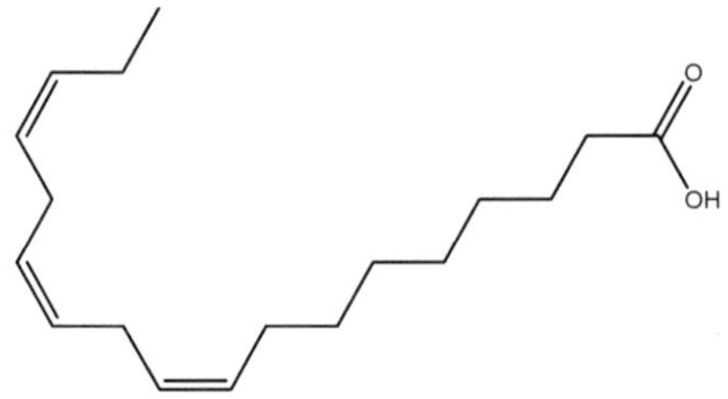

alpha-linolenic acid

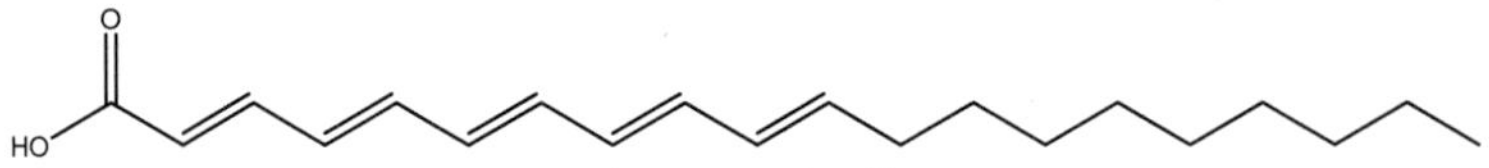

eicosapentaenoic acid

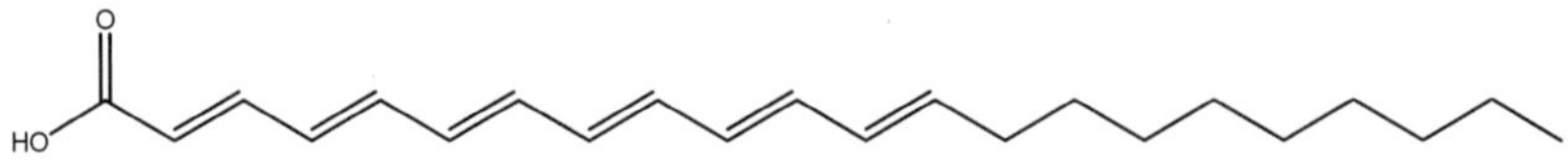

docosahexaenoic acid

Figure 4. Structures of the major PUFAs.

PUFAs of Vegetable Origin

LA is thought to be associated with a lower risk of cardiovascular disease mortality, probably through a cholesterol lowering effect and there have been many studies into the effects of n-6 PUFAs in this area. Many studies confirm beneficial effects and a reduction in mortality, while others report no benefit, or no relationship at all [38].

One study concluded that higher intake of LA protected against ischemic stroke. This was thought to be due to decreased blood pressure, reduced platelet aggregation and enhanced erythrocyte deformation, leading to improved microvascular circulation [39].

It is well known that LA has a cholesterol lowering effect, both total cholesterol and LDL is reduced by LA. This mechanism is possibly due to enhanced hepatic receptor-dependent clearance of LDL and a reduced LDL cholesterol production. LA intake must be above a certain critical threshold for this effect to be observed [35].

Overall there seems to be benefits in substituting saturated fats with n-6 PUFAs leading to a reduction in cardiovascular deaths, primarily through a cholesterol lowering effect.

ALA is thought to protect against cardiovascular disease. A study which looked at long-term increased intake of ALA and its effects on cardiovascular risk factors, found that long term ALA consumption was at least as effective as LA in reducing ischemic heart disease risk. Although in this case ALA increased serum triglycerides, it is thought that this effect is outweighed by the beneficial reduction in plasma fibrinogen concentration (and hence a possible antithrombotic effect) [40]. Another study carried out in Costa Rica found that there was a lower risk of non-fatal myocardial infarction when adipose tissue contained high levels on ALA. This was particularly true for individuals with a low dietary fish (and hence low EPA and DHA) consumption [41].

A recent study showed that higher consumption of ALA resulted in lower prevalence of carotid plaques and a reduced intima-media thickness of the carotid arteries. The mechanism by which this occurred was not known, but was thought to be as a result of the conversion of ALA to EPA and DHA [42]. The major problem with this type of study is that it is difficult to determine whether the results are due to ALA or other components of the diet.

A meta analysis of ALA in fatal coronary heart disease and prostate cancer concluded that ALA consumption might be associated with a reduced risk of coronary heart disease mortality, however it may also be associated with an increased risk of prostate cancer. At present this link has not been confirmed, it may be due to the consumption of ALA from different dietary sources, for example from meat intake, rather than a high vegetable oil intake, but evidence for this is so far contradictory. The protective effect of ALA on coronary mortality is thought to outweigh the risk of prostate cancer and in those at significant risk of cardiovascular disease, ALA consumption would still be recommended [43].

The mechanism of action of ALA is thought to be due to the influence of n-3 fatty acids on arrhythmias, inflammation and thrombosis, rather than on plasma lipids. ALA is not thought to be as effective as LA in modulating either LDL cholesterol production and clearance, or in increasing hepatic LDL receptor activity. ALA has however, been shown to reduce inflammatory markers associated with atherogenesis, such as C-reactive protein, interleukin-6 (IL-6) and serum amyloid A. The reported effects of ALA on thrombosis and platelet aggregation have so far been inconsistent [35].

The studies involving ALA suggest it does impart important protection from cardiovascular disease, however, it is still not certain whether the benefits of ALA are due to its inherent activity, or through its conversion to EPA and DHA [35].

PUFAs of Fish Origin

Fish is the main dietary source of EPA and DHA and fish consumption has consistently been shown to decrease risk of sudden cardiac death. One study looking into the relationship between fish consumption and heart rate saw a reduced heart rate in men who consumed fish. Adjusted heart rate was 67.5 beats per minute (bpm) in men who consumed fish less than once a week, but in those who consumed fish more than twice a week it was 65.6 bpm [44].

Other studies have found that n-3 PUFAs reduce pulse pressure and total vascular resistance [45] and DHA, but not EPA, was shown to reduce ambulatory blood pressure and heart rate [46]. Because an increased heart rate and high blood pressure are risk factors for sudden cardiac death this may explain the strong correlation between n-3 PUFAs and reduced cardiovascular mortality.

There have been numerous studies into the effects of n-3 PUFAs on cardiovascular mortality. One study found an increased intake of DHA, EPA and possibly ALA lowered the risk of fatal ischemic heart disease, but not non-fatal heart attacks. This was attributed to a possible antiarrhythmic action [47]. Further research concluded that fish oil derived PUFAs, reduce the risk of acute coronary events, but this effect may have been compromised by a high concentration of mercury present in some fish, which may increased the risk of myocardial infarction and accelerated atherosclerosis [48]. A meta-analysis of randomised controlled trials into this area suggested that a diet supplemented with n-3 PUFAs may decrease mortality due to myocardial infarction, sudden death and overall mortality in patients with coronary heart disease [49].

The protective effect of fish oils on cardiovascular mortality is thought to be due to several different mechanisms. EPA and DHA are antiarrhythmic agents which is due to the ability of n-3 fatty acids to prevent calcium overload in cardiac myocytes during periods of stress, where they have a membrane stabilising effect. In contrast to this the n-6 PUFAs are thought to be arrhythmogenic [50].

The decreased blood pressure and vascular resistance are due to an increased vascular function. EPA and DHA are thought to enhance NO production, NO is a potent vasodilator which relaxes arterial walls. It has also been shown that EPA and DHA reduce tumour necrosis factor-α and IL-6 and hence have an anti-inflammatory effect which may slow atherogenesis. In addition, EPA and DHA reduced atherosclerotic plaque development through the reduction of vascular adhesion molecules, for example vascular cell adhesion molecule-1 (VCAM-1). It is through a combination of these three mechanisms that EPA and DHA are thought to reduce coronary heart disease mortality [35].

The n-3 fatty acids have been shown to increase LDL cholesterol, but decrease very low density lipoprotein (VLDL) [51]. In addition EPA and DHA are hypotriacylglycerolemic agents, they have been shown to reduce plasma triglycerides through the inhibition of hepatic triglyceride and VLDL apoB secretion. For this reason it is thought that the other beneficial effects of n-3 PUFAs, rather than lipid metabolism, are responsible for the decreased risk of coronary mortality [35]. This is opposite to the proposed action of the n-6 fatty acids.

Finally, n-3 fish oil PUFAs have an antithrombotic effect, although at present this is not thought to contribute substantially to the antiatherogenic effect. A reduction of pro-aggregatory eicosanoids, such as thromboxane B2 occurs as a result of EPA competing in the arachidonic acid cascade, and prostacylin levels remain the same. Reduced platelet aggregation and reduced coagulation factors have also been observed, but the evidence to support this as a mechanism of reducing cardiovascular risk is contradictory at present [35].

In conclusion the n-3 PUFAs contribute to reducing mortality through several mechanisms, resulting in reduction in the risk factors such as raised blood pressure and cholesterol which are associated with cardiovascular diseases. An interesting finding in one study was that fish consumers were more educated, drank less alcohol, were less often smokers and were more physically active than non-consumers of fish. This indicates that there may be a combination of lifestyle factors which contribute to the reduced mortality in fish eaters [44]. It has been suggested that eating fish on a regular basis is responsible for most of the benefits of n-3 fatty acids [37]. However, for a person who consumes no fish in their diet it would presumably be advantageous to take a marine oil supplement.

The results of certain studies have been contradictory. Also it is thought ALA is associated with an increased risk of prostate cancer, but this link has not been found with the n-3 PUFAs from fish oils and it is thought these may even protect against prostate cancer [43]. For this reason fish should be the first recommended source of n-3 fatty acids, but possible high mercury content in fish may increase the risk of myocardial infarction. In people who do not want to consume fish oil, for example vegetarians, ALA would be a suitable alternative. One of the disadvantages of fish oil supplements is the fishy aroma they impart if not in soft capsules. Their use also has a burden on the environment, if used extensively it may lead to the depletion of certain fish species from the ocean. This would not be a problem with the plant derived ALA [43]. In all the trials the PUFAs have been well tolerated and no significant side-effects have been reported.

One of the main problems with the current studies in both the n-3 and n-6 PUFAs is that it cannot be determined whether the beneficial effects are due to the fatty acid directly or through its metabolic conversion, or whether the effects are due to improvements in lifestyle and diet, such as a reduction in saturated fat intake. As a high saturated fat intake is a specified risk factor for cardiovascular disease, substitution with alternative fatty acids such as PUFAs, may even lower this risk.

A range of structurally unrelated compounds have also been implicated in beneficial effects on CVD. These include coenzyme Q10, lycopene, policosanol, pycnogenol, melatonin and resveratrol, and their structures are shown in Figure 5.

Coenzyme Q10

Coenzyme Q10 (CoQ10), also known as ubiquinone, is an antioxidant, free radical scavenger and membrane stabiliser [50]. It is found endogenously in the body and is primarily located in the mitochondria of myocardium, liver and kidney cells [52]. It has been used for the treatment of cardiovascular diseases including heart failure, hypertension, angina and arrhythmias, but the evidence to support its use is contradictory.

Several studies indicate that CoQ10 may be moderately effective as a treatment for hypertension [53]. A trial in 1994 showed when the CoQ10 dose was adjusted to achieve a target blood concentration greater than $2\mu g/ml$, a significant reduction in blood pressure was obtained (159/94 to 147/85) and this suggested that some patients were able to discontinue their previous anti-hypertensive medications [53,54]. This study indicated that CoQ10 was

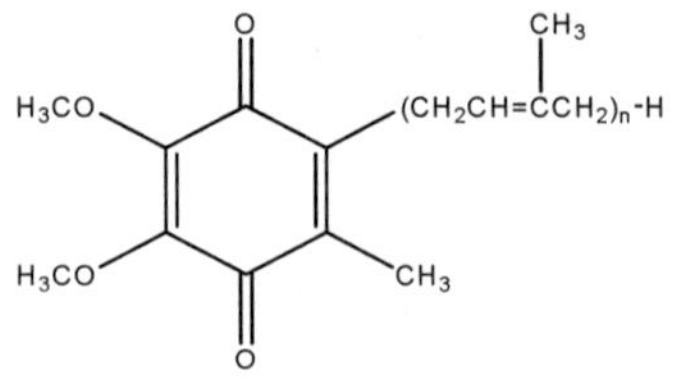

coenzyme Q10

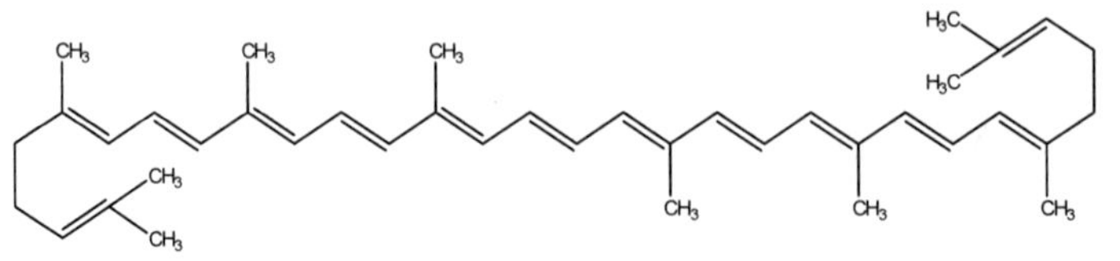

Lycopene

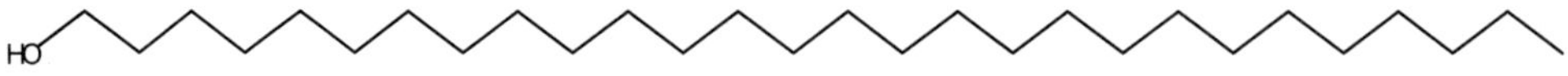

octacosanol

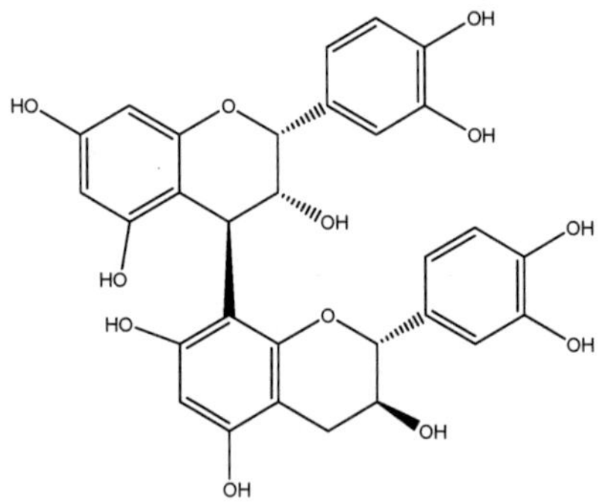

proanthocyanidin B3

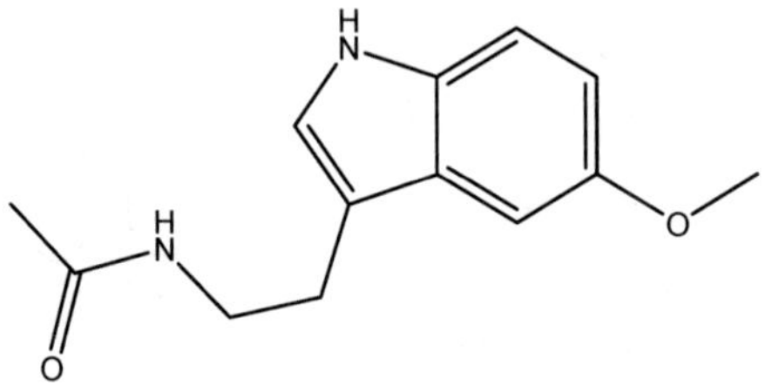

melatonin

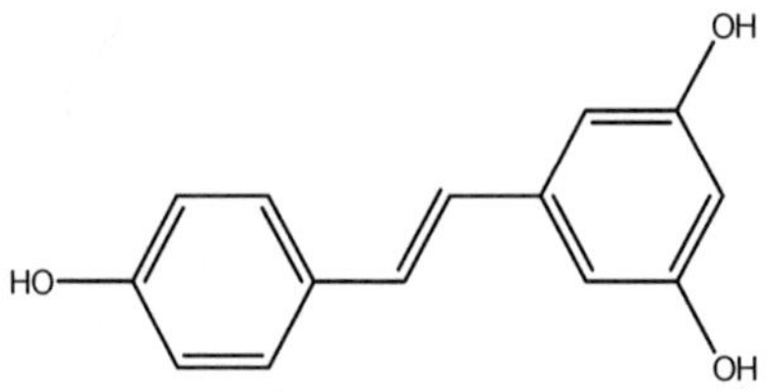

3,4',5-trihydroxystilbene

Figure 5. Coenzyme Q10, lycopene, policosanol, pycnogenol, melatonin and resveratrol, and their structures.

effective at lowering blood pressure, however, a mechanism of action has been more difficult to determine. It is thought that CoQ10 may decrease cytoplasmic redox potential by enhancing the efficiency of electron shuttle mechanisms, thereby optimising endothelial function by moderating the cytoplasmic NADH level [53]. More research is needed to prove or disprove this theory, but it is possible that CoQ10 may exert its beneficial effects through a variety of mechanisms.

It has been shown that patients with heart failure have lower levels of myocardial CoQ10 [52]. However the evidence is conflicting as to whether CoQ10 supplements are beneficial for patients with heart failure. One study claims that high dose CoQ10 administration will successfully manage refractory congestive heart failure. It showed that administration of CoQ10 improved the ejection fraction and functional status of the patient and it improved the patient's NYHA (New York Health Authority) heart failure classification. It also stated CoQ10 may improve quality of life, decrease cardiac complications and allow dose reduction in some of their other heart failure medications [55]. On the other hand, another study concluded that CoQ10 does not affect ejection fraction, peak oxygen consumption, or exercise duration in patients with congestive heart failure receiving standard medical therapy and it detected no objective benefit from CoQ10 supplementation [56]. In the former, more positive study, the dose was 300mg per day while in the latter study this was 200mg per day. There seems to be a large variation in the dosage that is needed to exert positive effects in different patients.

CoQ10 may also suppress arrhythmias. Reduced angina, improved ventricular function and reduced total arrhythmias were recorded as a result of administration of 120mg/day for 28 days [57].

Another trial looking at treatment of cardiomyopathy with CoQ10 reported symptomatic relief of dyspnoea, fatigue and chest pain and improvements in measurements of left ventricular thickness and diastolic function after administration sufficient to obtain CoQ10 levels greater than 2µg/ml. This is thought to be due to an improvement in cellular ATP production in cardiac myocytes [58].

Various studies consistently report that CoQ10 improves the recovery of the heart after stress. It appears CoQ10 improves the efficiency of mitochondrial energy production, so more energy is available for contractile function. Reduced troponin I release suggests CoQ10 reduces myocardial damage. Because of this it has been suggested that taking CoQ10 supplements prior to cardiac surgery is beneficial, it could result in increased cardiac recovery and reduced hospital stays [59].

In conclusion there seems to be contradictory evidence concerning the benefits of CoQ10 in many cardiovascular diseases. It is clear that more research is needed, involving larger numbers of people and the effects of increasing doses being investigated. There seems to be varying benefits in different people with lower doses, so it is suggested that serum blood levels should be at least 2.5µg/ml [60].

The potential benefits could be immense if CoQ10 proved to be efficacious, it is an endogenous compound, and no side-effects or tolerability problems have been reported. However, beta-blockers may reduce the efficacy of CoQ10, because they interfere with CoQ10 dependent enzymes [61] and statins have been reported to deplete CoQ10. Co-administration of CoQ10 with statins would counteract this depletion and may lead to an even greater reduction in cardiovascular disease and mortality [62].

It may also have benefits in other non-cardiovascular areas, it is thought CoQ10 deficiency may play a role in cerebellar ataxia [63]. CoQ10 could possibility be used prior to cardiac surgery, to increase cardiac recovery, decrease myocardial damage, prevent arrhythmias, decrease angina, lower blood pressure and overall improve the clinical outlook of the patient. If CoQ10 can successfully reduce some of the primary risk factors associated with cardiovascular disease, for example hypertension, it may help to prevent more serious complications, such as myocardial infarction.

Lycopene

Carotenoids are plant pigments which are found in many fresh fruits and vegetables, they are antioxidants and have long been considered to have protective effects in the body [64]. The carotenoid lycopene is an acyclic form of the antioxidant beta-carotene and it is thought to reduce the risks of coronary heart disease and cancer. This was originally attributed to its antioxidant properties, but further research has suggested other mechanisms, including modulation of intracellular gap junction communication; hormonal, immune system and metabolic pathways may also be involved [65].

Red fruits and vegetables are the most common sources of lycopene, for example tomatoes and tomato based products, watermelons, pink grapefruit and pink guava [64]. Lycopene is found in blood plasma and various tissues of the body, low levels of lycopene have been attributed to many chronic diseases. The recommended daily intake of lycopene is currently suggested to be 35mg daily [65]. A study on the lycopene content of tomatoes and tomato products and their contribution to dietary lycopene, concluded that most people do not meet the recommended daily intake requirements [66]. Hence there is the potential for lycopene to be used as a nutraceutical supplement.

To date, there has been limited research into the effects of lycopene in cardiovascular disease. A clinical trial in Finland, which investigated lycopene, atherosclerosis and coronary heart disease, concluded that men with low levels of serum lycopene have an increased intima-media thickness of the common carotid artery wall and an increased risk of acute coronary event or stroke. They concluded lycopene has a significant hypocholesterolemic effect [67], which is important as high cholesterol levels are a primary risk factor for cardiovascular disease. Another study looking at lycopene and myocardial infarction risk concluded that low levels of adipose tissue lycopene are associated with an increased risk of heart attacks [68].

Reactive oxygen species (ROS) and the oxidative damage they cause have been connected with the pathogenesis of various human chronic diseases, including atherogenesis and carcinogenesis [65]. Lycopene, because of its antioxidant and free radical scavenging activity is thought to slow the progression of atherosclerosis, through the inhibition of the oxidative processes which convert circulating LDL carrying cholesterol, to oxidised LDL. The oxidation of LDL is thought to be a key step in the atherogenic process, oxidised LDL is taken up by macrophages inside the arterial wall which leads to the formation of foam cells and atherosclerotic plaques [69].

Other mechanisms of action have also been proposed, including inhibition of hydroxymethylglutaryl coenzyme A (HMG-CoA) reductase and thereby inhibition of cholesterol synthesis, LDL degradation, alterations in the size and composition of LDL particles, plaque ruptures and altered endothelial functions [69]. More research is needed to determine what exact mechanisms of action this compound has.

In conclusion there is evidence to suggest lycopene is a beneficial compound in the prevention of coronary heart disease, which is most likely due to its antioxidant properties. However, there is a lack of studies looking specifically at lycopene and no studies have reported the tolerability, side-effects and drug interactions associated with this compound, particularly if taken in higher doses, although being an endogenous compound suggests these should be minimal. Further data is needed before this product could be considered for use clinically in the prevention of coronary heart disease. Trials are needed in subjects at high risk for cardiovascular disease, and in healthy individuals.

Policicosanol

Policosanol has been reported to lower plasma cholesterol. Elevated LDL cholesterol is a primary risk factor for cardiovascular disease and is a causative factor in atherosclerosis, which can lead to angina and/or myocardial infarction. It is important that patients with a serum cholesterol level above 5mmol/litre aim to lower this through dietary modification or lipid lowering drugs. Policosanol has the potential to be very important in this area and is thought to be just as effective as the currently available lipid lowering drugs, for example the statins [70]. Policosanol is already widely used in over 25 countries including Cuba, where it was developed, and in many Caribbean and South American countries [71].

Policosanol is a mixture of very long chain fatty alcohols and other constituents. It is obtained by solvent extraction and saponification mainly of sugarcane wax, but also of beeswax and spinach wax [72]. The main components are octacosanol, triacontanol and hexacosanol [71].

There have been more than 60 clinical trials to assess the effectiveness of policosanol as a lipid lowering agent and so far the results are very promising. One double-blind clinical trial undertaken in Cuba looking at the effect of policosanol in patients with type 2 hypercholesterolemia and additional coronary risk factors, showed policosanol 5 mg/day after 12 weeks of treatment significantly reduced serum LDL cholesterol by 18.2% and total cholesterol by 13.0%. In addition there was a significant increase in high density lipoprotein (HDL) cholesterol by 15.5%, and triglycerides remained unchanged [70]. These results are consistent throughout the various trials and people with hypercholesterolemia who took 5-10mg of policosanol per day for 6-8 weeks with dietary restrictions saw a reduction in LDL cholesterol by 18-22% and total cholesterol by 13-16%. Longer term studies show these cholesterol lowering effects were maintained for the length of the two year trial, with maximum reduction seen after 6-8 weeks of treatment. So far no trials with daily doses higher than 20mg per day have been undertaken, so the possibility that higher doses may have an even greater benefit is a possibility. Finally no rebound effects have been recorded after cessation [71].

The mechanism of action of policosanol is not well understood, but it is not thought to cause inhibition of HMG-CoA reductase, which is the main site of action of the statins. Experiments have shown that policosanol inhibits cholesterol biosynthesis from carbon-14 labelled acetate, but not from labelled mevalonic acid. This suggests cholesterol synthesis inhibition takes place at a step before mevalonate formation. In addition policosanol is thought to be involved in increasing hepatic LDL cholesterol uptake, through the increase in numbers of LDL receptors, and is believed to increase the serum LDL catabolic rates [70].

Other beneficial effects of policosanol have been reported, both animal experiments and human studies have shown that policosanol has an antiplatelet effect, by decreasing thromboxane B2 and increasing serum prostacyclin levels [70]. This might be the reason for the anti-ischemic effects of policosanol seen in animal studies. It has been suggested that the antiplatelet effect is equal to that of aspirin and a possible dual therapy use is a possibility, because it appears that policosanol has a different mechanism of action to that of aspirin [71]. This opens up new opportunities for further development of this nutraceutical.

In the clinical studies undertaken policosanol has been shown to be not only efficacious, but also well tolerated [70], and very few side-effects have been reported. During long term administration no clinical or biochemical adverse effects were identified; rarely weight loss, polyuria and headaches were described. Single doses of 1000mg have been given to healthy volunteers with no adverse events reported. In most of the trials the patients continued to take their usual medications (except lipid lowering drugs) and no drug interactions were reported, but no formal trials have been conducted into this area [71]. Overall policosanol is regarded as being safe, one trial demonstrated it as safe to use in non-insulin dependent diabetes mellitus patients [73]. Its use is not recommended in pregnancy or breast-feeding, or in children simply because of the lack of research into safety in this area [71].

In conclusion policosanol is a very promising supplement, which may have a use in many cardiovascular diseases. However further reliable clinical trials need to be undertaken to ensure that this product is safe and has no longer term side-effects (over many years), or serious drug interactions. Also a specified amount of each constituent needs to be decided, the formulations used in the trials so far have been variable, with differing amount of constituents being tested, making comparisons between the trials more difficult. With further research policosanol has the potential to be a very important natural drug therapy in the future.

Pycogenol

Pine bark has been used since the 4th century B.C. and Hippocrates mentioned its use against inflammatory diseases. More recently it has been reported to have cardiovascular effects, including vasorelaxant activity, angiotensin converting enzyme (ACE) inhibiting activity, and the ability to enhance microcirculation by increasing capillary resistance [74]. In a recent clinical trial it has also been shown to reduce LDL cholesterol [75].

Pycogenol is a specific blend of procyanidins, specifically oligomeric procyanidins such as proanthocyanidin B3, and other flavonoids and polyphenols, extracted form the bark of French marine pine (*Pinus maritima*). Its exact composition is unknown, but it seems to be the whole extract which is biologically effective, rather than any individual compound. There appears to be some synergistic interactions between the various components [74].

Pycogenol appears to have a wide variety of effects. A recent clinical trial showed supplementation with a pine bark extract increases the plasma antioxidant activity and alters the plasma lipoprotein profile. This study demonstrated that pycogenol has a significant antioxidant activity by increasing oxygen radical absorbance capacity (ORAC) in plasma. It also showed that pycogenol supplementation reduced LDL cholesterol and increased HDL cholesterol levels [41], therefore pycogenol has a role in reducing the risks of cardiovascular disease.

The reduction in LDL cholesterol levels is attributed to pycogenol's antioxidant activity. It inhibits LDL oxidation, in the same way that lycopene does [75].

Another trial showed that pycogenol improved the endothelial function of hypertensive patients. Supplementation with 100mg daily over 12 weeks helped to reduce the dose of nifedipine, a calcium channel antagonist, needed to control hypertension. It was thought that this antihypertensive effect was due to a variety of factors. After pycogenol was given, endothelin (a potent endogenous vasoconstrictor) levels decreased by 20%. There was also a decrease in thromboxane B2 levels, and an increase in the endothelial relaxing factor nitric oxide (NO). However there was no evidence to suggest that pycogenol acted as an ACE inhibitor [76]. The LDL cholesterol lowering action of pycogenol would also be of benefit in these patients.

One study investigating the effect of pycogenol in chronic venous insufficiency showed a significant reduction in the circumference of the lower limbs and improvement of subjective symptoms. This is due to pycogenol's stimulation of NO synthesis, leading to the relaxation of constricted blood vessels. By sealing leaky capillaries, due to the procyanidins' high affinity for proteins, pycogenol is thought to counteract edema [77].

An additional action of pycogenol is the inhibition of platelet aggregation induced by cigarette smoking. More studies are needed to determine the mechanism of action, but it is thought to be due to NO synthesis, induced by pycogenol, inhibiting thromboxane A2 production. Pycogenol is not thought to have the adverse effect on bleeding that aspirin has [74]. If pycogenol does not possess the side-effects associated with aspirin it could prove to be a valuable anti-aggregation agent.

Pycogenol has also been shown to stimulate lipolyis. Mature adipocytes exposed to pycogenol dispersed small (less than 20μm) lipid drops. This implies that pycogenol could be used to prevent obesity and therefore reduce another risk factor of cardiovascular disease [78].

In conclusion pycogenol has a wide variety of actions and has been shown to have positive effects on reducing many cardiovascular disease risk factors. It may also be beneficial in other areas, for example as an anti-inflammatory, in diabetic retinopathies or in Alzheimer's and Parkinson's disease. More clinical trials need to be conducted and safety data including side-effects, tolerability and drug interactions need to be investigated and a recommended dosage needs to be defined.

Melatonin

Research on animals, predominantly rats, has shown pharmacological doses of melatonin to overcome cardiac injury [79], and intraperitoneal doses as low as 75 µg/kg have been shown to be effective cardioprotectants when administered either before or during coronary occlusion [80]. Research carried out on humans supplemented with 3mg melatonin in tablet formulation, revealed significantly increased plasma melatonin concentrations peaking at 75minutes after ingestion (1830 ± 848 pg/ml), compared to 14 ± 11 pg/ml before ingestion. It was found that the melatonin attenuated the reflex sympathetic increases that occur in response to orthostatic stress, apparently mediated by melatonin induced changes to the baroreflexes [81].

Resveratrol

Resveratrol is a stilbene found in grapes and red wine, and has been shown to inhibit the peroxidation of LDL by both chelating and free radical scavenging mechanisms. The most widely accepted mechanism for resveratrol-mediated cardioprotection is its ability to inhibit platelet aggregation. At a physiological concentration of 3.6 µg/L, resveratrol was able to lower platelet aggregation by ~ 50% in healthy volunteers [82]. There is a possibility that the cardioprotective effects of resveratrol may be contributed to by the fact that it inhibits endogenous cholesterol biosynthesis, by inhibition of squalene monooxygenase [83].

Conclusion

The findings collated from the wide variety of *in vitro* experiments, animal studies and clinical trials previously discussed strongly suggest that supplementation of an individual's diet with certain of these nutraceuticals can have beneficial effects on cardiovascular health. Indeed, substantial evidence has been collected from studies involving soy protein supplementation of subjects' diets that the Food and Drug Administration gave their approval to the manufacturers of soy foods to use the health claim that consumption of at least 25g of soy protein per day is related to a reduced risk of developing CHD [55].

There are currently many different formulated green tea and soy nutraceutical products available for consumers to purchase. With the introduction of government campaigns like the '5-A Day' program, designed to increase public awareness of the need for a healthy lifestyle and diet, combined with ever-increasing knowledge of the potential health benefits attributable to certain dietary factors and the publication of new dietary recommendations, it is possible that such nutraceutical products will become commonplace adjuvants to many individuals' healthy lifestyles in the near future [38].

It is clear that there is the potential for benefit to be gained from the use of these nutraceutical supplements. Most are able to reduce various risk factors associated with cardiovascular diseases, such as cholesterol or hypertension, others are antiarrhythmic and therefore can reduce coronary heart disease mortality. However it is difficult to accurately define a recommended dosage, due to the fact that many of these nutraceuticals may be obtained as part of a healthy diet, resulting in some people having higher levels in their body compared to others. For effective cardiovascular protection, monitoring of plasma levels may be required before these products can be safely and effectively used to reduce cardiovascular disease.

References

[1]   Walker R, Edwards C. Clinical Pharmacy and Therapeutics. Third Edition. London: *Churchill and Livingstone; 2003.*

[2]   Merz-Demlow BE, Duncan AM, Wangen KE, Xu X, Carr TP, Phipps WR, Kurzer MS. Soy isoflavones improve plasma lipids in normocholesterolemic, premenopausal women. *American Journal of Clinical Nutrition 2000;* 71: 1462-1469.

[3]   Lichtenstein AH. Soy protein, isoflavones and cardiovascular disease risk. *Journal of Nutrition 1998*; 128: 1589-1592.

[4]   Kris-Etherton PM, Keen CL. Evidence that the antioxidant flavonoids in tea and cocoa are beneficial for cardiovascular health. *Current Opinion in Lipidology 2002*; 13: 41-49.

[5]   Hodgson JM, Puddey IB, Beilin LJ, Mori TA, Croft KD. Supplementation with isoflavonoid phytoestrogens does not alter serum lipid concentrations: a randomized controlled trial in humans. *Journal of Nutrition 1998*; 128: 728-732.

[6]   Maron DJ, Lu GP, Cai NS, Wu ZG, Li YH, Chen H, Zhu JQ, Jin XJ, Wouters BC, Zhao J. Cholesterol-lowering effect of a theaflavin-enriched green tea extract. A randomized controlled trial. *Archives of Internal Medicine 2003*; 163: 1448-1453.

[7]   Yang YC, Lu FH, Wu JS, Wu CH, Chang CJ. The protective effect of habitual tea consumption on hypertension. *Archives of Internal Medicine 2004*; 164: 1534-1540.

[8]   Vinson JA, Teufel K, Wu N. Green and black teas inhibit atherosclerosis by lipid, antioxidant, and fibrinolytic mechanisms. *Journal of Agriculture and Food Chemistry 2004*; 52: 3661-3665.

[9]   Mukhtar H, Ahmad N. Tea polyphenols: prevention of cancer and optimizing health. *American Journal of Clinical Nutrition 2000*; 71: 1698S-1702S.

[10]   Siddiqui IA, Afaq F, Adhami VM, Ahmad N, Mukhtar H. Antioxidants of the beverage tea in promotion of human health. *Antioxidants and Redox Signaling 2004*; 6: 571-582.

[11]   Davies MJ, Judd JT, Baer DJ, Clevidence BA, Paul DR, Edwards AJ, Wiseman SA, Muesing RA, Chen SC. Black tea consumption reduces total and LDL cholesterol in mildly hypercholesterolemic adults. *Journal of Nutrition 2003*; 133: 3298S-3302S.

[12]   Nakachi K, Matsuyama S, Miyake S, Suganuma M, Imai K. Preventive effects of drinking green tea on cancer and cardiovascular disease: epidemiological evidence for multiple targeting prevention. *BioFactors 2000*; 13: 49-54.

[13]   Vita JA. Tea consumption and cardiovascular disease: effects on endothelial function. *Journal of Nutrition 2003*; 133: 3293S-3297S.

[14] Hodgson JM, Puddey IB, Burke V, Watts GF, Beilin LJ. Regular ingestion of black tea improves brachial artery vasodilator function. *Clinical Science 2002*; 102: 195-201.

[15] Duffy SJ, Keaney JF Jr, Holbrook M, Gokce N, Swerdloff PL, Frei B, Vita JA. Short- and long-term black tea consumption reverses endothelial dysfunction in patients with coronary artery disease. *Circulation 2001;* 104: 151-156.

[16] Rietveld A, Wiseman S. Antioxidant effects of tea: evidence from human clinical trials. *Journal of Nutrition 2003*; 133: 3285S-3292S.

[17] Arts ICW, Hollman PCH, Feskens EJM, Bas Bueno de Mesquita H, Kromhout D. Catechin intake might explain the inverse relation between tea consumption and ischemic heart disease: the Zutphen Elderly Study. *American Journal of Clinical Nutrition 2001*; 74: 227-232.

[18] Geleijnse JM, Launer LJ, van der Kuip DAM, Hofman A, Witteman JCM. Inverse association of tea and flavonoid intakes with incident myocardial infarction: the Rotterdam study. *American Journal of Clinical Nutrition 2002*; 75: 880-886.

[19] Peters U, Poole C, Arab L. Does tea affect cardiovascular disease? A meta-analysis. *American Journal of Epidemiology 2001*; 154: 495-503.

[20] Mukamal KJ, Maclure M, Muller JE, Sherwood JB, Mittleman MA. Tea consumption and mortality after acute myocardial infarction. *Circulation 2002*; 105: 2476-2481.

[21] Lichtenstein AH, Jalbert SM, Adlercreutz H, Goldin BR, Rasmussen H, Schaefer EJ, Ausman LM. Lipoprotein response to diets high in soy or animal protein with and without isoflavones in moderately hypercholesterolemic subjects. *Arteriosclerosis, Thrombosis, and Vascular Biology 2002*; 22: 1852-1858.

[22] Setchell KDR, Brown NM, Lydeking-Olsen E. The clinical importance of the metabolite equol – a clue to the effectiveness of soy and its isoflavones. *Journal of Nutrition 2002*; 132: 3577-3584.

[23] Wangen KE, Duncan AM, Xu X, Kurzer MS. Soy isoflavones improve plasma lipids in normocholesterolemic and mildly hypercholesterolemic postmenopausal women. *American Journal of Clinical Nutrition 2001*; 73: 225-231.

[24] Sanders TAB, Dean TS, Grainger D, Miller GJ, Wiseman H. Moderate intakes of intact soy protein rich in isoflavones compared with ethanol-extracted soy protein increase HDL but do not influence transforming growth factor ($_1$ concentrations and hemostatic risk factors for coronary heart disease in healthy subjects. *American Journal of Clinical Nutrition 2002*; 76: 373-377.

[25] Potter SM, Baum JA, Teng H, Stillman RJ, Shay NF, Erdman JW Jr. Soy protein and isoflavones: their effects on blood lipids and bone density in postmenopausal women. *American Journal of Clinical Nutrition 1998*; 68: 1375S-1379S.

[26] Dewell A, Hollenbeck CB, Bruce B. The effects of soy-derived phytoestrogens on serum lipids and lipoproteins in moderately hypercholesterolemic postmenopausal women. *Journal of Clinical Endocrinology and Metabolism 2002*; 87: 118-121.

[27] Anthony MS, Clarkson TB, Williams JK. Effects of soy isoflavones on atherosclerosis: potential mechanisms. American Journal of Clinical Nutrition 1998; 68: 1390S-1393S.

[28] Nestel P. Role of soy protein in cholesterol-lowering. How good is it? *Arteriosclerosis, Thrombosis, and Vascular Biology 2002*; 22: 1743-1744.

[29] Han KK, Soares JM Jr, Haidar MA, Rodrigues de Lima G, Baracat EC. Benefits of soy isoflavone therapeutic regimen on menopausal symptoms. *Obstetrics and Gynecology 2002;* 99: 389-394.

[30] Mitchell JH, Collins AR. Effects of a soy milk supplement on plasma cholesterol levels and oxidative DNA damage in men – a pilot study. *European Journal of Nutrition 1999*; 38: 143-148.

[31] Teede HJ, Dalais FS, Kotsopoulos D, Liang Y, Davis S, McGrath BP. Dietary soy has both beneficial and potentially adverse cardiovascular effects: a placebo-controlled study in men and postmenopausal women. *Journal of Clinical Endocrinology and Metabolism 2001*; 86: 3053-3060.

[32] Anderson JW, Smith BM, Washnock CS. Cardiovascular and renal benefits of dry bean and soybean intake. *American Journal of Clinical Nutrition 1999*; 70: 464S-474S.

[33] Anthony MS, Clarkson TB. Association between plasma isoflavone and plasma lipoprotein concentrations. *Journal of Medicinal Food 1999*; 2: 263-266.

[34] Rivas M, Garay RP, Escanero JF, Cia P Jr, Cia P, Alda JO. Soy milk lowers blood pressure in men and women with mild to moderate essential hypertension. *Journal of Nutrition 2002*; 132: 1900-1902.

[35] Wijendran V, Hayes K. Dietary n-6 and n-3 fatty acid balance and cardiovascular health. *Annual Review of Nutrition 2004*; 24: 597-615.

[36] Hoffman DR. Fatty acids and visual dysfunction. *Food Science and Technology* (New York) (2000), 96(Fatty Acids in Foods and Their Health Implications (2nd Edition)), 817-841.

[37] Uauy R, Valenzuela A. Marine oils: Benefits of n-3 fatty acids. *Nutrition 2000*; 16: 680-684.

[38] Demaison L, Moreau D. Dietary n-3 polyunsaturated fatty acids and coronary heart disease-related mortality: a possible mechanism of action. *Cellular and Molecular Life Sciences 2002*; 59: 463-477.

[39] Iso H, Sato S, Umemura U, Kudo M, Koike K, Kitamura A, Imano H, Okamura T, Naito Y, Shimamoto T. Linoleic acid, other fatty acids and the risk of stroke. *Stroke 2002*; 33: 2086-2093.

[40] Bemelmans W, Broer J, Feskens E, Smit A, Muskiet F, Lefrandt J, Bom V, May J, Meyboom-de Jong B. Effect of an increased intake of α-linolenic acid and group nutritional education on cardiovascular risk factors: the Mediterranean Alpha-Linolenic Enriched Groningen Dietary Intervention (MARGARIN) study. *American Journal of Clinical Nutrition 2002;* 75: 221-227.

[41] Baylin A, Kabagambe E, Ascherio A, Spiegelman D, Campos H. Adipose tissue α-linolenic acid and non-fatal acute myocardial infarction in Costa Rica. *Circulation 2003;* 107: 1586-1591.

[42] Djoussé L, Folsom A, Province M, Hunt S, Ellison R. Dietary linolenic acid and carotid atherosclerosis: the National Heart, Lung and Blood Institute Family Heart Study. *American Journal of Clinical Nutrition 2003;* 77: 819-825.

[43] Brouwer I, Katan M, Zock L. Dietary α-linolenic acid is associated with a reduced risk of fatal coronary heart disease, but increased prostate cancer risk: a meta-analysis. *Journal of Nutrition 2004*; 134: 919-922.

[44] Dallongeville J, Yarnell J, Ducimetière P, Arveiler D, Ferrieres J, Montaye M, Luc G, Evans A, Bingham A, Hass B, Ruidavets J, Amouyel P. Fish consumption is associated with lower heart rates. *Circulation 2003*; 108: 820-825.

[45] Nestle P, Shige H, Pomeroy S, Cehun M, Raederstorff D. The n-3 fatty acids eicosapentaenoic acid and docosahexaenoic acid increase systemic arterial compliance in humans. *American Journal of Clinical Nutrition 2002*; 76: 326-330.

[46] Mori T, Bao D, Burke V, Puddey I, Beilin L. Docosahexaenoic acid but not eicosapentaenoic acid lowers ambulatory blood pressure and heart rate in humans. *Hypertension 1999*; 34: 253-260.

[47] Lemaitre R, King I, Mozaffarian D, Kuller L, Tracy R, Siscovick D. n-3 polyunsaturated fatty acids, fatal ischemic heart disease and non-fatal myocardial infarction in older adults: the Cardiovascular Health Study. *American Journal of Clinical Nutrition 2003*; 77: 319-325.

[48] Rissanen T, Voutilainen S, Nyyssönen K, Lakka T, Salonen J. Fish oil-derived fatty acids, docosahexaenoic acid and docosapentaenoic acid and the risk of acute coronary events. *Circulation 2000*; 102: 2677-2679.

[49] Bucher H, Hengstler P, Schindler C and Meier G. N-3 polyunsaturated fatty acids in coronary heart disease: A meta-analysis of randomised controlled trials. *The American Journal of Medicine 2002*; 112: 298-304.

[50] Chung M. Vitamins, Supplements, Herbal medicines, and Arrhythmias. *Cardiology in Review 2004*; 12: 73-84.

[51] Rivellese A, Maffettone A, Vessby B, Uusitupa M, Hermansen K, Berglund L, Louheranta A, Meyer B, Riccardi, G. Effects of dietary saturated, monounsaturated and n-3 fatty acids on fasting lipoproteins, LDL size and post-prandial lipid metabolism in healthy subjects. *Atherosclerosis 2003*; 167: 149-158.

[52] Witte K, Clark A, Cleland J. Chronic Heart Failure and Micronutrients. *Journal of the American College of Cardiology 2001*; 37:1765-1774.

[53] McCarty M. Coenzyme Q versus Hypertension: does CoQ decrease endothelial superoxide generation? *Medical Hypotheses 1999*; 53: 300-304.

[54] Langsjoen P, Langsjoen P, Willis R, Folkers K. Treatment of essential hypertension with coenzyme Q10. *Molecular Aspects of Medicine 1994*; 15: S265-S272.

[55] Sinatra S. Refractory congestive heart failure successfully managed with high dose coenzyme Q10 administration. *Molecular Aspects of Medicine 1997*; 18: S299-S305.

[56] Khatta M, Alexander B, Krichten C, Fisher M, Freudenberger R, Robinson S, Gottlieb S. The effect of coenzyme Q10 in patients with congestive heart failure. *Annals of Internal Medicine 2000;* 132: 636-640.

[57] Singh R, Wander G, Rastogi A, Shukla P, Mittal A, Sharma J, Mehrotra S, Kapoor R, Chopra R. Randomised, double-blind placebo-controlled trial of coenzyme Q10 in patients with acute myocardial infarction. *Cardiovascular Drugs and Therapy 1998*; 12: 347-353.

[58] Langsjoen P, Langsjoen A, Willis R, Folkers K. Treatment of hypertropic cardiomyopathy with coenzyme Q10. *Molecular Aspects of Medicine 1997*; 18: S145-S151.

[59] Rosenfeldt F, Pepe S, Linnane A, Nagley P, Rowland M, Ou R, Marasco S, Lyon W, Esmore D. Coenzyme Q10 protects the aging heart against stress, studies in rats human tissues and patients. *Annals of the New York Academy of Sciences 2002*; 959: 355-359.

[60] Langsjoen P, Folkers K, Lyson K, Muratsu K, Lyson T, Langsjoen P. Effective and safe therapy with coenzyme Q10 for cardiomyopathy. *Klinische Wochenschrift 1988;* 66: 583-590.

[61] Kishi T, Kishi H, Folkers K. Inhibition of cardiac CoQ10-enzymes by clinically used drugs and possible prevention. In: Folkers K, Yamamura Y eds. *Biomedical and Clinical aspects of Coenzyme Q. Vol 1.* Amsterdam: Elsevier/ North Holland Biomedical Press; 1977: 47-62.

[62] Preedy V, Mantle, D. Adverse effect on coenzyme Q10 levels. *Pharmaceutical Journal 2004*; 272:13.

[63] Lamperti C, Naini A, Hirano M, De Vivo D, Bertini E, Servidei S, Valeriani M, Lynch D, Banwell B, Berg M, Dubrovsky T, Chiriboga C, Angelini C, Pegoraro E, DiMauro S. Cerebellar ataxia and coenzyme Q10 deficiency. *Neurology 2003*; 60: 1206-1208.

[64] Rao A, Agarwal S. Role of lycopene as antioxidant carotenoid in the prevention of chronic diseases: A Review. *Nutritional Research 1999*; 19: 305-323.

[65] Rao A, Agarwal S. Role of antioxidant lyopene in cancer and heart disease. *Journal of the American College of Nutrition 2000*; 19: 563-569.

[66] Rao A, Waseem Z, Agarwal S. Lycopene content of tomatoes and tomato products and their contribution to dietary lycopene. *Food Research International 1998*; 31: 737-741.

[67] Rissanen T, Voutilainen S, Nyyssönen K and Salonen J. Lycopene, atherosclerosis and coronary heart disease. *Experimental Biology and Medicine 2002*; 227: 900-907.

[68] Kohlmeier L, Kark J, Gomez-Gracia E, Martin B, Steck S, Kardinaal A, Ringstad J, Thamm M, Masaev V, Riemersma R, Martin-Moreno J, Huttunen J, Kok F. Lycopene and myocardial infarction risk in the EURAMIC study. *American Journal of Epidemiology 1997*; 146: 618-626.

[69] Rao A. Lycopene, tomatoes and the prevention of coronary heart disease. *Experimental Biology and Medicine 2002*; 227: 908-913.

[70] Más R, Castaño G, Fernandez L, Illnait J, Fernandez J, Alvarez E. Effects of policosanol in patients with type II hypercholesterolemia and additional coronary risk factors. *Clinical Pharmacology and Therapeutics 1999*; 65: 439-447.

[71] Gouni-Berthold I and Berthold H. Policosanol: Clinical pharmacology and therapeutic significance of a new lipid lowering agent. *American Heart Journal 2002*; 143: 356-365.

[72] Hargrove J, Greenspan P, Hartle D. Nutritional significance and metabolism of very long chain fatty alcohols and acids from dietary waxes. *Experimental Biology and Medicine 2004*; 229: 215-226.

[73] Torres O, Agramonte A, Illnait J, Mas Ferreiro F, Fernandez L, Fernandez J. Treatment of hypercholesterolemia in NIDDM with policosanol. *Diabetes Care 1995*; 18: 393-397.

[74] Packer L, Rimbach G, Virgili F. Antioxidant activity and biologic properties of a procyanidin-rich extract from pine (*Pinus maritima*) bark, pycnogenol. *Free Radical Biology and Medicine 1999*; 27: 704-724.

[75] Devaraj S, Vega-López S, Kaul N, Schonlau F, Rohdewald P, Jialal I. Supplementation with a pine bark extract rich in polyphenols increases plasma antioxidant capacity and alters the plasma lipoprotein profile. *Lipids 2002*; 37: 931-934.

[76] Liu X, Wei J, Tan F, Zhou S, Würthwein G, Rohdewald P. Pycogenol, French maritime pine bark extract, improves endothelial function of hypertensive patients. *Life Sciences 2004*; 74: 855-862.

[77] Koch R. Comparative study of venostasin and pycnogenol in chronic venous insufficiency. *Phytotherapy Research 2002*; 16: S1-S5.

[78] Hasegawa N. Stimulation of lipolysis by pycnogenol. *Phytotherapy Research 1999*; 13: 619-620.

[79] Reiter R J, Tan D-X. Melatonin: a novel protective agent against oxidative injury of the ischemic/reperfused heart. *Cardiovascular Research 2003*; 58: 10-19.

[80] Chen Z, Chua C C, Gao J, Hamdy R C, Chua B H L. Protective effect of melatonin on myocardial infarction. *American Journal of Physiology 2003*; 284: H1618-H1624.

[81] Ray C A. Melatonin attenuates the sympathetic nerve responses to orthostatic stress in humans. *Journal of Physiology 2003*; 551: 1043-1048.

[82] Bhat K P L, Kosmeder J W II, Pezzuto J M. Biological effects of resveratrol. *Antioxidants and Redox Signaling 2001*; 3: 1041-1064.

[83] Laden B P, Porter T D. Resveratrol inhibits human squalene monooxygenase. *Nutrition Research 2001*; 21: 747-753.

In: Focus on Nutrition Research
Editor: Tony P. Starks, pp. 33-48

ISBN 1-59454-768-8
© 2006 Nova Science Publishers, Inc.

Chapter II

Protective Effect of Vitamin C against Protein Modification in Brain: Its Importance to Neurodegenerative Conditions

Concepción Sánchez-Moreno[1]* and Antonio Martín[†]
*Department of Plant Foods Science and Technology,
Instituto del Frío-CSIC, Madrid, Spain
[†] Nutrition and Neurocognition Laboratory,
Jean Mayer USDA-Human Nutrition Research Center
on Aging at Tufts University, Boston, MA, USA

Abstract

The debilitating consequences of age-related brain deterioration are extensive and extremely costly in terms of quality of life and longevity. One of the potential causes of age-related destruction of neuronal tissue appears to be caused by the free radicals-mediated toxic damage. Free radicals and other reactive oxygen species are derived either from normal essential metabolic processes in the human body or from external sources such as exposure to X-rays, ozone, cigarette smoking, air pollutants and industrial chemicals. The brain appears to be particularly susceptible to free radical attack because it generates more of these compounds per gram of tissue than any other organ in the body. Protein modification can be induced by several mechanisms including: oxidative cleavage of the peptide chain, oxidation of specific amino acid residues such as lysine, arginine, proline, and threonine, advanced glycation (reaction of reducing sugars with lysine). Protein modification results in cross-linking and aggregation, as well as loss of

[1] Corresponding author: Concepción Sánchez-Moreno, Department of Plant Foods Science and Technology, Instituto del Frío, Consejo Superior de Investigaciones Científicas (CSIC), C/ José Antonio Novais 10, Ciudad Universitaria, E-28040 Madrid, SPAIN, Tel.: +34 915492300 - +34 915445607, Fax: +34 915493627, E-mail: csanchezm@if.csic.es, Website: http://www.if.csic.es

enzyme activity. Oxidative modification of proteins has been implicated in various neurodegenerative conditions including Alzheimer's disease (AD) and Parkinson's disease (PD). Modified amino acid residues have been detected in brains from Alzheimer's patients. Recent studies have shown that various vitamin compounds with antioxidant-like properties can slow the progression of AD. In addition, vitamin C is also known to act as a scavenger of free radicals substances that play a role in causing diseases. Because of its redox potential, vitamin C, as an electron donor in biological systems, modulates several metabolic and enzymatic reactions. As a corollary of the "free radical hypothesis, oxidative modification, and cell function impairment", antioxidants that can inhibit protein oxidation may slow the progression of cognitive decline and neurodegenerative disease. In fact, significant reductions in vitamin C have been observed in patients with AD, vascular dementia (VD), and PD. Interestingly, vitamin C is present in brain's tissue at higher concentrations than any other tissue in the body. Therefore, better understanding of the roles of vitamin C in brain is important in the quest to improve its intake and recommendations.

Keywords: vitamin C, protein modification, neurodegeneration

Introduction

Vitamin C is one of the most fundamental vitamins for health and prevention of disease. Vitamin C (ascorbic acid), first identified in citrus fruits, prevents scurvy, one of the oldest scourges of mankind, and it is an essential micronutrient required for normal metabolic functioning of the body. The role of vitamin C and citrus fruits in conquering scurvy represents one of the most thrilling chapters in the development of nutrition as a science. All animal species appear to require vitamin C, but a *dietary need* is limited to humans, guinea pigs, and monkeys, among others, because these species lack the enzyme L-gulonolactone oxidase, which is necessary for vitamin C synthesis from 6-carbon sugars. Patients with scurvy usually have a plasma vitamin C level less than 0.1 mg/dL, equivalent to 6 μmol/L. These low blood levels of vitamin C are observed in only 2% of the patient population. However, there is evidence regarding low vitamin C levels in apparently healthy individuals, less than 0.35 mg/dL (lower than 20 μmol/L), which is common among elders and appears to be associated with detrimental effects on immunity responses and cognition [Foy et al., 1999, Ramakrishna, 1999, Rosenberg and Miller, 1992]. In fact, vitamin C concentrations have long been reported to decrease with age and with certain pathologic processes [Ramakrishna, 1999, Riviere et al., 1998, Rosenberg and Miller, 1992].

The molecular mechanisms of the vitamin C role in brain are poorly understood. Although vitamin C is a cofactor for several enzymes involved in the biosynthesis of collagen and neurotransmitters, vitamin C is the most efficient antioxidant in biological fluids. Vitamin C is used as a cofactor for the biosynthesis of catecholamines, in particular the conversion of dopamine to norepinephrine, which is catalyzed by β-monooxygenase. Interestingly, several changes in mood disorders and depression often occur during scurvy, which may be due to deficiency in dopamine hydroxylation.

Several studies have investigated the role of vitamin C in cognitive performance in humans and different animal models, and have found, for the most part, a positive association, with low levels correlated to low memory performance [Deschamps et al., 2001]. A few studies have looked at sex- and age-matched community-dwelling and hospitalized patients with severe AD, moderate AD, or no AD. When these studies evaluated the nutritional status of the subjects and measured their levels and intakes of vitamin C, they found that in patients with AD, plasma levels of vitamin C decreased in proportion to the severity of cognitive impairment, despite similar vitamin C intakes. Using the Mini Mental exam for psychological evaluation and plasma albumin to evaluate nutritional status, in general, hospitalized individuals with AD had lower Mini Mental exam scores than did community-dwelling subjects. Furthermore, nutritional evaluation of these patients indicated that, although their vitamin C intake was adequate, their plasma vitamin C concentration was lower than that of community-living subjects [Riviere et al., 1998]. Plasma levels of vitamin C have been reported by several studies to be lower in people with AD in proportion to the degree of cognitive impairment; and yet this observation is not explained by lower vitamin C intake. Some studies have suggested that this nutrient may be recommended in generous concentrations in persons with AD to modulate cells' response or perhaps to combat oxidative stress. Mounting evidence indicates that an increased intake of fruits and vegetables with high concentration of vitamin C is associated with a reduced risk of chronic diseases such as cancer, cardiovascular disease, and cataract, however, the mechanisms that mediate these benefits remain poorly understood; antioxidant mechanisms have been proposed as one of the key players of its actions.

Vitamin C is present in human tissues in significant concentrations and in some tissues, such as suprarenal gland and brain, its concentration reaches several fold higher than other tissues and blood. Vitamin C is present in the extracellular fluids at the μmol/L level and is transported across the membrane into the cell where it can be found in mmol/L concentration. This transport exhibits a saturable kinetics. Physiologically, ascorbate provides electrons for enzymes, for chemical compounds that are oxidants, and for other electron acceptors. Ascorbic acid is the most widely cited form of water-soluble antioxidant and prevents oxidative damage to cell membranes induced by aqueous radicals. In this process, vitamin C donates its two high-energy electrons to scavenge free radicals, much of the resulting dehydroascorbate may be re-reduced to vitamin C and therefore used repeatedly; this may suggest that only small amounts of vitamin C are necessary because of its repeated use. But then, why do levels of ascorbic acid in tissues with the highest metabolic activity, such as suprarenal gland and the brain, contain higher vitamin C than other tissues? This raises important questions about how much of the vitamin's role is antioxidant or has to do with other tasks independent of the antioxidant function. For example, vitamin C is a cofactor or cosubstrate for several enzymes including the hydroxylation of the amino acids involved in the synthesis of collagen and enzymes involved in the synthesis of neurotransmitters such as dopamine and norepinephrine. In addition, high concentrations of ascorbate reduce NAD(P)H and therefore can provide the high-energy electrons necessary to reduce the molecular oxygen used in the respiratory burst of phagocytes. In these functions, although a significant amount of ascorbate is wasted, necessary high-energy electron is provided in large amounts. This also suggests that the amount of vitamin C required to prevent disease, such as scurvy, may not be sufficient to provide optimum cell function and protect against neurodegenerative diseases (ND). In addition, human brain astrocytes supplemented with vitamin C showed increased intracellular concentrations and enhanced lysosomal protein degradation than non-supplemented cells [Martín et al., 2002].

In this review, we examine the potential role that protein oxidation may have in neurodegenerative diseases and what role vitamin C may play in preventing these conditions. We also address the question regarding the potential role that vitamin C may play under certain conditions as a pro-oxidant, contributing to the oxidative-mediated damage in brain and its relevance *in vivo*.

Protein Modification in Brain: Their Importance in Neurodegenerative Conditions

The implication of the low vitamin C concentration may contribute to the incidence or severity of age-associated ND is in general well supported, however, the mechanisms of this effect remain very poorly understood. Well-known examples of degenerative disease, whose frequency of occurrence increases with aging include AD and PD. These pathological processes are commonly associated with severe cognitive impairment. Aging of the brain is in general associated with functional changes in cells and tissues, which may be mediated by a combination of factors including inflammatory processes and damage inflicted by free radicals. Free radicals-mediated oxidative damage has been implicated in both the initiation and development of ND [Reiter, 1998, Reiter, 1995]. Studies in humans have demonstrated a significant increase in oxidized protein from brains of neurological normal individuals and from individuals with different neurological diseases, such as AD, PD and Huntington's disease [Beal, 2002, Carney and Carney, 1994, Chevion et al., 2000, Evans et al., 1999]. The free radical theory of aging proposes that aging occurs as a consequence of the deleterious effects of free radicals produced during cellular metabolism [Harman, 1981]. Among the main reasons offered to support the hypothesis of the oxidative damage in ND are the special characteristics of the brain composition and metabolic activity—the brain uses large amounts of molecular oxygen (O_2)—and proposes that the brain is highly vulnerable to attack by oxygen free radicals. Interestingly, the brain, which is approximately 2% of the body weight, uses 20% of the total inspired O_2 in a resting individual. It is the main use of this metabolism to generate energy in the form of adenosine triphosphate (ATP) from carbohydrates with a turnover of about $4x10^{21}$ molecules of ATP per minute in the complete brain and may contribute to the generation of free radicals. Furthermore, because only a small portion of the total O_2 used by the cells is used to produce ATP, the rest may be reduced to reactive oxygen species and, if not controlled properly, cause tissue damage. There are other factors that in conjunction with the high oxygen consumption may contribute to the neurologic damage in aging, including the rich brain's composition in polyunsaturated fatty acids, the presence of high contain of low molecular weight iron and cupper complexes that can catalyze free radical generation, the elevated levels of iron coupled with high concentrations of vitamin C in the brain, and the abundant presence of excitatory amino acid neurotransmitter in some regions of the brain. All these factors may constitute an optimum environment for the formation of free radicals.

It seems ironic that oxygen, an element indispensable for life, under certain situations may be involved in the formation of a number of chemical compounds, known as reactive oxygen species, which can cause deleterious effects in the human body. Many such reactive species are free radicals and have a surplus of one or more free-floating electrons rather than having matched pairs and are, therefore, unstable and highly reactive. Types of free radicals include the hydroxyl radical ($OH^{\bullet}$), the superoxide radical ($O_2^{\bullet-}$), the nitric oxide radical ($NO^{\bullet}$) and the lipid peroxyl radical ($LOO^{\bullet}$).

Pre-clinical models of neurological conditions such as AD and of cerebral ischaemia appears to indicate the presence of protein oxidation in the brain and it has been proposed to play a critical role in the initial and/or developmental steps of ND. While protein oxidation has been proposed to arise via a number of different biochemical processes, in many cases the formation of protein carbonyls has been linked to metal catalyzed (or site specific) oxidations [Refsgaard et al., 2000, Requena et al., 2001]. The oxidation of proteins in many cases is specific both to the protein and to the region of the protein that is damaged [Refsgaard et al., 2000].

In this sense, Alam and coworkers [Alam et al., 1997] studied the protein carbonyl assay to assess oxidative protein damage in postmortem brain tissue from patients with PD and age-matched controls. Carbonyl concentration was higher among brain areas associated with PD, such as substantia nigra, caudate nucleus, and putamen, than brains from healthy individuals. However, increased carbonyl levels were also found in areas of the brain not involved in PD. These findings suggest that protein carbonyl formation may be related to therapy with L-DOPA, which can exert pro-oxidant properties *in vitro* [Alam et al., 1997]. Consistent with this possibility, brain regions from individuals with incidental Lewy body disease (putative presymptomatic PD) showed no rise in carbonyls in any of the brain areas.

To investigate the issue of oxidative stress Odetti et al. 1998 [Odetti, 1998] analyzed the presence and amount of lipid and protein oxidation markers in Down's syndrome, which is associated with premature aging and progressive mental retardation and shares the pathological features of AD. Two forms of advanced glycation endproducts, which have been also localized in brain lesions of AD, have been identified in the brain of Down's syndrome patients. Protein modification results in cross-linking and aggregation. Aging and neurodegenerative disorders have been associated with the increase in protein oxidation, according to the data previously cited, and the decrease in the activities of several critical enzymes and structural proteins [Carney and Carney, 1994]. W/S ratio of MAL-6 spin-labeled synaptosomes, phenylhydrazine-reactive protein carbonyl content, glutamine synthetase activity and creatine kinase activity are four biomarkers of neuronal protein oxidation [Hensley et al., 1995]. These biomarkers were assessed in three brain regions (cerebellum, inferior parietal lobule and hippocampus) of AD-demented and age-matched control subjects [Hensley et al., 1995]. Hensley and coworkers concluded that the brain regional variation of these oxidation-sensitive biomarkers corresponds to established histopathological features of AD (senile plaque and neurofibrillary tangle densities) and is paralleled by an increase in immunoreactive microglia. These studies indicated that senile plaque-dense regions of the AD brain might represent environments of elevated oxidative stress.

Several papers during the last decade have been trying to shed new light on the role of oxidative damage in the development of ND. Interestingly, Smith et al., 1991 [Smith et al., 1991] provided evidence that the concentration of oxidatively modified proteins is increased in the aged brain. Post mortem frontal- and occipital-pole brain samples obtained from subjects with AD and controls were analyzed for protein oxidation products (carbonyl), and for the activity of two enzymes vulnerable to oxidation, including glutamine synthetase and creatine kinase. Smith and colleagues [Smith et al., 1991] demonstrated in this study a regional loss of glutamine synthetase activity in the brain of Alzheimer's patients. Glutamine synthetase is more sensitive to mixed-function oxidation than creatine kinase. Compared with young controls, researchers observed that both age groups, the Alzheimer and age-matched controls, had increased carbonyl content and decreased glutamine synthetase and creatine kinase activities. Because glutamine synthetase activity was differentially reduced in the frontal-pole in AD, they suggested that AD might represent a specific brain vulnerability to age-related oxidation [Smith et al., 1991]. More recent papers have discussed previous research looking for new support to confirm the importance of oxidative stress on ND and particularly in AD. While it is easy to get comfortable in the idea that neurons at risk of death in AD display extensive oxidative damage to all classes of biological macromolecules, including protein, lipids and nucleic acids, their appearance, role and significance in ND remains obscure. Interestingly, while it was thought before that oxidative stress and oxidized molecules were strong components of the plaques, new reports indicate that the primary site of oxidative damage is not neurofibrillary tangles or senile plaques but the cell bodies of vulnerable neurons [Perry et al., 2000]. Furthermore, examination of cellular changes in the brain of AD patients shows that oxidative stress appears to be an event that precedes the appearance of neurofibrillary tangles, one of the hallmark pathologies of the disease, but the initial source of the oxidative stress remains unclear [Rottkamp et al., 2000]. It appears that changes in the redox balance are altered in the disease [Smith et al., 2000], but the factors that contribute to these changes remain elusive. In fact, contrary to the *in vitro* findings, examination of the plaques and neurofibrillary tangles in relation to the extent of the oxidative stress has shown that oxidative damage is not a result of increasing lesion density. Moreover, the AD case with the greatest extent amyloid-beta (Aβ) deposition or neurofibrillary tangles formation shows the lowest amount of oxidative damage.

Therefore, the conclusion for some researchers is to assume that the lesions observed in the brain of AD, long thought as a deleterious process, may be working as a cytoprotective by reducing the formation of free radicals and tissue damage. This is a quite exocentric view of what the formation of an end product such as the plaques may represent in the brain. However, it has been documented that the milieu inside the cell has a large capacity for sequestering metal, and using the *in vitro* model it has been demonstrated that in the presence of albumin and/or other proteins, metal-mediated oxidation is prevented [Ohta et al., 2001]. Aβ protein binds copper stronger than other transition metals. However, this process may place additional charges to the lesion process by increasing the production of reactive oxygen species and neurotoxicity [Kontush, 2001]. Superoxide formation has been suggested to be one of the molecules produced by the amyloid-metal binding in addition to the auto-oxidation of catecholamines and thiols. Superoxide is formed when molecular oxygen acquires an additional electron.

$$O_2 + e^- \rightarrow O_2^-$$

Normally, the superoxide is short-lived and is converted to hydrogen peroxide by the enzyme superoxide dismutase (SOD) which maintains levels of superoxide at $<10^{-11}$. Ascorbic acid reacts with superoxide at a rate of 10^4-10^5 $M^1 s^1$. In this process, ascorbic acid is oxidized to dehydroascorbic acid by superoxide with a second-order rate constant of 2.8 x 10^4 $M^1 s^1$ to give oxalate ion and threonic acid [Bielski, 1985, Guaiquil et al., 2001]. Thus, the role of ascorbic acid in protecting molecules—proteins, lipids, and DNA—and cells from oxidative challenge may be important in the brain.

However, although some *in vitro* studies have been confounded by results of pro-oxidant effects of ascorbic acid, studies with cells have shown that vitamin C has an independent role in cellular protection against cell death induced by oxidative stress. In fact, mounting evidence, including our own studies [Martín et al., 2002, Sánchez-Moreno et al., 2003], has shown that vitamin C plays a relevant role in protecting cells against free radical-mediated oxidative damage [Blasiak and Kowalik, 2001]. In addition, oxidative stress-mediated calcium influx has been shown to play a relevant role in cell injury. Interestingly, a study using leukocytes demonstrated that intracellular vitamin C inhibited calcium influx into leukocytes and consequently contributed in helping to minimize cell damage [Ozturk et al., 2001]. Other studies using HL-60 cells as a model were able to show that vitamin C can protect cells against cell death induced by oxidative stress [Su et al., 2000].

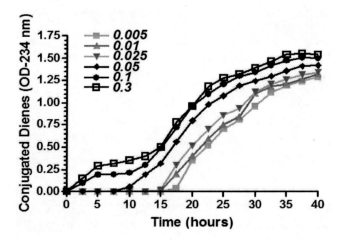

Figure 1. Oxidative modification of LDL (0.1 mg/mL) with different concentrations of copper (μmol/L).

Oxidative mechanisms play an important role in the pathogenesis of AD, PD and other neurodegenerative diseases. To assess whether proteins and proteins contained by lipids are susceptible to oxidative modification *in vitro*, we studied oxidation time-course for up to 100 h of human purified plasma low-density-lipoprotein (LDL) in the absence (autooxidation) or presence of exogenous oxidants. Autooxidation of diluted LDL in the presence of sterile and metal free buffer containing different concentrations of copper (μmol/L) was found to result in a slow accumulation of lipid peroxidation products. The time-course of lipid hydroperoxide accumulation revealed three consecutive phases, lag-phase, propagation phase and plateau phase (Figure 1).

Qualitatively similar time-course has been typically reported using human plasma and plasma lipoproteins. Autooxidation of LDL was accelerated by adding exogenous oxidants, delayed by adding antioxidants and completely inhibited by adding a chelator of transition metal ions.

The anodic electrophoretic mobility of LDL protein (0.1 mg/mL) following incubation with cooper for 18 h was assessed on agarose gels (Figure 2). For comparison, native LDL (nLDL) was also loaded into the gel (indicated by lanes 1 and 9 from the left). The arrowhead on the right side of the gel indicates the origin of LDL loading. Protein in the presence of low concentrations of Cu^{2+} remained unmodified. However, when the concentration of Cu^{2+} was 0.05 µmol/L or higher, protein shows anodic electrophoretic mobility (lanes 5, 6, and 7). LDL protein incubated with free-metal PBS (indicated by lane 8) is also shown.

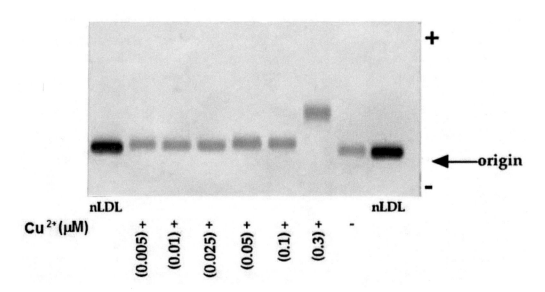

Figure 2. Effect of Cu2+ on oxidative modification of LDL (0.1 mg/mL) after 18 h of incubation in PBS.

Autooxidation of LDL also resulted in the consumption of endogenous ascorbate, alpha-tocopherol, urate and linoleic and arachidonic acids. Taking into account that (i) lipid peroxidation products measured in our study are known to be derived from fatty acids, and (ii) lipophilic antioxidants and fatty acids present in LDL are likely to be located in LDL lipoproteins, we conclude that lipoproteins of human LDL are modified *in vitro* during its autooxidation. This autooxidation appears to be catalyzed by transition metal ions, such as Cu^{2+} and Fe^{2+}, which are present in native CSF. This data suggests that the oxidation of proteins and/or lipoproteins might occur *in vivo* and may play a role in the pathogenesis of neurodegenerative diseases.

Similar to Figure 2, the anodic electrophoretic mobility of LDL protein (0.1 mg/mL) following incubation with cooper for 48 h was assessed on agarose gels (**Figure 3**). For comparison, native LDL (nLDL) was also loaded into the gel (indicated by lanes 1 and 9 from the left). Protein in the presence of Cu^{2+} shows a dose-response anodic electrophoretic mobility. LDL protein incubated with free-metal PBS (indicated by lane 8) remains unmodified. Results shown are representative of six experiments.

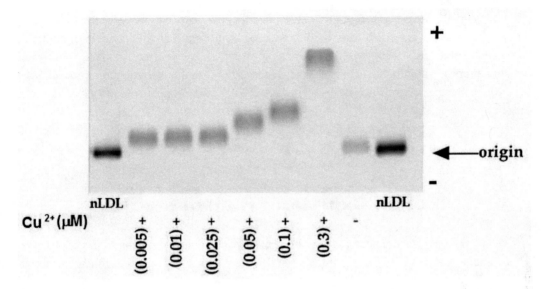

Figure 3. Effect of Cu2+ on oxidative modification of LDL (0.1 mg/mL) after 48 h of incubation in PBS.

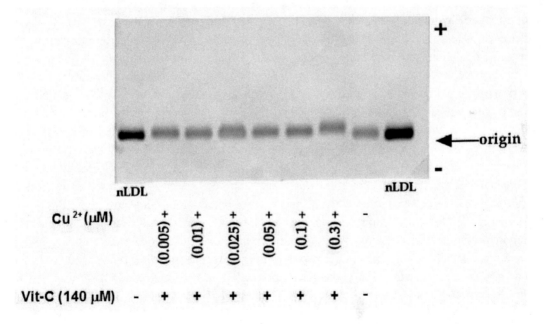

Figure 4. Effect of Cu2+ and vitamin C on oxidative modification of LDL (0.1 mg/mL) after 48 h of incubation in PBS.

In a series of studies designed to investigate the effects of metal ions on protein oxidation, experiment after experiment, we found that LDL-protein became oxidatively modified in a dose- and time-response manner (unpublished data). However in the presence of vitamin C LDL was protected and remained protected until the concentration of vitamin C was consumed. As shown in **Figure 4**, vitamin C present in 140 µmol/L exerted an antioxidant effect preventing LDL-protein from becoming modified following 48 h incubation in the presence of Cu^{2+} up to 0.1 µmol/L. However, LDL incubated in 0.3 µmol/L after 48 started showing changes as determined by the increased anodic electrophoretic mobility (Figure 4, lane 7). Interestingly compared with Figure 3, LDL-protein exhibited a significant protection when vitamin C was present in the buffer. In fact, sequential determination of vitamin C in the supernatant indicates that the electrophoretic mobility of the protein on the agarose gel is visible when the concentration of vitamin C is below 5 µmol/L.

In all the experiments described here vitamin C was determined using the method described by Martín and colleagues [Martín et al., 2002].

Protein Oxidation: Human Studies

Copper chaperones are necessary for intracellular trafficking of copper to target proteins. This is probably due to the fact the milieu inside the cell has a large capacity for sequestering this metal [Ohta et al., 2001].

Reactive oxygen species can attack amino acid residues (particularly histidine, arginine, and lysine) to produce carbonyl (C=O) functions that can be measured after reaction with 2,4-dinitrophenylhydrazine [Reznick and Packer, 1994]. Thus, the "carbonyl assay" has become the most widely used protocol to measure protein oxidation. Another potential mechanism of protein oxidation involves nitric oxide, with formation of the highly toxic radical, peroxynitrite, which can be measured by a nitrotyrosine assay. Because o-tyrosine and 3-nitrotyrosine are typical protein carbonyl end products, are stable to acid hydrolysis, and are not normally present in proteins, they have been largely used as markers of protein oxidative damage. Quantitative postmortem studies [Smith et al., 1991] found that brain carbonyl levels were increased with age, but no difference was observed between aged and AD brains. Likewise, AD brains had o-tyrosine levels, measured by high-performance liquid chromatography, similar to controls [Hayn et al., 1996]. Another study measured protein carbonyls by gas chromatography/mass spectrometry in AD brains and showed no difference [Lyras et al., 1997]. In contrast, Hensley et al., [Hensley et al., 1995, Hensley et al., 1998] reported that the brain regions, hippocampus and inferior parietal lobule, had higher protein carbonyl content than cerebellum in the same AD brain. A chemiluminescence assay to detect carbonyl groups has been used in one study in which it was reported that AD showed higher levels than controls [McIntosh et al., 1997]. Interestingly, the protein carbonyl assay was used as a "general" assay of oxidative protein damage [Smith et al., 1991]. Some studies have compared brain regions from different "batches" due to restrictions in the supply of material, and observed differences between patients and controls; however, one must be cautious in comparing levels in brain regions from a different set. Some studies have shown that the levels of protein carbonyls among different brain regions were higher in AD brains compared with control subjects in the hippocampus. In addition, the presence of protein carbonyls in neurofibrillary tangles, nontangle bearing neurons, and glia has been detected by using immunocytochemic techniques with *in situ* 2,4-dinitrophenylhydrazine labelling in AD but not in controls [Smith et al., 1996]. Other studies reported similar results by looking for immunohistologic evidence of nitrotyrosine, suggesting that peroxynitrite might be also involved in protein damage in AD [Good et al., 1996, Smith et al., 1997, Su et al., 1997]. Studies in humans have demonstrated a significant increase in oxidized protein from brains of neurological normal, and from individuals with different neurological diseases, such as Alzheimer's, Parkinson's and Huntington's disease [Carney and Carney, 1994].

Table 1. Effect of vitamin C on protein oxidation.

Author/Ref.	Year	Study Focus and/or Details of the Study
[Aldred and Griffiths, 2004]	2004	As LDL protein is the control point for LDL metabolism, the degree of oxidation and protection by antioxidants such as vitamin C is likely to be of great importance for (patho)-physiological uptake of LDL by monocytes
[Barja et al., 1994]	1994	Vitamin C and protein and lipid peroxidation. Dietary vitamin C decreases endogenous protein oxidative damage, malondialdehyde, and lipid peroxidation and maintains fatty acid unsaturation in the Guinea pig liver
[Carty et al., 2000]	2000	Dietary vitamin C supplementation can reduce certain types of oxidative protein damage in subjects with low basal antioxidant
[Ciorba et al., 1999]	1999	Nitric oxide, vitamin C and voltage-dependent K^+ channels. Channel protein is protected from methionine oxidation by the enzyme methionine sulfoxide reductase and the antioxidant vitamin C
[Farombi et al., 2004]	2004	Markers of oxidative stress may be modified by several mechanisms after feeding rats with complex dietary factors and that both pro- and antioxidant effects may consequently be observed simultaneously after short-term feeding of antioxidant-rich foods
[Gosiewska et al., 1996]	1996	Vitamin C deficiency and iron homeostasis. Gene expression of iron-related proteins during iron deficiency caused by scurvy in Guinea pigs
[Grant et al., 2005]	2005	The presence of ascorbate induces expression of brain derived neurotrophic factor in SH-SY5Y neuroblastoma cells after peroxide insult, which is associated with increased survival
[Hayn et al., 1996]	1996	AD brains had o-tyrosine levels, measured by HPLC, similar to controls
[Hensley et al., 1995]	1995	Biomarkers of neuronal protein oxidation. Senile plaque-dense regions of the AD brain may represent environments of elevated oxidative stress
[Hensley et al., 1998]	1998	AD pathogenesis may involve the activation of oxidant-producing inflammatory enzyme systems, including nitric oxide synthase
[Ivanov, 1997]	1997	Ascorbic acid and regulation of smooth muscle cell proliferation inside the arterial wall. Ascorbate affects proliferation of guinea-pig vascular smooth muscle cells by direct and extracellular matrix-mediated effects

Table 1. Effect of vitamin C on protein oxidation. (Continued)

Author/Ref.	Year	Study Focus and/or Details of the Study
[Kataoka, 1993]	1993	Vitamin C and patients with HTLV-I associated myelopathy. Efficacy of intermittent high-dose vitamin C therapy in patients with HTLV-I associated myelopathy
[Livesley, 1984]	1984	Vitamin C and plasma cholesterol. Vitamin C supplementation may have a greater role to play in preventing death from ischaemic heart disease
[Lyras et al., 1997]	1997	Increased damage to protein (especially in parietal lobe) strengthens the possibility that oxidative damage may play a role in the pathogenesis of AD
[Mahmoodian, 1999]	1999	Vitamin C and expression of type IV collagen, laminin and elastin in blood vessels. Vitamin C deficiency affects lowering expression of type IV collagen and elastin, but not laminin, in blood vessels of vitamin C-deficient guinea pigs
[McIntosh et al., 1997]	1997	There is increased susceptibility to ROS in the AD temporal cortex that may contribute to the pathogenesis of the disease
[Peterkofsky et al., 1991]	1991	Vitamin C and insulin-like growth factor-I (IGF-I). Existence of elevated activity of low molecular weight insulin-like growth factor-binding proteins in sera of vitamin C-deficient and fasted guinea pigs
[Polidori et al., 2004]	2004	Plasma antioxidant status, immunoglobulin G oxidation and lipid peroxidation in demented patients. Independent of its nature vascular or degenerative-dementia is associated with the depletion of a large spectrum of antioxidant micronutrients and with increased protein oxidative modification
[Pratico and Delanthy, 2000]	2000	Free radical injury appears to be a fundamental process contributing to the neuronal death seen in the disorder, and this hypothesis is supported by many studies using surrogate markers of oxidative damage
[Reznick and Packer, 1994]	1994	Carbonyl assay. Reactive oxygen species can attack amino acid residues to produce carbonyl functions that can be measured after reaction with 2,4-dinitrophenylhydrazine
[Smith et al., 1997]	1997	The widespread occurrence of nitrotyrosine in neurons suggests that oxidative damage is not restricted to long-lived polymers such as NFTs, but instead reflects generalized oxidative stress that is important in Alzheimer's disease
[Smith et al., 1991]	1991	Carbonyl levels. Brain carbonyl levels increased with age, but no difference was observed between aged and AD brains
[Smith et al., 1996]	1996	The presence of protein carbonyls in neurofibrillary tangles, nontangle bearing neurons, and glia has been detected by using immunocytochemic techniques with in situ 2,4-dinitrophenylhydrazine labelling in AD but no in controls
[Su et al., 1997]	1997	The neurons with DNA damage in the absence of tangle formation may degenerate by tangle-independent mechanisms and that oxidative damage may contribute to such mechanisms in AD

Porkkala-Sarataho et al. [Porkkala-Sarataho et al., 2000] studied the effects of vitamin C (500 mg of slow release ascorbate per day), vitamin E (182 mg of RRR-alpha-tocopherol acetate per day), and the combination of both antioxidants on urinary 7-hydro-8-oxo-2'-

deoxyguanosine, serum cholesterol oxidation products, and oxidation resistance of lipids in no depleted men. This study, in concordance with many similar approaches to investigate the role of antioxidants in protecting proteins from becoming modified, found that combination of vitamins E and C enhanced the oxidation resistance of isolated lipoproteins and total serum lipids. **Table 1** summarizes some studies regarding the effect of vitamin C on protein oxidation.

Conclusion

Antioxidants protect by contributing an electron of their own and in doing this they neutralize free radicals and help prevent cumulative damage in cells and tissues. In fact, a significant percentage of the total antioxidant activity of fruits and vegetables is related to their vitamin C content. They help prevent or repair the damage that is done to the body's cells by free radicals. This means that antioxidants replace free radicals in our body before they can cause any damage.

There is overwhelming evidence that eating 5 or more servings of fruits and vegetables a day protects against chronic disease and extends against cognitive decline. In fact, studies indicate that people who are generous in the intake of fruits and vegetables have half the risk of developing chronic disease as those who only eat 2 servings of fruits and vegetable each day.

Because of its redox potential, vitamin C modulates several metabolic and enzymatic reactions and protects proteins from becoming no functional. Therefore, further studies will be required to clarify the mechanisms by which the presence of high concentrations of vitamin C in brain low the capacity of brain proteins to become modified, thereby potentially slowing the ignition and progression of neurodegenerative diseases.

References

Alam, ZI; Daniel, SE; Lees, AJ; Marsden, DC; Jenner, P; Halliwell, B. A generalised increase in protein carbonyls in the brain in Parkinson's but not incidental Lewy body disease. *J Neurochem* 1997, 69, 1326-1329.

Aldred, S; Griffiths, HR. Oxidation of protein in human low-density lipoprotein exposed to peroxyl radicals facilitates uptake by monocytes; protection by antioxidants in vitro. *Environ Toxicol Pharmacol* 2004, 15, 111-117.

Barja, G; Lopez-Torres, M; Perez-Campo, R; Rojas, C; Cadenas, S; Prat, J; Pamplona, R. Dietary vitamin C decreases endogenous protein oxidative damage, malondialdehyde, and lipid peroxidation and maintains fatty acid unsaturation in the guinea pig liver. *Free Radic Biol Med* 1994, 17, 105-115.

Beal, MF. Oxidatively modified proteins in aging and disease. *Free Radic Biol Med* 2002, 32, 797-803.

Bielski, BHJ. Fast kinetic studies of dioxygen-derived species and their metal complexes. *Philos Trans R Soc B-Biol Sci* 1985, 311, 473-482.

Blasiak, J; Kowalik, J. Protective action of vitamin C against DNA damage induced by selenium-cisplatin conjugate. *Acta Biochim Pol* 2001, 48, 233-240.

Carney, JM; Carney, AM. Role of protein oxidation in aging and in age-associated neurodegenerative diseases. *Life Sci* 1994, 55, 2097-2103.

Carty, JL; Bevan, R; Waller, H; Mistry, N; Cooke, M; Lunec, J; Griffiths, HR. The effects of vitamin C supplementation on protein oxidation in healthy volunteers. *Biochem Biophys Res Commun* 2000, 273, 729-735.

Chevion, M; Berenshtein, E; Stadtman, ER. Human studies related to protein oxidation: protein carbonyl content as a marker of damage. *Free Radic Res* 2000, 33, S99-S108.

Ciorba, MA; Heineman, SH; Weissbach, H; Brot, N; Hoshi, T. Regulation of voltage-dependent K^+ channels by methionine oxidation: effect of nitric oxide and the vitamin C. *FEBS lett* 1999, 442, 48-52.

Deschamps, V; Barberger-Gateau, P; Peuchant, E; Orgogozo, JM. Nutritional factors in cerebral aging and dementia: epidemiological arguments for a role of oxidative stress. *Neuroepidemiology* 2001, 20, 7-15.

Evans, P; Lyras, L; Halliwell, B. Measurement of protein carbonyls in human brain tissue. *Methods Enzymol* 1999, 300, 145-156.

Farombi, EO; Hansen, M; Ravn-Haren, G; Moller, P; Dragsted, LO. Commonly consumed and naturally occurring dietary substances affect biomarkers of oxidative stress and DNA damage in healthy rats. *Food Chem Toxicol* 2004, 42, 1315-1322.

Foy, CJ; Passmore, AP; Vahidassr, MD; Young, IS; Lawson, JT. Plasma chain-breaking antioxidants in Alzheimer's disease, vascular dementia and Parkinson's disease. *QJM-Int J Med* 1999, 92, 39-45.

Good, PF; Werner, P; Hsu, A; Olanow, CW; Perl, DP. Evidence for neuronal oxidative damage in Alzheimer's disease. *Am J Pathol* 1996, 149, 21-28.

Gosiewska, A; Mahmoodian, F; Peterkofsky, B. Gene expression on iron-related proteins during iron deficiency caused by scurvy in guinea pigs. *Arch Biochem Biophys* 1996, 325, 295-303.

Grant, MM; Barber, VS; Griffiths, HR. The presence of ascorbate induces expression of brain derived neurotrophic factor in SH-SY5Y neuroblastoma cells after peroxide insult, which is associated with increased survival. *Proteomics* 2005, 5, 534-540.

Guaiquil, VH; Vera, JC; Golde, DW. Mechanism of vitamin C inhibition of cell death induced by oxidative stress in glutathione-depleted HL-60 cells. *J Biol Chem* 2001, 276, 40955-40961.

Harman, D. The aging process. *Proc Natl Acad Sci USA* 1981, 78, 7124-7128.

Hayn, M; Kremser, K; Singewald, N; Cairns, N; Nemethova, M; Lubec, B; Lubec, G. Evidence against the involvement of reactive oxygen species in the pathogenesis of neuronal death in Down's syndrome and Alzheimer's disease. *Life Sci* 1996, 59, 537-544.

Hensley, K; Hall, N; Subramaniam, R; Cole, P; Harris, M; Aksenov, M; Aksenova, M; Gabbita, SP; Wu, JF; Carney, JM; Lovell, M; Markesbery, WR; Butterfield, DA. Brain regional correspondence between Alzheimer's disease histopathology and biomarkers of protein oxidation. *J Neurochem* 1995, 65, 2146-2156.

Hensley, K; Maidt, ML; Yu, ZQ; Sang, H; Markesbery, WR; Floyd, RA. Electrochemical analysis of protein nitrotyrosine and dityrosine in the Alzheimer brain indicates region-specific accumulation. *J Neurosci* 1998, 18, 8126-8132.

Ivanov, VO; Ivanova, SV; Niedzwiecki, A. Ascorbate affects proliferation of guinea-pig vascular smooth muscle cells by direct and extracellular matrix-mediated effects. *J Mol Cell Cardiol* 1997, 29, 3293-3303.

Jacques, PF. Effects of vitamin C on high-density lipoprotein cholesterol and blood pressure. *J Am Coll Nutr* 1992, 11, 139-144.

Kataoka, A, Imai, H., Inayoshi, S., Tsuda, T. Intermittent high-dose vitamin C therapy in patients with HTLV-I associated myelopathy. *J Neurol Neurosurg Psychiatry* 1993, 56, 1213-1216.

Kontush, A. Amyloid-beta: an antioxidant that becomes a pro-oxidant and critically contributes to Alzheimer's disease. *Free Radic Biol Med* 2001, 31, 1120-1131.

Livesley, B. Vitamin C and plasma cholesterol. *Lancet* 1984, 2, 1275.

Lyras, L; Cairns, NJ; Jenner, A; Jenner, P; Halliwell, B. An assessment of oxidative damage to proteins, lipids, and DNA in brain from patients with Alzheimer's disease. *J Neurochem* 1997, 68, 2061-2069.

Mahmoodian, F; Peterkofsky, B. Vitamin C deficiency in guinea pigs differentially affects the expression of type IV collagen, laminin, and elastin in blood vessels. *J Nutr* 1999, 129, 83-91.

Martín, A; Joseph, JA; Cuervo, AM. Stimulatory effect of vitamin C on autophagy in glial cells. *J. Neurochem.* 2002, 82, 538-549.

McIntosh, LJ; Trush, MA; Troncoso, JC. Increased susceptibility of Alzheimer's disease temporal cortex to oxygen free radical-mediated processes. *Free Radic Biol Med* 1997, 23, 183-190.

Odetti, P; Angelini, G; Dapino, D; Zaccheo, D; Garibaldi, S; Dagna-Bricarelli, F; Piombo, G; Perry, G; Smith, M; Traverso, N; Tabaton, M. Early glycoxidation damage in brains from Down´s syndrome. *Biochem Biophys Res Commun* 1998, 243, 849-851.

Ohta, Y; Shiraishi, N; Inai, Y; Sook I; Lee, M; Iwahashi, H; Nishikimi, M. Ascorbate-induced high-affinity binding of copper to cytosolic proteins. *Biochem Biophys Res Commun* 2001, 287, 888-894.

Ozturk, G; Mulholland, CW; Hannigan, BM. Vitamin C decreases intracellular calcium level in human lymphoid cells. *J Physiol Pharmacol* 2001, 52, 285-292.

Perry, G; Nunomura, A; Hirai, K; Takeda, A; Aliev, G; Smith, MA. Oxidative damage in Alzheimer's disease: the metabolic dimension. *Int J Dev Neurosci* 2000, 18, 417-421.

Peterkofsky, B; Palka, J; Wilson, S; Takeda, K; Shah, V. Elevated activity of low molecular weight insulin-like growth factor-binding proteins in sera of vitamin C deficient and fasted guinea pigs. *Endocrinology* 1991, 128, 1769-1779.

Polidori, MC; Mattioli, P; Aldred, S; Cecchetti, R; Stahl, W; Griffiths, H; Senin, U; Sies, H; Mecocci, P. Plasma antioxidant status, immunoglobulin G oxidation and lipid peroxidation in demented patients: relevance to Alzheimer disease and vascular dementia. *Dement Geriatr Cogn Disord* 2004, 18, 265-270.

Porkkala-Sarataho, E; Salonen, JT; Nyyssonen, K; Kaikkonen, J; Salonen, R; Ristonmaa, U; Diczfalusy, U; Brigelius-Flohe, R; Loft, S; Poulsen, HE. Long-term effects of vitamin E, vitamin C, and combined supplementation on urinary 7-hydro-8-oxo-2'-deoxyguanosine, serum cholesterol oxidation products, and oxidation resistance of lipids in nondepleted men. *Arterioscler Thromb Vasc Biol* 2000, 20, 2087-2093.

Pratico, D; Delanty, N. Oxidative injury in diseases of the central nervous system: focus on Alzheimer's disease. *Am J Med* 2000, 109, 577-585.

Ramakrishna, T. Vitamins and brain development. *Physiol Res* 1999, 48, 175-187.

Refsgaard, HH; Tsai, L; Stadtman, ER. Modifications of proteins by polyunsaturated fatty acid peroxidation products. *Proc Natl Acad Sci USA* 2000, 97, 611-616.

Reiter, RJ. Oxidative damage in the central nervous system: protection by melatonin. *Prog Neurobiol* 1998, 56, 359-384.

Reiter, RJ. Oxidative processes and antioxidative defense mechanisms in the aging brain. *FASEB J.* 1995, 9, 526-533.

Requena, JR; Chao, CC; Levine, RL; Stadtman, ER. Glutamic and aminoadipic semialdehydes are the main carbonyl products of metal-catalyzed oxidation of proteins. *Proc Natl Acad Sci USA* 2001, 98, 69-74.

Reznick, AZ; Packer, L. Oxidative damage to proteins: spectrophotometric method for carbonyl assay. *Methods Enzymol* 1994, 233, 357-363.

Riviere, S; Birlouez-Aragon, I; Nourhashemi, F; Vellas, B. Low plasma vitamin C in Alzheimer patients despite an adequate diet. *Int J Geriatr Psychiatr* 1998, 13, 749-754.

Rosenberg, IH; Miller, JW. Nutritional factors in physical and cognitive functions of elderly people. *Am J Clin Nutr* 1992, 55, S1237-S1243.

Rottkamp, CA; Nunomura, A; Raina, AK; Sayre, LM; Perry, G; Smith, MA. Oxidative stress, antioxidants, and Alzheimer disease. *Alzheimer Dis Assoc Dis* 2000, 14, S62-S66.

Sánchez-Moreno, C; Paniagua, M; Madrid, A; Martín, A. Protective effect of vitamin C against the ethanol mediated toxic effects on human brain glial cells. *J Nutr Biochem* 2003, 14, 606-613.

Smith, CD; Carney, JM; Starkereed, PE; Oliver, CN; Stadtman, ER; Floyd, RA; Markesbery, WR. Excess brain protein oxidation and enzyme dysfunction in normal aging and in Alzheimer disease. *Proc Natl Acad Sci USA* 1991, 88, 10540-10543.

Smith, MA; Perry, G; Richey, PL; Sayre, LM; Anderson, VE; Beal, MF; Kowall, N. Oxidative damage in Alzheimer's. *Nature* 1996, 382, 120-121.

Smith, MA; Harris, PLR; Sayre, LM; Beckman, JS; Perry, G. Widespread peroxynitrite-mediated damage in Alzheimer's disease. *J Neurosci* 1997, 17, 2653-2657.

Smith, MA; Rottkamp, CA; Nunomura, A; Raina, AK; Perry, G. Oxidative stress in Alzheimer's disease. *Biochim Biophys Acta* 2000, 1502, 139-144.

Su, JH; Deng, G; Cotman, CW. Neuronal DNA damage precedes tangle formation and is associated with up-regulation of nitrotyrosine in Alzheimer's disease brain. *Brain Res* 1997, 774, 193-199.

Su, Y; Sun, CM; Chuang, HH; Chang, PT. Studies on the cytotoxic mechanisms of ginkgetin in a human ovarian adenocarcinoma cell line. *Naunyn Schmiedebergs Arch Pharmacol* 2000, 362, 82-90.

In: Focus on Nutrition Research　　　　　　　　　　ISBN 1-59454-768-8
Editor: Tony P. Starks, pp. 49-70　　　　　　　　© 2006 Nova Science Publishers, Inc.

Chapter III

Food Restriction Effects on Plasma Amino Acids, Myofibrillar Protein Profiles, Plasma and Muscle Free and Sterified Fatty Acids on Monogastric and Ruminants: A Review

André Martinho de Almeida[*], *Sofia van Harten*
and Luís Alfaro Cardoso
Instituto de Investigação Científica Tropical – Tropical Research Institute,
CVZ, Lisboa, Portugal

Abstract

Undernutrition is a major setback of animal production in the tropics. Progressive weight loss is characterized by a mobilization of body depots, especially fat and to a lesser extent protein. Muscle and therefore protein breaks down in order to supply amino acid as an energy source, generating a vast array of responses in serum free amino acid concentrations, myofibrillar protein (with special reference to Myosin Heavy Chains, Actin, Protein C, α Actinin and Tropomyosin + Troponin T) profiles and free fatty acids and fatty acids incorporated in triacylglycerol as a consequence of several factors: animal species and the severity of food restriction. The objective of this work is to present a review regarding these very important aspects of undernutrition. Several domestic animals species, both ruminant and monogastric will be considered with significance to both laboratory and farm animals. Special relevance will be given to works conducted at our group particularly on two experiments, first with laboratory rats and in a latter point *Boer goat* bucks in an applied prospective.

---

[*] [a]Author for correspondence: André de Almeida, Tropical Research Institute, FMV, Rua Prof. Cid dos Santos, 1300-477 Lisboa, Portugal.

Introduction

Contrary to temperate environments, most tropical climates are characterized by the existence of two distinct seasons: dry and rainy, with the latter showing higher average temperatures than the first one. Such marked difference between seasons leads to a strong conditioning of local pasture production and hence animal science. Rainy season pastures are available in higher quantities and show good nutritional quality whereas dry season's pastures have poor nutritional quality with high fibre and low protein contents (Butterworth, 1984).

It is frequent in extensive or traditional management systems, the lack of supplementation during the dry season which leads to a seasonal weight loss of 20-40 % as demonstrated by several authors (Preston and Leng, 1987; Clariget et al., 1998). Pasture shortage hence significantly affects animal production in tropical nations such as Mali (Wilson, 1987), Brazil (Abdalla et al., 1999), The Philippines (Alejandrino et al., 1999) or South Africa (Luswetti, 2000), reflecting on all aspects of animal production.

In situations of pasture shortage as described above, strong modifications on animal metabolism are observed. Such physiological modifications are essentially characterized by the mobilization of body depots, especially lipids and to a lesser extent protein (Belkhou et al., 1991) which therefore affects aspects reviewed in this paper: serum amino acids, myofibrillar protein profiles, plasma and muscle free and sterified fatty acids.

Undernutrition and Plasma Free Amino Acid (PFAA) Concentrations in Ruminants

Severe undernutrition or food deprivation in the form of long or short term fasting in ruminants seems to lead to vast array of responses in the profiles of Plasma Free Amino acid. Such responses could be different, if not antagonist, depending on the severity or type of food restriction, the species, age or productive state of the animals in study or even the type of diet provided. In this section, we briefly review alterations described in PFAA as a consequence of undernutrition in domestic ruminants: Cattle, Sheep and Goat.

The level of concentrate on ruminants diet (consequently affecting protein and energy content) necessarily affects PFAA concentrations. Prior et al. (1981) studied the effects of high levels of concentrate on PFAA in sheep and Steers by comparison with control animals fed standard hay. They observed decreased concentrations of the amino acids Glu, Val, Ile and His and increased concentrations of Ser and Gly in sheep, whereas in steers reduced concentrations of Val and Ile and increased concentrations in Gly were observed. In both cases the remaining amino acids seem to show similar levels for both experimental groups. In a similar manner, forages of poor quality also seem to affect PFAA concentrations with an increase in Ser and Ile concentrations in sheep fed low quality forages (Goetsch et al., 1998). The two cited works seem to indicate an influence of food quality and level on PFAA concentrations, an influence that could be extrapolated to fasting and more severe food restriction.

During food restriction, muscle proteins are degraded rendering them available for animal metabolism. According to Bergen (1979) such situations lead to a significant increase of the concentration of most PFAA.

An analysis of circadian variations in PFAA concentrations, as done by Ndibualonji et al. (1997) in dairy cows fed twice a day allowed the detection of an increase in concentrations of Ala, Glu, Gly, Arg, His, Ile, Leu, Met, Phe and Val as blood sampling was done several hours post-feeding, while Tyr and Asp are reduced and Ser, Pro, Lys and Thr are kept constant.

In 27 h fasting periods in ewes a decrease in Gly concentration was detected along with an increase in Ile, Leu, Phe, Lys, Tyr and Glu, while Thr, Met, His, Arg, Asp, Ser and Ala maintained concentrations similar to control animals (Cross et al., 1975). Such results do not coincide with those of Heitman and Bergman (1980) where higher concentrations of Gly, Leu, Ile and Val and lower concentrations of Cit in underfed sheep were observed while Ala, Glu, Ser, Arg, Thr, Lys, Phe, Tyr and Orn had similar results in both experimental groups (3 days fasting and control). Extended fasting period (six days) again leads to different results from the previously mentioned as demonstrated by Pell and Bergman (1983): increased concentrations of Asp, Ile, Leu, Lys and Tau and a decrease of Ser, Cit and Tyr concentrations, while those of Thr, Glu, Pro, Gly, Ala, Val, Phe and Orn remained constant.

In *Holstein* cows under short fasting periods (20 hours), higher concentrations of plasma Ala and Ser were registered while Asp and Gly showed similar levels (Ndibualonji et al., 1993). In a prolonged fasting (Ndibualonji et al., 1997) higher concentrations of Arg, Gly, His, Leu, Lys, Ser and Val were detected while Thr, Phe, Ile, Ala and Asp were kept constant and Glu, Met, Pro and Tyr decreased as fasting progressed. In weight losing dairy cows caused by high production, Piva et al., (1994) detected and increase of the concentrations of Lys, Gly, Arg, Orn, His, Ala and Val as lactation progressed, while Met, Ile, Leu and Asp were kept similar to the beginning of lactation and Phe and Glu concentrations decreased. Opposite results were described in similar conditions by Meijer et al., (1995) that observed a decrease of Arg, His, Ile, Leu, Lys, Met, Phe, Tyr and Glu, an increase in Val, Ala, Cit, Pro, Ser and Tau and maintenance of Trp, Orn, Thr, Asp and Cys.

In Boer goat bucks, under food restriction (86 % of estimated daily protein needs), animals showed higher concentrations of Val, Ile, Leu, Thr, Met, Lys, Tau, Orn, and Hyp, similar concentrations of Gly, Ser, Asp, Glu, Arg, His and Pro and lower concentrations of Ala, Tyr and Cit (Almeida et al., 2004), such experiences will be the subject of a latter section of this paper.

Undernutrition and Plasma Free Amino Acid (PFAA) Concentrations in Monogastrics

Like in the previous section regarding ruminants, in monogastrics, apparently there seems not to be a standard profile of plasma amino acid profiles as a consequence of undernutrition. Again, there seems to different responses according to type of undernutrition (fasting or short/long tern undernutrition), the quality of feed, the species, breed or productive performance of the animal involved.

In adult horses, Johnson and Hart (1974) studied PFAA concentrations in several timings during a 48 hours fasting. In the first 18 hours PFAA concentrations remained stable, after which most amino acids increased their concentrations (Arg, Ile, Leu, Lys, Met, Phe, Thr, Val, Ala, Cys, Glu, Gly and Pro) as His, Ser, Tyr and Gla kept similar levels to the beginning of the experiment. Such results are partially coherent with those provided by Russel et al., (1986) also in adult horses. According to such authors in the first 4-6 hours post-feeding there is an increase in Glu, Gla, Ala, Leu and Ile, decreasing in the following six hours to values very similar to the initial ones. Such concentrations are maintained for a 20 – 26 h period, after whereas an increase in concentrations is observed as a result of protein catabolism. In newborn foals, a ten-hour fasting period seems to lead to an increase in the concentrations Ala, Arg, Gly, Hpr, Phe and Ser, decrease in Cit, Glu, His, Ile, Leu, Orn, Pro, Trp, Tyr and Val and maintenance of Asp, Cys, Lys, Met, Tau and Thr (Zicker and Rogers, 1994).

The effect of a 23-day fasting period PFAA was determined by Cuperlovic and Stosic (1970) in swine. In such study, all essential amino acids (Thr, Val, Met, Ile, Leu, Phe, Lys and His) and Ser, Cit, Tyr and Arg showed increased concentrations, while Pro, Glu, Gly, Ala and Orn had lower concentrations than those registered in control group. In protein deficiency situations and in similar animals most PFAA (Thr, Val, Ile, Leu, Lys, Pro, Glu, Gly, Ala, Tyr, Orn and Arg) decreased their concentrations with protein restriction (Cuperlovic and Stosic, 1970). In pregnant sows a protein restriction conduced to higher concentrations of Ala, Asp, Glu and Lys then adequately fed animals (Wu et al., 1998).

A six-week food restriction period effect on PFAA was studied in domestic cats by Biourge et al., (1994a). A progressive decline in the concentrations of Ala, Thr, Pro, Arg, Tau, Phe, Met, Trp and Cit and an increase in Gla, Glu and Orn concentrations was observed, while most of the remaining amino acid in study registered unaltered concentrations. Comparing these results with those obtained in young cats fed according to their maintenance needs can mean that plasma concentrations of His, Ile, Leu, Lys, Phe, Thr, Trp and Val are higher in adult animals (Biourge et al., 1994b).

Bloxam (1972) studied PFAA concentrations in the laboratory rat at 24 and 72 hours fasting periods. A significant decrease was registered in Asp, Arg, Pro, Ser, Gly and Ala; a minor increase in the first days of Lys and Thr, followed by marked descent and maintenance of Glu, Phe, Met, Tau, Cit, His and Tyr levels. During progressive weight loss, as described by Moldawer et al., (1981) an increase in Gly and Glu was registered as well as similar Ala concentrations. Divino Filho et al. (1999) studied the effect of food restriction of protein restriction in adult rats. According to these authors most PFAA (Thr, Ala, Cit, Glu, Gla, Gly, His, Orn, Ser and Tau) increased their concentrations while Met, Trp, Phe, Tyr and Lys decreased their levels and those of Val, Ile, Leu and Arg were kept throughout the experiment. Almeida et al., (2002) analyzed the effects of severe undernutrition (34 % weigh loss) on the PFAA: Ser, Glu, Thr, Ile, Met, Gly, Ala, Cys, Val, Leu, Phe, His, Orn and Lys, and higher levels were registered in food-restricted animals for Ser, Thr, Ile, Met, Cys and Phe. Such experiences will be described in detail in a following section.

Undernutrition and Tri-Methylhisitidine

Tri-Methylhisitidine (Me3His) is an analogue to the amino-acid histidine, found predominantly in muscle actin and myosin (Wassner et al., 1980). As it cannot be reused, it is quickly excreted in urine (Wassner et al., 1980) being an indicator of muscle protein breakdown (Ward and Buttery, 1980). In dairy cows, plasma concentrations of Me3His increased post-partum as nitrogen and energy balances dropped to negative values. Contrary, as balances increased to positive values, a decrease in Me3His concentration was also observed (Blum et al., 1984). Such results are in accordance with those of Ndibualonji et al. (1997) as Me3His concentrations increase as a consequence of fasting. Identical results can also be observed in Boer goat bucks (Almeida et al., 2004) where an extremely high increase was observed as a consequence of undernutrition (approximately 5 times control animals) as it will be seen in a following section.

Undernutrition and Myofibrillar Protein Profiles

Undernutrition has a significant effect on muscle characteristics of animal species. Such an effect is visible at the level of muscle mass (Mosoni et al., 1999 and Ameredes et al., 1999) or muscle fibres (Bedi et al., 1982). As reported by Wassner et al., (1977), there seems to be a growing degradation rate of muscle protein in the rat subjected to increasing fasting periods. Such data are in accordance with Ogata et al., (1978), also in rats and where myofibrillar protein catabolism in underfed animals is six times the one of normally fed animals. Undernutrition also seems to affect protein synthesis, significantly lower in animals fed below maintenance needs (Mosoni et al., 1999).

As it promotes protein catabolism, undernutrition also affects catabolism of each of the myofibrillar proteins itself (Fong et al., 1989). In myofibrillar protein degradation situations (and hence higher plasma concentrations of Me3Hist), Iñarrea et al., (1990) reported a reduction of the quantities of Troponin C, Troponin I and Myosin light chains in breast muscles of the chicken.

Bates et al., (1983) studied Myosin and Actin synthesis rates in underfed and *ad libitum* fed rats. According to this researcher, the relation between synthesis of underfed and ad libitum fed are 50 % for myosin and 25% for Actin. Synthesis rates of Actin and myosin heavy chains in fed and underfed rats were studied by Clark and Wildenthal (1986) at the level of skeletal and cardiac muscles. Their results imply a drop of 20 to 35 % in Myosin Heavy Chains and 40 to 60 % in Actin. Such data are in accordance with Samarel et al., (1987) in rabbits. Such authors determined myocardium atrophy, associated to undernutrition and high degradation rates of Actin and Myosin Heasvy Chains. Fong et al., (1989) obtained similar results for Actin, Myosin Heavy and Myosin Light Chains synthesis rates in rats under growing food deprivation. Although synthesis and degradation rates are clearly influenced by undernutrition, an actual significant alteration on protein quantities is seldom reported in monogastric animals. Almeida et al., (2002) studied myofibrillar protein profiles in fed and underfed rats (loss of 40 % of initial body weight) and noticed no significant difference on profiles of undernourished and control animals. In ruminants the effect of undernutrition on myofibrillar protein profiles seems to be more defined. Almeida et al., (2004) working with Boer goat bucks determined a loss in Protein C and α - actinin in underfed animals with a weight loss of 20 %. Such experiments will be the object of the next two following sections.

Undernutrition Effect on PFAA and Myofibrillar Protein in *Rattus Norvegicus*: No Preferable Amino Acid Degradation and Lack of Alterations in Gastrocnemius Myofibrillar Protein at High Body Weight Loss

This experiment was conducted at our laboratory in the Tropical Research Institute (Lisboa, Portugal) and was published previously (Almeida et al., 2002). Sixteen adult male rats (380 g) were divided in two groups (n = 8): CR (Control) and RR (Underfed). Group CR animals were fed *ad libitum*, while RR group animals were fed restrictively to 34 and 55 % of the Energetic and Protein maintenance requirements at the beginning of the experiment (5 g / day). After 23 days of experiment trial group had lost 34 % of the initial body weight and were sacrificed. Animals were bled by jugular cut, and blood samples and the gasterocnemius muscle collected. Plasma amino acid profile determination was accomplished using Ion Exchange Chromatography in amino acid analyser *Pharmacia Biotech Biochrom 20* (Peapack, NJ, USA). Gastrocnemius muscles were prepared using the methods described by Parrish Jr. et al., (1973) for the determination of myofibrillar protein extract. Electrophoresis of myofibrillar proteins was done on SDS-PAGE electrophoretic gels at 160 volts. Gels were fixed and coloured with Coomassie. Gels were digitised and analysed for band areas of the myofibrillar proteins: Myosin Heavy Chains, Protein C, α - Actinin, Tropomyosin + Troponin T, Actin and also the injected pattern Bovine Sera Albumin.

Relative areas of the peaks of the amino acids Ser, Glu, Thr, Ile, Met, Gly, Ala, Cys, Val, Leu, Phe, Hys, Orn and Lys are presented on Figure 1. Phe, Ser, Thr, Cys, Ile and Met relative areas of group control animals were respectively 32% 36% 53% 17% and 14% of those registered in restricted fed animals. No difference was observed for the rest of the amino acids. Areas for myofibrillar proteins Myosin Heavy Chains, Protein C, α - Actinin, Tropomyosin + Troponin T and Actin are shown on Figure 2 and results were similar for both groups.

Regarding essential amino acids for the rat (Leu, Ile, Val, Lys, Thr, Met, Phe and His), only Ile, Thr, Phe and Met were affected in the underfed group. The results obtained in our experiment, regarding non essential amino acids for the rat (Ser, Ala, Cys, Gly, Asp, Glu, Arg, Tyr, Pro, Orn, Cit and Tau), seem to be contrary to the observations of other authors (Divino Filho et al., 1999). These results indicate an increase in the concentrations of non-essential amino acids as a consequence of undernutrition. Higher concentrations in the serum of most essential amino acids were also observed in other monogastric species, and are a direct consequence of body protein depletion.

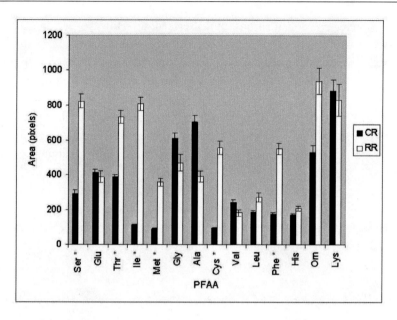

Figure 1. PFAA profiles in underfed laboratory rats. Amino acids with * indicate statistical significance; CR – Control; RR – Restricted Feeding (Almeida et al., 2002).

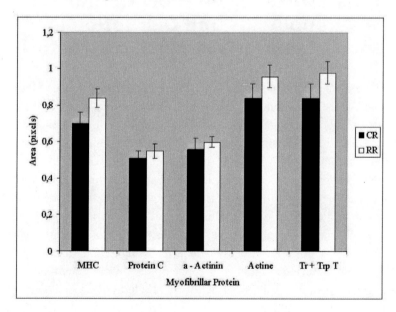

Figure 2. Myofibrillar Protein profile in underfed laboratory rats. CR – Control; RR – Restricted Feeding (Almeida et al., 2002).

An analysis of the degradation pathway shows that undernutrition affected two amino acid degraded by the Succinyl CoA (Ile and Met - increased concentrations in the underfed group), and three of the Pyruvate (Thr, Cys and Ser – increased concentrations in the underfed animals) pathways. Band areas of amino acid degraded by Acetoacetyl CoA and α Ketoglutarate pathways are very similar in both experimental groups, with the exception of Pro. The obtained PFAA profiles seem to indicate that, there is not preferable amino acid catabolism as a response to situations of underfeeding. However, amino acid pool is a dynamic event. It could therefore be considered that the absence of individual amino acid lower peak areas between control and restricted fed animals could be due to the differences in the balances of serum amino acid flux input (protein catabolism) and output (amino acid degradation). According to Lobley (1992), in monogastric species, low intracellular concentrations of ATP such as those caused by undernutrition causes the start of the enzyme BCOADH (Branched Chain Oxo-acid Dehydrogenase) thus motivating branched chain amino acid catabolism and hence lower their concentrations and explaining results obtained for Val and Leu.

Myofibrillar protein profiles obtained were alike in both groups, and no distinction was registered concerning relative quantity of each protein. Consequently there is no preferable protein catabolism as a response to undernutrition, thus maintaining myofibrillar protein proportions and arrangement of the gasterocnemius muscle in the rat.

Undernutrition Effect on PFAA and Myofibrillar Protein in *Capra Hircus* (Boer Goat Breed): Higher Efficiency of Short Carbon Chain Amino Acids and Disruption of Semi-Membranous Muscle Structure

This experiment was conducted at the Department of Animal Science of the University of the Orange Free State (Bloemfontein, South Africa) and at our laboratory in the Tropical Research Institute (Lisboa, Portugal) and was published in detail by Almeida et al., (2004).

Fifteen Boer Goat intact young bucks (28 ± 0.2 kg) were divided in two weight-matched groups: CG (n = 7; Control group) and RG (n = 8; Underfed). RG animals received 500 g of red grass (*Themeda trianda*) hay, cut in middle August, during dry season (80 and 86 % of daily metabolisable energy and crude protein NRC requirements respectively) daily. The CG animals received 600 g of red grass hay, plus 170 g of maize, 44 g Molasses and 15 g Urea per day a nutritional plane above maintenance needs. After a 28-day period animals were slaughtered. Blood was collected weekly and after slaughtering, the semi-membranosus muscle samples were collected. Amino acid concentrations were determined using a HPLC and Beckman Coulter Amino Acid Analyser 7300 (Fullerton, CA, USA), with a Lithium buffer system. The semi-membranosus muscle samples were prepared using the methods described earlier.

CG animals increased in bodyweight by 3.8 kg (10 % increase), while the RG group lost 5.6 kg (20 % decrease). At the end of the experiment, significant differences between CG and RG were observed in the following amino acids: Ala, Tyr and Cit (21, 32 and 50% respectively higher concentrations than in the Control group on the last day) and Val, Leu, Ile, Thr, Met, Lys, Tau, Orn, Hyp and Me3His (52, 57, 30, 29, 61, 91, 41, 55, 300 and 560% higher concentrations in the Underfed group, compared to the CG group on day 28). The concentrations of Gly, Ser, Asp, Glu, Arg, His, Pro and Ser(P) were generally similar for both groups at this stage. Results for amino acids at the end of experimental period are presented in Figures 3a and 3b. Band areas for the myofibrillar protein Myosin Heavy Chains, Protein C, α - Actinin, Tropomyosin + Troponin T and Actin are presented in Figure 4. Both groups exhibited similar band areas for each of the proteins, with the exception of Protein C and α - Actinin that had higher band areas in the CG animals (16 and 32 % respectively).

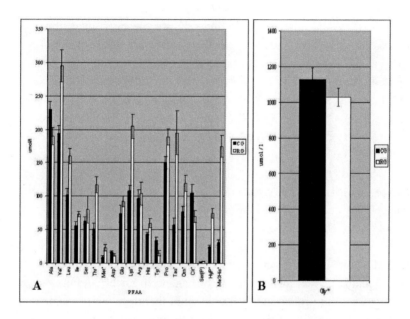

Figure 3. PFAA profiles in underfed Boer Goat Bucks at day 28. A – All amino acids except Gly; B – Amino acid Gly. Amino acids with * indicate statistical significance; CG – Control; RG – Restricted Feeding (Almeida et al., 2004).

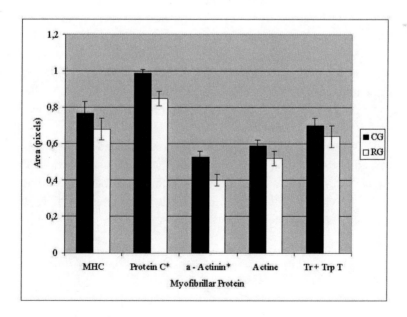

Figure 4. Myofibrillar Protein profile in underfed Boer Goat bucks. Myofibrillar Proteins with * indicate statistical significance; CG – Control; RG – Restricted Feeding (Almeida et al., 2004).

The results obtained in this trial point that an increase in amino acid concentrations is associated with thedegradation of the Succinyl CoA and Acetoacetyl CoA pathways. Amino acids that generally degraded by the α Ketoglutarate, Pyruvate and Oxaloacetate pathways, maintain similar concentrations in both groups. These results are parallel to those before reported in ruminants (Cross et al., 1975, Ndibualonji et al., 1997). As demonstrated by Wolff and Bergman (1972), Ala, Glu, Ser, Asp and Gly are the most vital gluconeogecic amino acids, indicative of 8-9 % of the total glucose formed in sheep (the correspondent to all residual amino acids) for maintenance situations. In this experiment the amino acids Ala, Glu, Ser, Asp and Gly, in the RG group, established similar levels during the experimental stage with no significant disparity to the CG animals. These results are in agreement with Heitman and Bergman, (1980), Cascino et al. (1995) and Leij-Halfwerk (2000) and could be caused by a quicker degradation of glucose synthesis of these amino acids, which stop accretion in blood, unlike Val, Leu, Ile, Thr, Met, Lys and His that accumulated. In situations of undernutrition, amino acids with a additional Carbon atoms (Val, Leu, Ile, Thr, Met, Lys and His) have increased levels in the serum, while amino acids with not as much Carbon atoms have similar concentrations to those observed at the beginning of the undernutrition period and the control group of animals.

In ruminants, catabolism of branched chain amino acids, and leucine, is lower due to the enzyme BCOADH that is less important than in monogastric, such as rodents (Lobley, 1992). This perhaps explains higher concentrations of leucine in underfed animals. Branched chain amino acid (from muscle protein catabolism) would therefore tend to cumulate in the blood stream, due to a lower activity of BCOADH in ruminants. Concerning the amino acids of the urea cycle (Arg, Cit and Orn), CG animals had superior concentrations of Cit, and lower of Orn by contrast. Alike concentrations of Arg were registered for the two groups, possibly as this amino acid results from the degradation of Asp, through the formation of Arginino-succinate (Umbarger and Zubay, 1988) no significant difference was registered in the last amino acid. In conditions of undernutrition, urea excretion tends to diminish as a nitrogen saving mechanism (Edmonds and Baker, 1987). This could give good reason for the increase in Orn concentration as a consequence of underfeeding (Moyano et al., 1998), as Orn is also a product of Arg degradation (Umbarger and Zubay, 1988). A lower concentration of Cit in the RG animals could be connected to the decline of the concentrations of Carbomoyl Phosphate, stimulated by a fall of NH_3 availability.

A significant decrease in the concentrations of protein C and α - Actinin were recorded in all underfed animals. According to Bandman (1994), Protein C is present at the level of the second third of each half of the A band, while α - Actinin is located in the Z line, acting as a cementing matrix. A change in the proportions of these proteins seems to contribute to a change in muscle structure at the level in these regions.

Undernutrition and Free Fatty Acids (FFA) and Fatty Acids Incorporated in Triacylglycerols (TGA) in Muscle and Plasma of Ruminants

Several authors, leading, however, to an unclear situation regarding ruminants, studied the influence of different levels of food restriction on muscle FFA and TGA.

The effect of two distinct diets (more energetic *versus* less energetic) on muscle free fatty acids of bovines was studied by Clemens et al. (1973). The authors observed an increase in the concentration of C18:0 (stearic acid) when animals were fed with the hipocaloric diet. The same conclusion was noticed by Williams et al. (1983) in cows fed with forage in comparison with grain. They also showed an increase in C14:0 (myristic acid), in C18:2 (linoleic acid) and a decrease in C18:1 (oleic acid). In a similar study, also in cows fed with forage, (Marmer et al., 1984), opposite results were found regarding C18:1 (increase) and C18:2 (decrease) and the same result as to C18:0 (increase). Enser et al. (1998) showed the same results as the latter authors and also an increase in C16:0 (palmitic acid) in cows fed a forage versus concentrate diet.

Soppela and Nieminen (2002) studied the effect of moderate undernutrition on muscle FFA composition of reindeer. In animals who lost 16% of their initial body weight due to feed unavailability during wintertime, C18:1 was significantly higher and C18:2 was lower compared to well-nourished reindeer.

In a previous study of the same authors (Soppela and Nieminen, 2001) a significant reduction of C18:1 and C18:2 incorporated in triacylglycerols were found in undernourished reindeer calves. The authors referred the suggestion of selective mobilization of these fatty acids during the impairment of the nutritional status.

Studies on plasma free fatty acids of ruminants also revealed an unclear situation regarding the influence of undernutrition on these lipids. Dunshea et al. (1988) worked with goats fed a hipocaloric diet (35 KJ ME) versus a more energetic one (70 KJ ME). They obtained an increase in C18:1 and a decrease in C18:2 in the undernourished animals' plasma. A similar decrease in the same fatty acid was determined by Speake et al. (1997) in obese and lean sheep. Both groups suffered a reduction in the proportion of linoleic acid after being fasted for two days. Rukkwamsuk et al. (2000) obtained a decrease in C16:0, C18:0 and C18:1 when working with cows submitted to feed restriction (44 MJ/d of NE) in comparison with cows overfed (96MJ/d of NE).

Undernutrition in plasma of Boer goat bucks (fed 80% of energy maintenance needs) led to an increase in C16:0 (FFA) and a decrease in free C18:2 (van Harten et al., 2003b). In the same study, C18:2 incorporated in triacylglycerols revealed an increase, whereas C18:1, also associated to triacylglycerols, was found to increase in the restricted group, being both fatty acids determined in the muscle.

Undernutrition and Free Fatty Acids (FFA) and Sterified Fatty Acids (TGA) in Muscle and Plasma of Monogastrics

The influence of different levels of weight loss on fatty acids concentrations (free and triacylglycerols incorporated forms) was studied by several authors in monogastric species.

The results did not reveal a clear situation relatively to free fatty acids: Yaffe et al. (1980) observed an increase in C18:0, C18:1 and C18:2 (linoleic acid) in rats decreasing nearly 30% of body weight during 7 days of fasting. On the other hand, Hardy et al. (2002) observed in plasma of energy-restricted rats (60% of *ad libitum* intake) a decrease in C14:0 (myristic acid), C16:0 and C18:0. Nawrocki et al. (1999) working with diabetic rats noticed an increase in C18:2, when these suffered an involuntary glucose restriction.

In pigs fed only 20% of the *ad libitum* feeding level, Lopez–Pedrosa et al. (1998) observed a diminution in plasma' saturated, mono–unsaturated and poli–unsaturated fatty acids (not specified), when a decrease of 57% body weight was achieved.

In the muscle, Nawrocki et al. (1999) reported an increase in free fatty acids (C18:1 and C18:2) when an influence of involuntary glucose restriction was observed in diabetic rats. Cefalu et al. (2000) also noticed an increase in C18:1, in C16:0 and C18:0 in the muscle of rodents when subjected to feed restriction of 60% of *ad libitum* intake while C18:2 suffered a decrease.

In a work mentioned above (Hardy et al. 2002) a decrease in stearic and miristic acid incorporated in triacylglycerols was observed in rats fed only with 60% of *ad libitum* intake, while palmitic acid associated with triacylglycerols suffered an increase. Nawrocki et al. (1999) also showed changes in fatty acids incorporated in triacylglycerols of the muscle in diabetic rats. According to their results, C14:0, C16:0 and C18:0 decreased and C18:2 revealed an increase.

In feed restricted rats, (34% of energy maintenance needs), free C14:0 was found increased in plasma while C18:1 (FFA) was found decreased in plasma and muscle of the undernourished group (van Harten et al., 2003a). Also in the muscle, C18:0 suffered an increase in its free and in its sterified form as did C16: 0 associated to triacylglycerols.

Our experiments mentioned above with the references van Harten et al. (2003a; 2003b) will now be described, so as to highlight the utilized methodologies.

Muscle and Plasma Free Fatty Acids and Fatty Acids from Triacylglycerols in Underfed Animals: Experiments with the Laboratory Rat (*Rattus Norvegicus*)

Our work concerned the characterisation of the profile of muscle and plasma free fatty acids and fatty acids from triacylglycerols in underfed animals, with a level of weight loss (45%) simulating practical conditions of livestock feeding resources during seasonal droughts in tropical countries (van Harten et al., 2003a). Assays were conducted in the Tropical Research Institute (Lisbon, Portugal).

As a model, rats were used in the study. Sixteen Whister male rats (360g) were divided in 2 groups (n=8): C (control) fed *ad libitum* and R (restricted feeding) fed 34% of the energy and 55% of protein maintenance requirements, simulating weight loss in frequent drought periods. Animals were slaughtered at day 23 of the experimental period and samples were taken from plasma and gastrocnemius muscle. The profile determination of free fatty acids and fatty acids of triacylglycerols was accomplished using a gas chromatograph (*Hewlett Packard* 5890). The identification of the fatty acids was done using standards obtained by Sigma–Aldrich (Química, S.A.) The internal normalization method was used to determine percentages of fatty acid present in the muscle and plasma (ISSO 5508, 1990). Gastrocnemius muscles were prepared using the methods described by Maxwell et al., (1980) for the determination of lipid extraction. The same extraction was effectuated in plasma, but according to the method of Folch et al., (1957). Derivatization of muscle and plasma samples was effectuated by the same method (ISSO 5509, 2000) to determine free fatty acids and fatty acids incorporated in triacylglycerols, with separated preparations for each analysis.

Results are presented in Figures 5 and 6. Undernutrition significantly induced the increase of % free C14:0 content in the plasma (59%) and decreased the % C16:0 incorporated in triacylglycerols of muscle fat (27%). In underfed rats, C18:0 suffered a relative increase in its free (92%) and in its sterified form (223%) in the adipocytes of the muscle. Food restriction decreased the % of C18:1 as free fatty acid in the muscle (39%) and in plasma (29%).

In our results C14:0 free fatty acid relative increase in plasma reflects a degradation priority over other fatty acids. Our results of C16:0 partially coincide with the observations by Nawrocki et al. (1999), since they also noticed a decrease in triacylglycerol C16:0 when working with undernourished rats. These latter authors also observed no alteration in the free form of C18:0 in the plasma in diabetic rats, coinciding with our results. However, in this experience, opposite to our findings the authors showed a decrease in C18:0 in the triacylglycerols in the adipocytes of the muscle and no alteration in its free form. Stearic acid is a fatty acid with great energy capacity requiring 8 cycles of ß–oxidation (Koolman et al., 1996) and this fact can be related to our findings concerning its % increase in the free and sterified forms in the muscle, readily available for hydrolysis in extreme conditions.

Concerning the decrease of free C18:1 in muscle and in plasma of underfed rats, our results do not agree with those showed by Nawrocki et al. (1999), which describe an increase in C18:1 in the muscle and no effect of energy restriction on its plasmatic concentration in diabetic rats, nor with Yaffe et al. (1980) who also demonstrated opposite results in rats with 30% body weight loss. These authors explanation of such an increase is related with a small existence of stored fat, where mobilization of fatty acids is still in progress, despite the level of undernutrition.

Relatively to C18:2 no statistical significant effect of undernutrition was found in our work, in contrast with the studies of Yaffe et al. (1980) and Nawrocki et al. (1999). Both their works found increases in free form of this fatty acid in the plasma. The latter author also found in muscle an increase of C18:2 free and sterified form. Yaffe et al. (1980) again explained their results in the plasma with the existence of adipose tissue as the probable source of the essential fatty acid while our results might be explained with a possible preservation of this essential fatty acid.

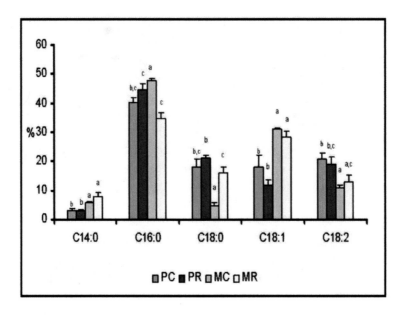

Figure 5. Rat plasma and muscle TGA %; PC-plasma control; PR-Plasma restricted; MC-Muscle control; MR - muscle restricted. Bars with different superscripts indicate statistical significance (van Harten et al., 2003a).

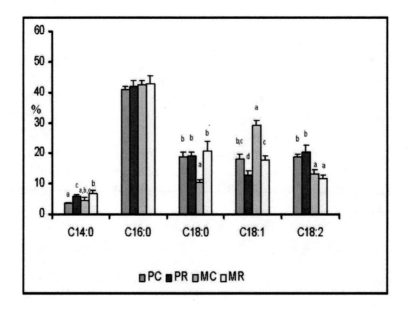

Figure 6. Rat plasma and muscle FFA %; PC-plasma control; PR-Plasma restricted; MC-Muscle control; MR - muscle restricted. Bars with different superscripts indicate statistical significance (van Harten et al., 2003a).

Our results show a priority in the hydrolysis of long chain fatty acids of great energy potential (C18:0 and C18:1) in animals with losses of 45% of their initial weight. These results suggest that the supplementation of long chain fatty acids will enhance the recover of deep organic depletion due to food restriction.

Muscle and Plasma Free Fatty Acids and Fatty Acids from Triacylglycerols in Underfed Animals: Experiments with Boer Goat Bucks (*Capra Hircus*)

The trial with Boer goats was conducted at Bloemfontein (South Africa) as described in van Harten et al. (2003b). Fifteen bucks weighting 28 kg were organised in two groups: control group (C) fed *ad libitum* (n=7) and a restricted group (R) fed 80% of energetic maintenance needs (n=8). After 30 days of experiment, animals were slaughtered in a standard small ruminant line in a commercial abattoir. Blood was collected using vacuum Heparine – Lithium test tubes and syringes (both vacumtainer® type) and then centrifuged using a *Hettich Rotanta R* centrifuge. Plasma was separated and placed in plastic test tubes and kept at –20°C for further analysis. After slaughtering, semimembranous muscle samples were collected with a lancet and kept at -75°C for further analysis. Plasma and muscle were prepared using the methods described earlier.

The content of blood and muscle free fatty acids fatty acids in the fraction of triacylglycerols was studied and results are presented in Figures 7 and 8. Percentage of C16:0 as free fatty acid in the plasma suffered a significant effect of undernutrition (increase of 6%) and C18:1 showed a relative decrease in muscle fatty acid incorporated in triacylglycerols in underfed goats (19%). C18:2 revealed a relative increase in muscle fatty acid incorporated in triacylglycerols (337%) and a relative decrease in free fatty acid in the plasma in the restricted group (17%).

In our results the percentages of free C16:0 in the plasma increased, revealing a higher level of degradation of this fatty acid. Rukkwamsuk et al. (2000) found opposite results. One reason why it is the only free fatty acid that suffered a relative increase in the plasma of underfed bucks may be due to it being considered one of the most abundant fatty acid in nature (Christie, 1989).

Oleic acid is an unsaturated fatty acid and due to its double bond, its degradation goes through several steps, including the need for an isomerase transforming a cis–conformation into a trans–conformation (Koolman et al., 1996). This fact may explain its relative decrease as a reserve constituent, as it free form does not reveal any effect of undernutrition thus it does not seem to be preferred as an energy source.

The results of C18:2 as a free fatty acid coincide with those presented by Dunshea et al. (1988) in goats, Speake et al. (1997) in sheep and Rukkwamsuk et al. (2000) in cows. C18:2 is an essential fatty acid (McDonald et al., 1988), therefore its relative increase as a reserve constituent and its relative decrease as an energy source may indicate a conservation trend of this fatty acid in cases of undernutrition.

Our results show that the retention of linoleic acid in the muscle triacylglycerols is in agreement with the accumulation of an essential fatty acid reserve in low undernutrition conditions. Muscle functionality can thus be preserved. The variation of the levels in the rest of the fatty acids studied does not reveal a conclusive intervention of the effect of low undernutrition in these animals. C16:0 was the only fatty acid which presented a relative increase in its free fatty acid form in the plasma in the underfed animals, suggesting a priority in the hydrolysis of this fatty acid in the restricted fed group.

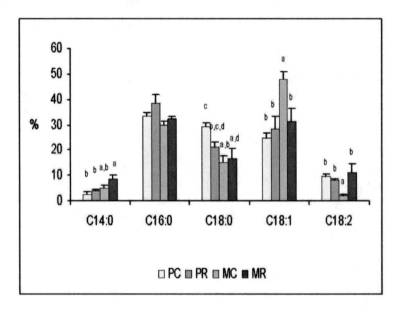

Figure 7. Boer goat plasma and muscle FFA %; PC-plasma control; PR-Plasma restricted; MC-Muscle control; MR - muscle restricted. Bars with different superscripts indicate statistical significance (van Harten et al., 2003b).

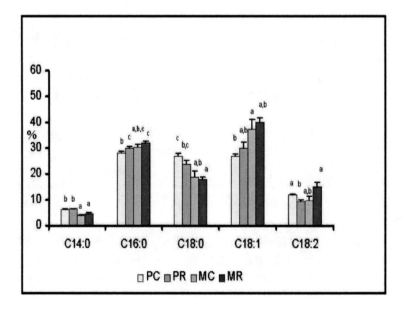

Figure 8. Boer goat plasma and muscle TGA %; PC-plasma control; PR-Plasma restricted; MC-Muscle control; MR - muscle restricted. Bars with different superscripts indicate statistical significance (van Harten et al., 2003b).

These results indicate the need of further studies concerning the recover of deep organic depletion due to food restriction.

Conclusion

In underfed monogastric and ruminants, it is visible from the cited references that, in both types of animals, show an extremely varied pattern regarding PFAA concentrations. Such variation can be due to a vast array of factors: severity and duration of food deprivation; type of restriction (mineral, protein or energy deficiency) and also the animal species, sex, productive state or finally age. Our results in laboratory rats indicate that no preferable amino acid degradation pathway is preferred. On the contrary, our assays with Boer goat bucks point to an increase in the concentrations of long carbon chain amino acids while smaller carbon chain amino acids are similar to control animals. These results indicate a superior energetic efficiency of the latter.

As a consequence of undernutrition, there seems to be a tendency to increase myofibrillar protein catabolism and lower or stop protein synthesis. However reports of preferable myofibrillar protein catabolism are relatively rare, thus indicating maintenance of muscle structure and functionality. An exception seems to be our results with Boer goat bucks that, under 20 % weight loss in 30 days, had lower amounts of Protein C and α - Actinin indicating a disruption of muscle structure where those proteins are located.

No significant conclusion could be made relatively to the influence of undernutrition on free and sterified fatty acids in plasma and muscle regarding monogastric and ruminants due to several contradictions found in the different studies here reviewed. These contradictions may be due to differences in the level of undernutrition undertaken by the authors.

Our results show a priority in the hydrolysis of long chain fatty acids of great energy potential (C18:0 and C18:1) in the animals with losses of 45% of their initial weight. These results suggest that the supplementation of long chain fatty acids will enhance the recover of deep organic depletion due to food restriction.

Acknowledgements

Authors thank Fundação para a Ciência e a Tecnologia for financing A.M. Almeida (Praxis XXI/BM/17921/98) and S. van Harten (Praxis XXI/BM/20753/99). We would also like to thank Elevier Science for allowing inclusion of data from Almeida et al. (2002); Almeida et al. (2004); Van Harten et al. (2003a) and Van Harten et al. (2003b) in this publication.

References

Abdalla, A.L., Louvandini, H., Bueno, I.C., Vitti, D.M., Meireles, C.F. and Gennari, S.M. (1999). Constraints to milk production in grazing dairy cows in Brazil and management strategies for improving their productivity. *Prev. Vet. Med. 38*(2-3): 217-230.

Alejandrino, A.L., Assad, C.O., Malabayabasm B., De Vera, A.C., Herrera, M.S., Deocaris, C.C., Ignacio, L.M. and Palo, L.P. (1999). Constraints on dairy cattle productivity at the smallholder level in the Philippines. *Prev. Vet. Med. 38*(2-3): 167-178.

Almeida, A.L., Schwalbach, L.M.J., deWaal H.O., Greyling, J.P.C. and Cardoso, L.A. (2004). Serum amino acid and myofibrillar protein profiles in Boer goat following undernutrition. *Small Ruminant Research 55*: 141-147.

Almeida, A.L., Van Harten, S. and Cardoso, L.A. (2002). Serum amino acid and myofibrillar protein profiles of fed and underfed laboratory rats. *Nut Res 22*: 1453-1459.

Ameredes, B.T., Watchko, J.F., Daood, M.J., Rosas, J.F., Donahoe, M.P. and Rogers, R.M. (1999). Growth hormone improves body mass recovery with refeeding after chronic undernutrition-induced muscle atrophy in aging male rats. *J. Nutr*. 129: 2264-2270.

Bandman, E. (1994). Química de los tejidos animales: Parte I - Proteínas. In J.F. Price and B.S. Schwegert (Eds.); *Ciencia de la carne y de los productos cárnicos* (2nd Edition, pp 581), Zaragoza (Spain): Editorial Acríba.

Bates, P.C., Grimble, G.K., Sparrow, M.P. and Millward, D.J. (1983). Myofibrillar protein turnover – Synthesis of protein bound 3-methylhistidine, actin, myosin heavy chain and aldolase in rat skeletal muscle in the fed and starved states. *Biochem. J*. 214: 593-605.

Bedi, K.S., Birzgalis, A.R., Mahon, M., Smart, J.L. and Wareham, A.C. (1982). Early life undernutrition in rats 1. Quantitative histology of skeletal muscles from underfed young and refed adult animals. *Br. J. Nutr*. 47: 417-430.

Belkhou, R., Cherel, Y., Heitz, A., Robin, J.P. and Le Maho, Y. (1991). Energy contribution of proteins and lipids during prolonged fasting in the rat. *Nut Res* 11: 365-374.

Bergen, W.G. (1979). Free amino acids in blood of ruminants – Physiological and nutritional regulation. *J Anim Sci,* 49(6): 1577-1589.

Biourge, V., Groof, J.M., Fisher, C., Bee, D., Morris, J.G. and Rogers, Q.R. (1994a). Nitrogen balance, plasma free amino acid concentrations and urinary orotic acid excretion during long term fasting in cats. *J. Nutr. 124*: 1094-1103.

Biourge, V., Groof, J.M., Morris, J.G. and Rogers, Q.R. (1994b). Long term fasting in adult obese cats: Nitrogen balance, plasma free amino acid concentrations and urinary orotic acid excretion. *J. Nutr. 124*: 2680S-2682S.

Bloxam, D.L. (1972). Nutritional aspects of amino acid metabolism 2. The effects of starvation on hepatic portal-venous differences in plasma amino acid concentration and on the liver amino acid concentrations in the rat. *Br. J. Nutr*. 27: 233-247.

Blum, J.W., Reding, T., Jans, F., Wanner, M., Zemp, M. and Bachmann, K. (1984). Variations of 3-Methylhistidine in blood of dairy cows. *J. Dairy Sci*. 68: 2580-2587.

Butterworth, M.H. (1984). *Beef cattle nutrition and tropical pastures* (1st Edition), London (England): Longman.

Cascino, A., Muscaritoli, M., Cangiano, C., Conversano, L., Laviano, A., Ariemma, S., Meguid, M.M. and Fanelli Rossi, F. (1995). Plasma amino acid imbalance in patients with lung and breast cancer. *Anticancer Res 15*(2): 507-10.

Cefalu, W.T., Wang, Z.Q., Bell-Farrow, A.D., Terry, J.G., Sonntag, W., Waite, M. and Parks, J. (2000). Chronic caloric restriction alters muscle membrane fatty acid content. *Exp. Ger.* 35: 331—341.

Christie W.W. (1989). A pratical guide. 2nd ed. *The Oily Press Ltd.*

Clariget, R.P., Forsberg, M. and Rodriguez-Martinez, H. (1998). Seasonal variation in live weight, testes size, Testosterone, LH secretion, Melatonin and Thyroxine in Merino and Corriedale rams in SubTropical climate. *Acta vet. Scand.* 39: 35-47.

Clark, A.F. and Wildenthal, K. (1986). Disproportionate reduction of Actin Synthesis in hearts of starved rats. *The Journal of Biological Chemistry 261*(28): 13168- 13172.

Clemens, E., Arthaud, V., Mandigo, R. and Woods, W. (1973). Fatty acid composition of bulls and steers as influenced by age and dietary energy level. *Journal of Animal Science 37*: 1326-1331.

Cross, D.I., Boling, J.A. and Ely, D.G. (1975). Plasma amino acids in fed and fasted wethers. *J Anim Sci 41*(4): 1164-1169.

Cuperlovic, M. and Stosic, D. (1970). Some effects of protein deficiency in young growing pigs II. Blood plasma free amino acids. *Acta vet. Scand.* 11: 1-15.

Divino Filho, J.C., Hazel, S.J., Anderstam, B., Bergström, J., Lewitt, M. and Hall, K. (1999). Effect of protein intake on plasma and erythrocyte free amino acids and serum IGF-I and IGFBP-1 levels in rats. *Am. J. Physiol. 277*: E693-E701.

Dunshea, F.R., Bell, A.W. and Trigg, T.E. (1988). Relations between plasma non–esterified fatty acid metabolism and body tissue mobilization during chronic undernutrition in goats. *British Journal of Nutrition 60*:633-644.

Edmonds, M.S. and Baker, D.H.(1987). Effects of fasting on tissue amino acid concentrations and urea cycle enzymatic activities in young pigs. *J Anim Sci 65*: 1538-52.

Enser, M, Hallett, K.G., Hewett, B., Fursey, G.A.J., Wood, J.D. and Harrington, G. (1998). Fatty acid content and composition of UK beef and lamb muscle in relation to production system and implications for human nutrition. *Meat Science 49*: 329-341.

Folch J, Lees M, Stanley G.H.S. (1957). A simple method for the isolation and purification of total lipids from animal tissues. *J Biol Chem 226*: 497-509.

Fong, Y.F., Moldawer, L.L., Marano, M.A., Wei, H., Barber, A., Fischman, D.A. and Lowry, S.F. (1989). Starvation leads to decreased levels of mRNA for myofibrillar proteins. *Journal of Surgical Research 46*: 457-461.

Goetsch, A.L., Galloway Sr., D.L. and Patil, A.R. (1998). Arterial amino acid concentrations in sheep consuming forage diets. *Small Ruminant Research 29*: 51-60.

Hardy, R.W., Meckling-Gill, K.A., Williford, J., Desmond, R.A. and Wei, H. (2002). Energy restriction reduces long-chain saturated fatty acids associated with plasma lipids in aging male rats. *J Nutr 132*: 3172-3177.

Iñarrea, P., Gonzalez, J., Andrades, M.S. and Palacios, J. (1990). Changes in breast muscle composition in the young chick. *Poultry Science 69*: 1325-1330.

ISSO 5508:1990 (E). (1990). Animal and vegetable fats and oils–Analysis by gas chromatography of methyl esters of fats acids.

ISSO 5509:2000 (E). (1990).Animal and vegetable fats and oils-Preparation of methyl esters of fatty acids.

Johnson, R.J. and Hart, J.W. (1974). Influence of feeding and fasting on plasma free amino acids in the equine. *J Anim Sci 38*(4): 790-794.

Jordan, D.J. and Le Feuvre, A.S. (1989). The extent and cause of perinatal lamb mortality in 3 flocks of Merino sheep. *Australian Veterinary Journal 66*(7): 198-201.

Koolman J, Röhm KH. Color atlas of biochemistry. *Thieme*, (1996).

Leij-Halfwerk, S., Dagnelie, P.C., van Den Berg, J.W., Wattimena, J.D., Hordijk-Luijk, C.H. and Wilson, J.P. (2000). Weight loss and elevated gluconeogenesis from alanine in lung cancer patients. *Am J Clin Nutr 71*(2): 583-9.

Lobley, G.E. (1992). Control of the metabolic fate of amino acids in ruminants: a review. *J. Anim. Sci. 70*: 3264-3275.

Lopez–Pedrosa, J.M., Torres, M.I., Fernández, M.I., Ríos, A. and Gil, A. (1998). Severe malnutrition alters lipid composition and fatty acid profile of small intestine in newborn piglets. *J. Nutr 128*: 224-233.

Lusweti, E.C. (2000). The performance of the Nguni, Afrikander and Bonsmara cattle breeds in developing areas of Southern Africa. *South African Journal of Animal Science* 30 (S1): 28-29.

Marmer, W.N., Maxwell, R.J. and Williams, J.E. (1984). Effects of dietary regimen and tissue site on bovine fatty acid profiles. *Journal of Animal Science 59*: 109-121.

Maxwell R.J, Marmer W.N, Zubillaga M.P, Dalickas G.A. (1980). Determination of total fat in meat and meat products by a rapid, dry column method. *J Assoc Of Anal Chem 63*: 600-3.

McDonald P, Edwards R.A, Greenhalgh J.F.D. (1988). *Animal Nutrition,* 4th ed. London: Longman Group,. p. 543.

Meijer, G.AL., Van der Meulen, J., Bakker, J.G.M., Van der Koelen, C.J. and Van Vuuren, A.M. (1995). Free amino acids in plasma and muscle of high yelding dairy cows in early lactation. *J. Dairy Sci.* (78): 1131-1141.

Moldawer, L.L., Bistrian, B.R. and Blackburn, G.L. (1981). Factors determining the preservation of protein status during dietary protein deprivation. *J. Nutr.111*: 1287-1296.

Mosoni, L., Malmezat, T., Valluy, C., Houlier, M.L., Attaix, D. and Patureau Mirand, P. (1999). Lower recovery of muscle protein lost during starvation in old rats despite a stimulation of protein synthesis. *Am. J. Physiol. 277*: E608-E616.

Nawrocki, A., Górska, M., Zendzian-Piotrowska, M. and Górski, J. (1999). Effect of Streptozotocin Diabetes on fatty acid content and composition in different lipid fractions of rat skeletal muscle. *Horm Metab Res 31*: 252-256.

Ndibualonji, B.B., Debue, B, Dehareng, D. and Godeau, J.M. (1993). Effect of short-term fasting on plasma amino acids, glucose and insulin in non-pregnant and non-lactating Friesian cows. *Ann Zootech 42*: 212.

Ndibualonji, B.B., Dehareng, D. and Godeau, J.M. (1997). Influence de la mise à jeun sur l'amidoacidémie libre, l'urémie et la glycémie chez la vache laitière. *Ann Zootech 46*: 163-174.

Ogata, E.S., Foung, S.K.H. and Holliday, M.A. (1978). The effects of starvation and refeeding on muscle protein synthesis and catabolism in the young rat. *J. Nutr.* 108: 759-765.

Parrish Jr., F.C., Young, R.B., Miner, B.E. and Andersen, L.D. (1973). Effect of postmortem conditions on certain chemical morphological and organoleptic properties of bovine muscle. *Journal of food science* 38: 690-695.

Pell, J.M. and Bergman, E.N. (1983). Cerebral metabolism of amino acids and glucose in fed and fasted sheep. *Am. J. Physiol.* 244: E282-E289.

Piva, G., Masoero, F., Fiorentini, L. and Moschini, M. (1994). Pre and post calving plasma free amino acids in high yelding dairy cows. *Ann Zootech* 43: 306.

Preston, T.R. and Leng, R.A. (1987). Matching ruminant production systems with available resources in the Tropics and Sub-Tropics (1st Edition). *Armindale* (New South Wales, Australia): Penambul Books.

Prior, R.L., Huntington, G.B. and Britton, R.A. (1981). Influence of diet on amino acid absorption in beef cattle and sheep. *J. Nutr. 111*: 2212-2222.

Rukkwamsuk, T., Geelen, M.J.H., Kruip, T.A.M. and Wensing, T. (2000). Interrelation of fatty acid composition in adipose tissue, plasma and liver of dairy cows during the development of fatty liver postpartum. *J. Dairy Sci.* 83: 52-59.

Russel, M.A., Rodiek, A.V. and Lawrence, L.M. (1986). Effect of meal schedules and fasting on selected plasma free amino acids in horses. *J. Anim. Sci.* 63: 1428-1431.

Samarel, A.M., Parmacek, M.S., Magid, N.M., Decker, R.S. and Lesch, M. (1987). Protein synthesis and degradation during starvation induced cardiac atrophy in rabbits. *Circulation Research 60*: 933-941.

Soppela, P. and Nieminen, M. (2001). The effect of wintertime undernutrition on the fatty acid composition of leg bone marrow fats in reindeer (*Rangifer tarandus tarandus* L.). *Comp Biochem Physiol B-Biochem and Mol Biol 128*: 63-72.

Soppela, P. and Nieminen, M. (2002). Effect of moderate wintertime undernutrition on fatty acid composition of adipose tissues of reindeer (*Rangifer tarandus tarandus* L.). *Comp Biochem Physiol A-Mol and Int Physiol 132*: 403-409.

Speake, B.K., Noble, R.C., Bracken, J. and Bishop, S.C. (1997). Responses in plasma free fatty acid composition to divergent selection for predicted carcass lean content in sheep. *Journal of Agriculture Science 129*: 193-198.

van Harten, S., Almeida, A.M., Morais, Z and Cardoso, L.A. (2003a). Free fatty acids and fatty acids of triacylglycerols profiles in muscle and plasma of fed and underfed laboratory rats. *Nutr. Res. 23*: 1685-1690.

van Harten, S., Almeida, A.M., Morais, Z, Schwalbach, L.M., Greyling, J.P., de Waal, H.O. and Cardoso, L.A. (2003b). Free fatty acids and fatty acids of triacylglycerols profiles in muscle and plasma of fed and underfed Boer goats. *Nutr. Res. 23*: 1447-1452.

Ward, L.C. and Buttery, P.J. (1980). Dietary protein intake and 3-Methylhistidine excretion in the rat. *Br. J. Nutr. 44*: 381-392.

Wassner, S.J., Orloff, S. and Holliday, M.A. (1977). Protein degradation in muscle: response to feeding and fasting in growing rats. *Am. J. Physiol. 233*(2): E119-E123.

Wassner, S.J., Schlitzer, J.L. and Li, JB. (1980). A rapid, sensitive method for the determination of 3-Methylhistidine levels in urine and plasma using High-Pressure Liquid Chromatography. *Analytical Biochemistry 104*: 284-289.

Williams, J.E., Wagner, D.G., Walters, L.E., Horn, G.W., Waller, G.R., Sims, P.L. and Guenther, G.W. (1983). Effect of production systems on performance, body composition and lipid and mineral profiles of soft tissue in cattle. *Journal of Animal Science 57*: 1020-1028.

Wilson, R.T. (1987). Livestock production in Central Mali: Factors influencing growth and liveweight in agro-pastoral cattle. *Trop Anim Health Prod 19*(2):103-14.

Wolff, J.E. and Bergman, E.N. (1972). Gluconeogenesis from plasma amino acids in fed sheep. *Am. J. of Physiol. 223*(2): 455-460

Wu, G., Pond, W.G., Ott, T. and Bazer, F.W. (1998). Maternal dietary protein deficiency decreases amino acid concentrations in fetal plasma and allantoic fluid of pigs. *J. Nutr. 128*: 894-902.

Yaffe, S., Gold, A. and Sampugna, J. (1980). Effects of prolonged starvation on plasma free fatty acid levels and fatty acid composition of myocardial total lipids in the rat. *J Nutr 110*: 2490-2496.

Zicker, S.C. and Rogers, Q.R. (1994). Concentrations of amino acids in plasma and whole blood in response to food deprivation and refeeding in healthy two day old foals. *Am J Vet Res 55*(7):1020-1027.

In: Focus on Nutrition Research
Editor: Tony P. Starks, pp. 71-120

ISBN 1-59454-768-8

Chapter IV

Food and Weight-Related Behaviours: Do Beliefs Matter More than Nutrition Knowledge?

Madeleine Nowak[1], Petra G. Buettner[1],
David Woodward[2] and Anna Hawkes[3]

[1]School of Public Health and Tropical Medicine, within the North Queensland Centre for
Cancer Research, James Cook University, Townsville, Australia,
[2]School of Medicine, University of Tasmania, Hobart, Australia and
[3]Currently, Viertel Centre for Research in Cancer Control, Queensland Cancer Fund,
Fortitude Valley, Australia

Abstract

Western societies are faced with two diametrically opposed weight-related problems.
Firstly, the average weight of their populations is rising, together with the health, social
and economic problems associated with overweight and obesity. The rise in weight is
probably due to a combination of: time constraints; readily available inexpensive
prepared foods, beverages and snack foods; and lower activity levels due to energy
saving devices and more sedentary leisure activities. Secondly, the slim image, prevalent
in these societies, results in weight loss measures even among those who are not
overweight. This unnecessary and unrealistic 'striving for slimness' may result in poor
eating habits, inadequate dietary intake, needless psychological pressure, and eating
disorders. Preoccupation with a slim body image and restrictive eating practices is not
solely an issue among adult populations, but is also alarmingly prevalent in adolescents.

In order to better understand some of these issues, we have examined the food,
nutrition, weight and shape-related beliefs and behaviours of a group of adolescents in
Northern Australia. In this chapter we: report on a study showing that beliefs of
adolescents predict their weight loss behaviour; review information from the same
population showing that beliefs are a better predictor of food choice than nutrition
knowledge; and propose a model for food and weight related behaviour, which

incorporates the individual's beliefs into the well established Transtheoretical Model of Change.

Introduction

Western societies are faced with two diametrically opposed weight-related problems. Firstly, the average weight of their populations is rising [1-5] together with the health, social and economic problems associated with overweight and obesity [6,7]. Secondly, the slim image, prevalent in these societies, results in weight loss measures even among those who are not overweight [8,9]. This unnecessary and unrealistic "striving for slimness" may result in poor eating habits, inadequate dietary intake, needless psychological pressure, and eating disorders. Preoccupation with a slim image and restrictive eating practices are not solely an issue among adults, but are alarmingly prevalent among adolescents [10-12].

In previous studies of food and weight-related behaviour of adolescents from northern Australia we found that the majority of students in Year 8 were dissatisfied with their bodies, with approximately 40% reporting being "happy with the way my body looks" [13]. So many of the girls (52%) wanted to lose weight, including some who did not consider themselves overweight, that we suspected that wanting to lose weight among females may have become a fashion. In contrast, equal numbers of boys wanted to lose or gain weight, with 54% reporting they did not want to change their weight.

There were significant changes in the level of body satisfaction across school years with males becoming increasingly more satisfied while females became increasingly less satisfied [14]. Both males and females were concerned about their body shape and their weight, however there were major gender differences across school years. More males in higher school years than lower years thought their calves, thighs, chests and lower arms were too thin and consequently wanted to "bulk up". In contrast, more females in higher than lower years thought their hips, stomachs, thighs and buttocks were too fat and hence they reported wanting to lose weight.

More females (66%) than males (24%) had attempted weight loss, and older females were more likely to attempt weight loss than younger ones, but there was little change in the proportion of males attempting weight loss across school years. Among those who wanted to lose weight, the females were more likely to manipulate their food intake while the males were more likely to exercise. However, among those who attempted weight loss, hazardous methods of weight loss were used equally by males and females (10%). While there were no significant changes in the frequency of hazardous weight loss methods used by males across school years, more females in higher than lower years used diuretics and laxatives to manipulate their weight.

These adolescents reported a poor intake of core foods, with only one in four eating fruit, vegetables, a dairy product and a core cereal food daily [15]. They also reported a high intake of fatty and sugary foods. Thus foods high in fat and sugar appeared to be replacing these core foods in the diets of these adolescents. The fruit intake was particularly low, with only 41% of females and 35% of males eating fruit daily. Furthermore, 19% of students did not consume dairy products daily. Adolescents who ate three main meals per day were more likely than others to eat all four core foods daily.

There were significant gender differences in food intake and food related behaviour amongst these adolescents. The females ate fruit and vegetables more often and high fat savoury foods and high sugar foods less often than the males. However, the females also ate core cereal foods less often than the males, possibly because they considered these foods to be fattening.

Although the females were more concerned about their health than the males and reported trying to eat well, they tended to reduce their intake of bread, milk and meat when attempting weight loss. Furthermore, the lower intake of bread and milk persisted beyond the weight loss attempt as did the tendency to eat breakfast and lunch less often [15].

The major changes in food intake and exercise behaviour across school years were that females in the higher school years tended to exercise less often and were less likely to consume bread and milk every day than females in lower school years. The females in higher school years also ate between meal snacks less often, which correlated with their lower intake of some high fat and high sugar snack foods: potato crisps and high fat extruded snacks, ice cream, muesli bars, candies and chocolates, and soft drinks. In contrast, the males in higher school years consumed between meal snacks more often than those in lower school years [15].

The majority of these adolescents reported an association between eating and negative food-related emotions [15]. Overall, 70% of the males and 94% of the females reporting at least one of the following behaviours: eating more when depressed; eating from boredom; or associating guilt with eating. There were no significant changes across school years in the proportion of students reporting at least one of these behaviours. This type of emotional eating was reported more frequently by both males and females who had tried to lose weight than by students who had not tried to lose weight.

Most of these adolescents were aware of the relationship between their current food intake and the risk of future ill-health, however, future health was not particularly important to them [16]. When asked about a series of issues relating to looks, health and well being, they ranked issues of current looks and energy more highly than issues relating to future ill health, with looks and energy being even more important in higher school years. This ranking was not gender specific, although more females assigned the highest rank to their weight whereas more males assigned the highest rank to their fitness.

In this chapter we: explore the relationship between beliefs and behaviours relating to weight loss attempts; review information from the same population showing that beliefs are a better predictor of food choice than nutrition knowledge; and propose a model which can be used to both understand and change food and weight related behaviour.

Predictors of Weight Loss Attempts among Adolescents

The objective of the present study was to explore the relationships between weight and shape related beliefs and behaviours among these Australian adolescents, and to identify predictors of attempting weight loss. In addition to exploring these data with the more traditional multiple logistic regression analysis, we used Classification and Regression Tree (CART)- analysis [17-20] to provide more insight into the relationship between the variables and to identify specific risk groups.

Table 1. Description and bivariate results of potential predictors of weight loss attempts during previous year for boys.

Predictor	Weight loss attempts		p-value
	No (n=364)	Yes (n=114)	
Demographics			
Mean age (± SD) in years	15.0 (±1.5)	15.0 (± 1.6)	p=0.7570
Boarder	4.7%	4.5%	p=0.9188
Mother at work	67.9%	74.6%	p=0.1771
Father at work	93.0%	90.9%	p=0.4576
Body image			
Body mass index (± SD) in kg/m²	20.0 (±2.6)	22.3 (±3.3)	p<0.0001
Median number of body parts regarded too fat	0; IQR=0-0*	2; IQR=1-4	p<0.0001
"I see myself as being overweight"	12.7%	57.5%	p<0.0001
"I am happy with the way I look"	59.6%	35.1%	p<0.0001
"I would like to lose weight"	8.1%	67.3%	p<0.0001
"Others think I am too fat"	4.7%	28.8%	p<0.0001
Beliefs about body image			
Median rank of importance of weight	5; IQR=3-8	3; IQR=2-5	p<0.0001
"Slim people have more friends"	15.6%	23.2%	p=0.0635
"Slim people are most attractive"	55.9%	51.8%	p=0.4488
"Being thin is more important for a women"	56.7%	62.2%	p=0.3087
"Overweight women are not attractive for men"	54.9%	48.6%	p=0.2505
"To be fashionable a women must be thin"	46.1%	38.4%	p=0.1510
"Overweight people should blame themselves"	33.4%	37.3%	p=0.4573
"Fat people are lazy"	39.7%	36.0%	p=0.4861
"Overweight people are not healthy"	40.5%	42.9%	p=0.6585
Negative emotions			
"I eat more when I feel depressed"	20.0%	42.1%	p<0.0001
"Sometimes I eat because I am bored"	55.6%	72.8%	p=0.0011
"I often eat too much and feel guilty"	12.5%	41.2%	p<0.0001
Exercise			
Median number of days exercised last week	6; IQR=3-7	6; IQR=3-7	p=0.8751

*IQR = Inter-quartile range

CART-analysis is an explorative method of data analysis that was developed in the 1960s and 1970s [17-20]. The general aim of a CART-analysis is to define the most homogeneous subgroups of a data set with respect to an outcome variable. This is achieved by a step-wise procedure. In the first step, the entire data set is analysed by bivariate analysis of all potentially important predictors against the outcome variable. The strongest predictor is identified and the data set is divided into subgroups according to this predictor. In all subsequent steps of the analysis, the first step is repeated using the newly defined subgroups as the entire data set. CART-analysis is free from some of the restrictive assumptions inherent in many classical multivariate models and has been shown in other epidemiological research to provide important insights into the structure of data [21-23]. In particular, CART-analysis: provides a graphical display of the data with respect to the target variable; identifies interactions between variables; and defines prognostic groups or risk groups. CART-analysis has been rarely used previously in nutrition literature although Woodward used a similar technique to explore predictors of intakes of energy, nutrients and food-categories [24,25].

Table 2. Description and bivariate results of potential predictors of weight loss attempts during previous year for girls.

	Weight loss attempts		
Predictor	No (n=142)	Yes (n=273)	p-value
Demographics			
Mean age (± SD) in years	14.7 (±1.7)	15.2 (± 1.6)	p=0.0030
Boarder	20.6%	24.3%	p=0.3972
Mother at work	67.9%	70.2%	p=0.6219
Father at work	89.7%	88.6%	p=0.7461
Body image			
Body mass index (± SD) in kg/m^2	18.4 (±2.2)	21.2 (±3.1)	p<0.0001
Median number of body parts regarded too fat	1; IQR=0-3*	5; IQR=3-6	p<0.0001
"I see myself as being overweight"	14.5%	70.8%	p<0.0001
"I am happy with the way I look"	50.0%	15.5%	p<0.0001
"I would like to lose weight"	27.0%	91.2%	p<0.0001
"Others think I am too fat"	1.4%	28.0%	p<0.0001
Beliefs about body image			
Median rank of importance of weight	5; IQR=3-6	2; IQR=1-5	p<0.0001
"Slim people have more friends"	8.6%	11.1%	p=0.4213
"Slim people are most attractive"	27.9%	38.6%	p=0.0303
"Being thin is more important for a women"	51.4%	61.0%	p=0.0600
"Overweight women are not attractive for men"	16.9%	25.3%	p=0.0523
"To be fashionable a women must be thin"	13.4%	30.4%	p=0.0001
"Overweight people should blame themselves"	18.6%	20.2%	p=0.6899
"Fat people are lazy"	16.9%	16.9%	p=0.9979
"Overweight people are not healthy"	30.7%	31.3%	p=0.9114
Negative emotions			
"I eat more when I feel depressed"	45.1%	57.4%	p=0.0174
"Sometimes I eat because I am bored"	73.2%	83.2%	p=0.0171
"I often eat too much and feel guilty"	32.6%	70.0%	p<0.0001
Exercise			
Median number of days exercised last week	3; IQR=1-7	4; IQR=2-6	p=0.6410

*IQR = Inter-quartile range

In this study, data were collected using a questionnaire (Appendix 2), administered by teachers during a single school period and answered anonymously. The participants were 902 high school students attending Grades 8, 10, 11, and 12 (age range 12-20 years) at four of the six non government schools in Townsville, which is an Australian tropical coastal city with a population of approximately 145,000. Students in Grade 9 were not included in the sample because some of them had participated in a similar survey the previous year. The questions used for this component of the study included demographic information, questions relating to weight behaviour, weight-related beliefs and attitudes, perceptions of body weight and shape, and personal ranking of the importance of issues of weight, shape and health (Appendix 2). Data analyses included both stepwise multiple logistic regression analysis (backward) and CART-analysis (Appendix 1).

Table 3. Result of multiple logistic regression identifying predictors of attempted weight loss during the previous year, among boys (n = 456).

| Predictor | Weight loss attempts | | | |
	No (n=348)	Yes (n=108)	POR [95%-CI]*	p-value
How do you see yourself?				
Underweight/Okay/Don't think about it	307	45	1	
Overweight	41	63	3.0 [1.5, 6.0]	=0.0024
*Number of body parts regarded too fat***				
No body parts too fat	254	22	1	
1-3 body parts too fat	55	37	4.8 [2.3, 9.8]	<0.0001
4-12 body parts too fat	10	33	10.2 [3.5, 30.4]	<0.0001
*Rank importance of weight***				
Lower ranking (4-10)	226	45	1	
Higher ranking (1-3)	80	51	2.4 [1.3, 4.3]	=0.0046
"I eat more when I feel depressed"				
Disagree/not sure	276	62	1	
Agree	72	46	2.3 [1.2, 4.2]	=0.0082
Number of days exercised last week				
less than 6 days				
6 or 7 days	170	50	1	
	178	58	2.4 [1.3, 4.3]	=0.0045

* POR [95%-CI] = Prevalence odds-ratio and 95%-confidence interval.
** This model was adjusted for missing data in the answers to numbers of body parts regarded as too fat (45 missings) and ranking of importance of weight (54 missings).

Predictors of Attempting Weight Loss

A total of 902 students (54% males) with a mean age of 15 years (SD ± 1.6 years) participated in the study. Of these students 43.3% (23.8% boys; 65.8% girls) had attempted weight loss during the previous year. The mean body mass index (BMI) of all students was 20.3 kg/m^2 (SD ± 3.0 kg/m^2) with no significant gender difference (p = 0.298). Analysis of predictors of attempted weight loss was stratified by gender, as gender was identified as the strongest predictor of weight loss attempts, and because the authors hypothesised that predictors of attempts of weight loss are different for males and females.

Table 4. Result of multiple logistic regression identifying predictors of attempted weight loss during the previous year, among girls (n = 385).

Predictor	Weight loss attempts			
	No (n=129)	Yes (n=256)	POR [95%-CI]*	p-value
How do you see yourself?				
Underweight/Okay/ don't think about it	111	75	1	
Overweight	18	181	5.8 [2.9, 11.9]	<0.0001
Number of body parts regarded too fat				
None or 1 body part too fat	76	29	1	
2 or more body parts too fat	53	227	2.8 [1.4, 5.5]	=0.0027
*Rank importance of weight***				
Lower ranking (4-10)	79	78	1	
Higher ranking (1-3)	39	152	2.8 [1.6, 5.1]	=0.0007
"Other people think I am too fat"				
Disagree/not sure	127	183	1	
Agree	2	73	9.8 [2.2, 44.1]	=0.0030
"I often eat too much and feel guilty"				
Disagree/not sure	88	78	1	
Agree	41	178	2.4 [1.3, 4.2]	=0.0037

* POR [95%-CI] = Prevalence odds-ratio and 95%-confidence interval.
** This model was adjusted for missing data in the answer to ranking of importance of weight (40 missings).This model was also adjusted for the confounding effect of the belief "Slim people have more friends". The model correctly predicts 82.6% of the cases

For both sexes, weight loss attempts were strongly and significantly (p<0.0001; bivariate analyses) related to: BMI; a number of measures of personal body image; ranking of the importance of weight; and the negative emotions "I eat more when I feel depressed" (boys only), and "I often eat too much and feel guilty" (Table 1, Table 2). However, weight loss attempts were not related to a range of other general beliefs about body image or the frequency of undertaking exercise (Table 1, Table 2). Further descriptive information about the way these students ranked a number of issues relating to health, looks, and energy have been previously reported [16].

Logistic Regression Analyses

For both boys and girls, the independent predictors of weight loss attempts included: the number of body parts regarded as too fat; considering themselves overweight; and their ranking of the importance of weight. For boys the strongest predictor was the number of body parts they believed were too fat, with a significantly increased odds ratio of 10.2 (95%-CI = [3.5, 30.4]; $p < 0.0001$) for more than three body parts compared to none. The final logistic model for boys also included "I eat more when I feel depressed" ($p = 0.0082$), and the number of days of exercise during the previous week ($p = 0.0045$; Table 3). For female students, the strongest predictor of trying to lose weight was believing that others thought they were too fat (POR = 9.8; 95%-CI = [2.2, 44.1]; $p = 0.0030$). The additional predictor for girls was another negative emotion "I often eat too much and feel guilty" ($p = 0.0037$; Table 4). There were no significant interactions in either model.

This model was also adjusted for the confounding effects of body mass index, the negative emotion "I often eat too much and feel guilty", and the body image issue "Others think I am too fat". The model correctly predicts 83.3% of the cases.

CART-Analysis for Male Students

The end point of the CART was a tree-like structure of subgroups which are represented by boxes. The upper most box represents the entire data set, which consisted of 419 boys of whom 23.4% had tried to lose weight. The area of this box represents the sample size (n = 419), and the placement of the middle of this box relates to the scale of "percentage of boys who tried to lose weight."

The following explanation is intended to help the reader understand the analysis using Figure 1 and Table 5. As shown in Table 5 ("split 1"), boys who reported trying to lose weight differed in several characteristics from those who did not. They had a higher BMI, and were more likely to have unfavourable attitudes to their body. For example, they were more likely to see themselves as overweight; and less likely to see themselves as underweight; they were less likely to be happy with their body's appearance, and more likely to see multiple parts of their body as too fat; they gave a higher importance rating to body weight, and were more likely to report that other people consider them too fat. They were also more likely to have unfavourable eating behaviours: eating associated with boredom, depression or guilt. Statistically, the strongest association of attempted weight loss was with perceiving oneself as overweight, and for the next stage of the CART-analysis we analysed the "I'm overweight" and the "I'm not overweight" groups separately.

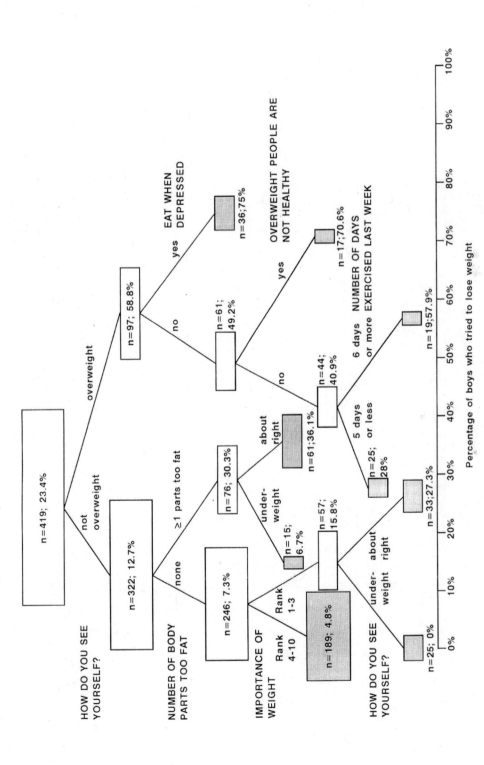

Figure 1. The CART-analysis for male students (n = 419) resulted in 9 homogenous subgroups for weight loss attempts. For each subgroup, the sample size and the percentage of boys who tried to lose weight are given. The area of a box refers to the sample size of the subgroup and the boxes are placed along the scale of percentage of boys attempting weight loss. Filled boxes mark end groups.

Table 5. Result of Classification and Regression Tree (CART)- analysis identifying predictors, among boys (n = 456), of attempted weight loss during the previous year.

	1. Split n = 419	2. Split n = 322	3. Split n = 97	4. Split n = 246	5. Split n = 76	6. Split n = 61	7. Split n = 57	8. Split n = 44
	Whole sample	I'm not over weight	I'm over weight	I'm not over weight; no body part too fat	I'm not overweight; 1+ body parts too fat	I'm over weight, don't eat more if sad	I'm not overwt; no body part too fat; weight is important	I'm overwt, don't eat more if sad; don't think overwt = unhealthy
Demographic variables								
Class (8 vs ≥10)	ns	ns	ns	ns	ns	ns	p=0.0208	ns
Age (≤13 yr vs > 13 yr)	ns	ns	ns	ns	ns	ns	p=0.0208	ns
Body size and exercise								
BMI (<18 kg/m² vs ≥18 kg/m²)	p=0.0126	ns	ns	ns	ns	/	ns	/
BMI (<20 kg/m² vs ≥20 kg/m²)	p=0.0003	ns	ns	ns	ns	ns	ns	ns
BMI (<22 kg/m² vs ≥22 kg/m²)	p<0.0001	p=0.0413	ns	ns	ns	ns	p=0.0478	ns
Days exercising last week (0-5 vs more)	ns	ns	ns	ns	ns	ns	ns	p=0.0457
Attitudes to own eating								
Sometimes I eat because I am bored (agree vs disagree/unsure)	p=0.0085	ns	ns	ns	ns	ns	ns	ns
I eat more when I feel depressed (agree vs disagree/unsure)	p<0.0001	p=0.0267	p=0.0126	ns	ns	ns	ns	ns
I often eat too much and feel guilty (agree vs disagree/unsure)	p<0.0001	p=0.0002	ns	ns	ns	ns	ns	ns
Attitudes to body size in general								
People who are overweight have only got themselves to blame (agree vs disagree/unsure)	ns	ns	p=0.0296	ns	ns	ns	ns	ns

Table 5. Continued

	1. Split n = 419 Whole sample	2. Split n = 322 I'm not over weight	3. Split n = 97 I'm over weight	4. Split n = 246 I'm not over weight; no body part too fat	5. Split n = 76 I'm not overweight; 1+ body parts too fat	6. Split n = 61 I'm over weight, don't eat more if sad	7. Split n = 57 I'm not overwt; no body part too fat; weight is important	8. Split n = 44 I'm overwt, don't eat more if sad; don't think overwt = unhealthy
Attitudes to body size in general (cont'd)								
Overwt people are not healthy (agree vs disagree/unsure)	ns	ns	p=0.0181	ns	ns	p=0.0376	ns	ns
Attitudes to own body size								
I see myself as overweight (yes vs no)	p<0.0001	/	/	/	/	/	/	/
I see myself as underweight (yes vs no)	p<0.0001	p=0.0003	/	p=0.0133	p=0.0264	/	p=0.0071	/
I feel happy with the way my body looks (agree vs disagree/unsure)	p<0.0001	ns	ns	ns	ns	ns	ns	ns
Other people think that I am too fat (agree vs disagree/unsure)	p<0.0001	ns	p=0.0300	ns	ns	ns	/	ns
Ranking of importance of weight (rank 1-3 vs rank 4-10)	p<0.0001	p=0.0016	ns	p=0.0090	ns	ns	/	ns
No. of body parts described as too fat								
(0 vs more)	p<0.0001	p<0.0001	ns	/	/	ns	/	ns
(0,1 vs more)	p<0.0001	p<0.0001	ns	/	ns	ns	/	ns
(0-2 vs more)	p<0.0001	p<0.0001	ns	/	ns	ns	/	ns
(0-3 vs more)	p<0.0001	p<0.0001	ns	/	ns	ns	/	ns
(0-4 vs more)	p<0.0001	p=0.0008	ns	/	ns	ns	/	ns
(0-5 vs more)	p<0.0001	p=0.0171	ns	/	ns	ns	/	ns

Table 5. Continued

	1. Split n = 419	2. Split n = 322	3. Split n = 97	4. Split n = 246	5. Split n = 76	6. Split n = 61	7. Split n = 57	8. Split n = 44
	Whole sample	I'm not over weight	I'm over weight	I'm not over weight; no body part too fat	I'm not overweight; 1+ body parts too fat	I'm over weight, don't eat more if sad	I'm not overwt; no body part too fat; weight is important	I'm overwt, don't eat more if sad; don't think overwt = unhealthy
No. of body parts described as too fat (continued)								
(0-6 vs more)	p=0.0116	p=0.0171	ns	/	ns	ns	/	ns
(0-7 vs more)	p=0.0128	p=0.0171	ns	/	ns	ns	/	ns
(0-8 vs more)	p=0.0128	p=0.0171	ns	/	ns	ns	/	ns
(0 −9 vs more)	p=0.0128	p=0.0171	ns	/	ns	ns	/	ns
(0 −10 vs more)	ns	p=0.0171	/	/	ns	ns	/	ns
(0 −11 vs 12)	ns	p=0.0171	/	/	ns	ns	/	ns

Footnote 1 to Table 5:

P-values (approximate or exact; ns = not significant) for potential predictors (coded as dummy variables) refer to their relation to "trying to lose weight". The "splits" refer to the branches of the CART presented in Figure 1 (from left to right and from top to bottom).

Footnote 2 to Table 5

The following dummy variables were also tested, but were not significant in the whole sample or any of the sub-groups shown (or, for some sub-groups, were not applicable):

Demographic variables: Boarder (yes vs no); Mother is working (yes vs no); Father is working (yes vs no);

Body size and exercise: BMI missing (yes vs no); Days exercising last week (none vs some days);

Attitudes to body size in general: Slim people have more friends (agree vs disagree/unsure); Being thin is more important for a woman than a man (agree vs disagree/unsure); People who are overweight have only themselves to blame (agree vs disagree/unsure); Most people who are fat are lazy; (agree vs disagree/unsure); Overweight people are not healthy; (agree vs disagree/unsure);

Attitudes to own body size: Ranking of importance of weight (missing vs valid value)

No. of body parts described as too fat Number of body parts described as too fat (missing vs valid value); (0 −11 vs 12); Number of body parts described as too fat; (0 −11 vs 12)

Footnote 3 to Table 5:

Within a column, more than one dummy variable may achieve a p<0.0001. The DV chosen for the split was the one with the highest chi-square statistic value, and is denoted in each column by the use of bold type. (The chi-square values themselves have been omitted to save space.)

The "I'm not overweight" sub-group comprised 322 boys, of whom 13% had attempted weight loss; the "I'm overweight" comprised 97 boys, of whom 59% had attempted weight loss. In these two sub-groups analysed separately, we no longer find in either group a significant impact for a number of the predictors noted in the previous paragraph (eg, two of the BMI dummy variables, link of eating with boredom, dissatisfaction with body), suggesting that these predictors form a tight cluster with self-perceived overweight. (Table 5, splits 2 and 3). Awareness of such a cluster could allow more holistic intervention strategies.

Among Those Who Did Not Consider Themselves Overweight

Some of the predictors mentioned above were significant in the whole sample, but not in the "I'm overweight" group – suggesting that their impact in one of the two sub-groups was strong enough to prevent it being "diluted out" by the other sub-group in the whole sample of boys. In the "I'm not overweight" sub-group, those who had attempted weight loss had a higher BMI, were less likely to see themselves as underweight, more likely to see multiple parts of their body as too fat, and consider body weight more important; and they were also more likely to report associating eating with depression or guilt. Regarding at least one body part as too fat had the strongest impact: 30% had attempted weight loss, compared to 13% of those who did not consider any body part too fat. However, the factors mentioned in this paragraph may be considered a cluster, to be collectively targeted in interventions specifically aimed at boys who do not consider themselves overweight.

Among Those Who Considered Themselves Overweight

In the "I'm overweight" sub-group, those who had attempted weight loss were more likely to report eating associated with depression and that other people considered them too fat, and were more likely to display negative attitudes to overweight people ("only have themselves to blame", "not healthy"). Once again, the factors mentioned in this paragraph may be regarded as a cluster to be addressed collectively in interventions specifically aimed at boys who consider themselves overweight.

The End-Product of the CART-Analysis for Boys

The remaining steps of the CART-analysis are outlined in Table 5 and Figure 1 above. The final result of the CART-analysis (Fig 1) is the identification of nine homogeneous risk groups among boys for attempting weight loss. The key characteristics are: whether they thought they were overweight; whether they thought their body parts were too fat; whether weight was an important issue for them; whether they reported eating more when depressed; the number of days they had exercised during the previous week; and their attitudes to overweight people ("overweight people are not healthy"). At one end of the spectrum, boys who did not think they were overweight or that any of their body parts were too fat, and who gave a low rating to the importance of weight (n=189), were least likely to have attempted weight loss in the previous year (4.8%, 95%-CI = [1.8%, 7.8%]). Interestingly, even among the group of 33 boys who considered themselves to be about the right weight and did not feel

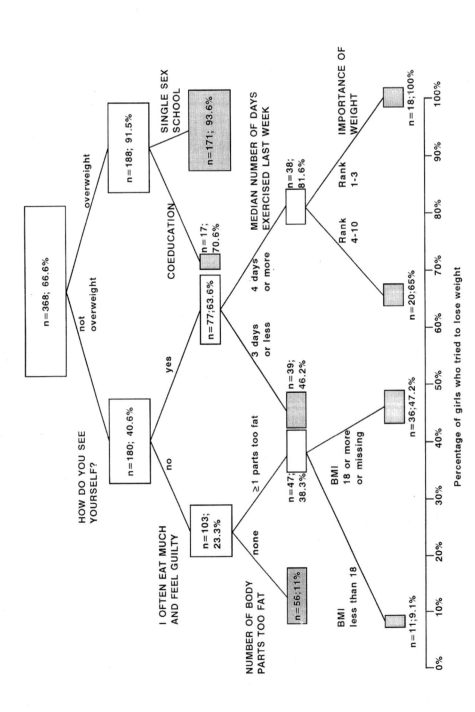

Figure 2. The CART-analysis for female students (n = 368) resulted in 8 homogenous subgroups for weight loss attempts. For each subgroup, the sample size and the percentage of girls who tried to lose weight are given. The area of a box refers to the sample size of the subgroup and the boxes are placed along the scale of percentage of girls attempting weight loss. Filled boxes mark end groups.

Table 6. Result of Classification and Regression Tree (CART)- analysis identifying predictors, among girls (n = 368), of attempted weight loss during the previous year.

	1. Split n = 368 Whole sample	2. Split n = 180 I'm not over weight	3. Split n = 188 I'm overweight	4. Split n = 103 I'm not overwt, not guilty about over-eating	5. Split n = 77 I'm not overwt, am guilty about over-eating	6. Split n = 47 I'm not overwt, not guilty about over-eating, 1+ body parts too fat	7. Split n = 38 I'm not overwt, feel guilty about over-eating, exercise 4+ d/w
Demographics							
Type of school (single sex vs co-education)	p=0.0002	ns	p=0.002	ns	ns	ns	ns
Class (8 vs ≥10)	p=0.0008	ns	ns	ns	ns	ns	ns
Class (8 or 10 vs 11 or 12)	p=0.0156	p=0.0481	ns	ns	ns	ns	ns
Class (8, 10, 11 vs 12)	p=0.0083	ns	ns	ns	ns	ns	ns
Age (≤13 years vs > 13 years)	p=0.0011	ns	ns	ns	ns	ns	ns
Age (≤15 years vs > 15 years)	p=0.0209	p=0.0353	ns	ns	ns	ns	ns
Age (≤16 years vs > 16 years)	p=0.0407	ns	ns	ns	ns	ns	ns
Body size							
BMI (<18 kg/m² vs ≥18 kg/m²)	ns	ns	ns	ns	ns	p=0.0324	ns
BMI (<20 kg/m² vs ≥20 kg/m²)	p=0.0117	ns	ns	ns	ns	ns	ns
BMI (<22 kg/m² vs ≥22 kg/m²)	p<0.0001	ns	ns	ns	ns	ns	ns
Days exercising last week							
(0, 1 vs more)	ns	ns	ns	ns	p=0.0410	ns	/
(0-2 vs more)	ns	ns	ns	ns	p=0.0021	ns	/
(0-3 vs more)	ns	ns	ns	ns	p=0.0006	ns	/
(0-4 vs more)	ns	ns	ns	ns	p=0.0100	ns	ns
(0-5 vs more)	ns	ns	ns	ns	p=0.0200	ns	ns
(0-6 days vs more)	ns	ns	ns	ns	p=0.0447	ns	ns

Table 6. Continued

	1. Split n = 368	2. Split n = 180	3. Split n = 188	4. Split n = 103	5. Split n = 77	6. Split n = 47	7. Split n = 38
	Whole sample	I'm not over weight	I'm overweight	I'm not overwt, not guilty about over-eating	I'm not overwt, am guilty about over-eating	I'm not overwt, not guilty about over-eating, 1+ body parts too fat	I'm not overwt, feel guilty about over-eating, exercise 4+ d/w
Attitudes to own eating							
Sometimes I eat because I am bored (agree vs disagree/unsure)	$p=0.0171$	ns	ns	ns	ns	ns	ns
I eat more when I feel depressed (agree vs disagree/unsure)	$p=0.0174$	ns	ns	ns	ns	ns	ns
I often eat too much and feel guilty (agree vs disagree/unsure)	$p<0.0001$	$p<0.0001$		/	/	/	/
Attitudes to body size in general							
Slim people are most attractive (agree vs disagree/unsure)	$p=0.0303$	ns	ns	ns	ns	ns	ns
Overweight women are not attractive to men (agree vs disagree/unsure)	ns	ns	$p=0.0248$	ns	ns	ns	ns
To be fashionable and look nice a woman must be thin (agree vs disagree/unsure)	$p=0.0001$	ns	ns	ns	ns	ns	ns

Table 6. Continued

	1. Split n = 368	2. Split n = 180	3. Split n = 188	4. Split n = 103	5. Split n = 77	6. Split n = 47	7. Split n = 38
	Whole sample	I'm not over weight	I'm overweight	I'm not overwt, not guilty about over-eating	I'm not overwt, am guilty about over-eating	I'm not overwt, not guilty about over-eating, 1+ body parts too fat	I'm not overwt, feel guilty about over-eating, exercise 4+ d/w
Attitudes to own body size							
I see myself as overweight (yes vs no)	**p<0.0001**	/	/	/	/	/	/
I see myself as underweight (yes vs no)	p<0.0001	p=0.0126	/	ns	ns	ns	ns
I feel happy with the way my body looks (agree vs disagree/unsure)	p<0.0001	p=0.0091	ns	ns	ns	ns	ns
Other people think that I am too fat (agree vs disagree/unsure)	p<0.0001	p=0.0002	p=0.0245	ns	p=0.0237	ns	ns
Ranking of importance of weight (rank 1-3 vs rank 4-10)	p<0.0001	p=0.0002	ns	ns	p=0.0090	ns	**p=0.0096**
No. body parts considered too fat							
(0 vs more)	p<0.0001	p<0.0001	/	**p=0.0018**	ns	/	ns
(0,1 vs more)	p<0.0001	p<0.0001	ns	p=0.0023	ns	ns	ns
(0-2 vs more)	p<0.0001	p<0.0001	ns	ns	ns	ns	ns
(0-3 vs more)	p<0.0001	p=0.0003	ns	ns	p=0.0337	ns	ns
(0-4 vs more)	p<0.0001	p=0.0007	ns	ns	p=0.0222	ns	ns
(0-5 vs more)	p<0.0001	p=0.0395	ns	ns	ns	ns	ns
(0-6 vs more)	p<0.0001	ns	ns	/	ns	/	ns
(0-7 vs more)	p=0.0002	ns	ns	/	ns	/	ns
(0-8 vs more)	p=0.0054	ns	ns	/	ns	/	ns
(0 –9 vs more)	p=0.0034	ns	ns	/	ns	/	ns
(0 –10 vs more)	p=0.0315	/	ns	/	/	/	/

*Refer to footnotes for Table 5

that even one of their body parts was too fat, but for whom weight was an important issue, 27.3% (95%-CI = [13.3, 45.5]) had tried to lose weight. At the other extreme, 75% (95%-CI = [57.8, 87.9]) of the 36 boys who thought they were overweight and who reported eating more when depressed, had tried to lose weight in the previous year.

CART-Analysis for Female Students

As shown in Table 6 ("split 1"), girls who reported trying to lose weight differed in several characteristics from those who did not. The strongest association with attempted weight loss was self-perceived overweight: only 41% of the girls who saw themselves as not being overweight had attempted weight loss, compared to 92% of those who saw themselves as being overweight. Further analysis, therefore, focussed on the sub-groups 'I'm overweight" and "I'm not overweight".

Several other characteristics (higher BMI, eating because of boredom or depression, believing that slimness is linked to being attractive and fashionable) were also associated with attempted weight loss among girls as a whole, but were not significant in the two sub-groups. These would appear to form a cluster with self-perceived overweight, and intervention strategies aimed at girls as a whole might sensibly focus on these collectively.

Among Those Who Did Not Consider Themselves Overweight

A number of characteristics significant in the whole sample of girls retained significance only among those who did not consider themselves overweight (higher year at school, older, being guilty about eating, not seeing herself as underweight, not being happy with her body, placing greater importance on weight, seeing several body parts as too fat). Their impact in the whole sample may therefore be regarded as an artefactual side-effect of their impact in the "I'm not overweight" sub-group. The factor with greatest impact in this sub-group was guilt: 64% of those who felt guilty about over-eating had attempted weight loss, compared with 23% of those who didn't. Several other factors mentioned in the previous paragraph - higher year at school, older, not seeing herself as underweight, not being happy with her body – did not reach significance in either the "guilty" or the "not guilty" sub-group; these would appear to form a cluster with guilt about over-eating, and intervention strategies aimed at girls who did not consider themselves overweight might sensibly focus on these collectively.

Among Those Who Considered Themselves Overweight

One characteristic, which was significant in the whole sample of girls retained significance only among those who considered themselves overweight: 94% of those at single-sex schools had attempted weight loss, compared to 71% of those at coeducational schools. This finding suggests that intervention strategies focussed on those who consider themselves overweight are particularly relevant to single-sex schools.

The End-Product of the CART-Analysis for Girls

Once again, it would be tedious to continue this description step by step. But the final result of the CART-analysis (Fig 2) is the identification of eight homogeneous risk groups for attempting weight loss. The key characteristics are: whether they thought they were overweight; whether they reported feeling guilty about over-eating; whether they attended a single-sex or coeducational school; whether they thought their body parts were too fat; their BMI; the number of days they had exercised during the previous week; and whether weight was an important issue for them. At one end of the spectrum, weight loss had been attempted by only 9% of those girls who did not think they were overweight or feel guilty about over-eating, had at least one body part they considered too fat but had a BMI less than 18 (9.1%; 95%-CI = [0.2, 41.3]). At the other extreme, weight loss had been attempted by 100% of those who did not think they were over-weight but felt guilty about over-eating, exercised more than four days per week and regarded weight as important (100%; 95%-CI = [81.5, 100.0]).

Logistic Regression and CART-Analysis are Complementary

For both male and female students, the predictors identified using logistic regression analysis were also evident in CART-analysis. For male students, CART-analysis provided additional information about: (1) "eating when depressed" which was particularly important for boys who believed they were overweight; (2) the number of days of exercise which was only important for a small group of boys who thought they were overweight but did not have negative emotions relating to food or negative attitudes to overweight people; and (3) the most extreme groups were identified by an association between food and negative emotions and the belief that "overweight people are not healthy". A relationship between eating and negative emotions was also of importance for girls who did not think they were overweight. Unlike the boys, believing that "overweight people are not healthy" did not affect weight loss attempts among girls.

As logistic regression and CART-analyses were conducted on the same data sets, one would expect both approaches to identify the same major predictors. However, CART-analysis creates subgroups where variables, which are less important in the whole sample can become influential and vice versa. Examples of both can be found in the CART-analysis for females. For example, believing that others thought them "too fat" did not constitute a risk factor within the CART-analysis, although it had the strongest impact on attempting weight loss in regression analysis.

In general, regression models and CART-analyses have different but complementary roles. Regression models identify risk factors and assess their impacts, whereas CART-analyses provide risk groups. In the present study, results of logistic regression analyses for boys and girls were relatively simple with only five predictors in each model. Nevertheless, these models would initially define 48 different groups of male and 32 groups of female students and, to the authors' knowledge, there is no simple solution for combining these groups into meaningful risk groups. CART-analyses directly provide such risk groups, and furthermore, can easily identify "outlier groups". For example, overall only 23.4% of the male students had attempted weight loss, however, the CART-analysis identified three relatively small groups in which more than 70% of the boys had attempted weight loss. Multiple logistic regression also enables the identification of extreme groups by using multiplication of effects. For example, the boys who: saw themselves as overweight; felt that four to 12 body parts were too fat; considered weight an important issue; reported eating more when depressed; and had exercised for at least six days in the previous week, would have a prevalence odds-ratio of 405.4 for trying to lose weight, compared with boys in the baseline categories for those predictors. In the present data set, this extreme group consisted of three boys. However, in many multiple logistic regression models, these groups are a mere theoretical concept and, consequently, estimates based on them must be considered weak. In contrast, groups identified by CART-analysis are always obvious in the CART diagrams of the data set.

Weight Loss Behaviours are Linked to Student Beliefs

Beliefs about their own weight and shape and the importance that they placed on weight were identified in our multiple logistic regression analyses as the major predictors of attempting weight loss for both male and female students. For both boys and girls these were essentially personal beliefs, however, girls were also more likely to attempt weight loss if they believed that others considered them too fat.

In boys, extreme groups from CART-analysis were associated with negative emotions surrounding eating behaviour and the belief that "overweight people are not healthy", while a substantial number of girls who did not consider themselves overweight, but associated eating with feelings of guilt were also likely to attempt weight loss. An association between eating and depression or negative emotions is recognised in the clinical literature in obese individuals [26], especially binge eaters [27,28], and those with eating disorders [29]. The results of this study suggest that such an association also occurs in the wider adolescent population. While adolescents have greater mood fluctuations than adults and may describe emotions as "depression", "boredom", "anxiety", or "guilt" when those a little older would merely report mild mental discomfort, adolescents do nevertheless report eating more in association with these feelings.

As stress and anxiety levels rise [30] in affluent societies with ready access to food, it may become increasingly difficult to moderate the food intake in a population, which turns to food for comfort and nurturing. Awareness of the variety of issues which are important to young people attempting weight loss may be helpful when designing population based interventions to moderate weight loss behaviour among adolescents. In the present study the beliefs that these students held about their own weight and shape were identified as the major predictors of weight loss behaviour. Therefore, interventions, which either promote weight loss or attempt to prevent unnecessary weight loss among adolescents, should address their beliefs and concerns about body weight and shape. On the other hand, adolescence may be a time when dealing with negative emotions is a more appropriate method of weight control than emphasising food restriction. However, negative emotions and believing there is a link between ill health and being overweight were only important in some subgroups. Thus, more tailor-made approaches seem warranted when tackling weight related behaviour in adolescents.

Food and Weight Beliefs and Behaviours of Adolescents

A study in the same population found strong associations between concerns about constituents of food and the consumption of those foods [31]. Males who expressed concern about the fat in food ate fried and takeaway foods less often than those who did not have this concern (p<0.0022). This relationship did not hold for the females who generally ate these foods less often than the males. In addition, students who were concerned about the fat in food ate high fat savoury foods less often than other students (p=0.0001). Furthermore those reporting concern about the sugar in foods ate high sugar foods less often than other students, while those concerned about the salt in food added salt to their food less often than students who did not hold this belief (p=0.0001). However, no relationship was found between concerns about the vitamin content of food and the frequency of intake of vitamin supplements, possibly because it is likely to be parents who purchase vitamin supplements and encourage their use.

Relationships between beliefs about food and the consumption of those foods were also highly significant. Students who reported that "eating fried food is bad for your health" were less likely to eat fried foods (p=0.0014), while those who believed that "most takeaway foods contain a lot of fat" ate fried and takeaway less often than students who did not hold that belief. Moreover, those who reported that "you should not eat the fat on meat" reported eating the fat on meat less often than other students (p=0.0001). However, there was no significant difference in the frequency of consumption of red meat between students who did or did not believe that "red meat is bad for you (p=0.0779).

The adolescents who reported trying "to eat foods I know are good for me" ate fruit more often (p=0.0001) and were more likely to eat fruit daily (p=0.0005) than other students. In addition, those who reported that "everyone needs to add salt to their food" added salt to their meals more often than those that did not hold this belief (p=0.0001). Furthermore, those who believed that "most people need to take vitamin and mineral supplements" were more likely to do so (p=0.0001).

Similarly, there was a strong relationship between beliefs about weight or weight reduction and the related behaviour. More students who agreed with the statement "I think I am overweight" also reported having tried to lose weight (p=0.0005). Among students who had tried to lose weight, those who believed that "exercise is important for weight loss" were more likely to have exercised for weight loss than those who did not hold this belief (p=0.002). Furthermore, among those who had attempted weight loss during the previous year, girls (but not boys) who believed that "skipping meals is a good way to lose weight" were more likely to also report having skipped meals as a weight loss measure (girls p=0.0005; boys p=0.1090).

However, among the adolescents who reported trying to lose weight at the time of the survey, the only significant association (of 16 options) between knowledge of foods to reduce when attempting weight loss and consumption of those foods, was that those who knew that high fat takeaway foods should be reduced ate those foods less often than students without that knowledge (p=0.0120).

It was concluded that beliefs about food and weight may be more important than knowledge in determining food related behaviour.

Development of a Food and Weight Behaviour Model

The Importance of Beliefs

Beliefs about weight and shape and the importance that these adolescents placed on their weight in relation to other issues of health and well-being were the strongest predictors of whether they would try to lose weight. Furthermore, there were significant relationships between their beliefs about the effectiveness of specific weight loss behaviours and their use of that behaviour. For example, those who believed that "skipping meals is a good way to lose weight" were more likely to miss meals when attempting weight loss than those who did not hold this belief. Therefore, any attempt to reduce the level of unnecessary weight loss attempts among adolescents should address issues of beliefs. Although beliefs were the major predictors of weight loss attempts, other issues were important in some subgroups, suggesting that it may be valuable to add specifically targeted interventions when designing weight loss programs.

There were also strong relationships between concerns about specific food components and the consumption of the relevant foods (such as sugar, fat and salt). Similarly, there were significant relationships between beliefs about foods and the consumption of those foods. However, there were few relationships between the knowledge of foods to eat for weight loss and the consumption of those foods by adolescents attempting weight loss. Hence, changing beliefs about foods to eat when attempting weight loss may have more impact on changing food related behaviour, than providing knowledge alone.

The consistent relationship between beliefs and behaviours for food intake and weight manipulation suggests that beliefs have a major role in explaining and changing such behaviour, at least in this adolescent population. While beliefs were the major predictors of weight loss behaviour, emotional eating and negative attitudes to overweight people were also important in some subgroups. The multifaceted nature of such behaviour must be acknowledged when designing population based programs.

The importance of beliefs in determining health behaviour has been previously incorporated into models of health behaviour such as the Health Belief Model [32,33], the Theory of Reasoned Action [34] and the Social Learning Theory [35]. These models recognise the importance of a number of personal, environmental and psychosocial factors in determining health behaviour. These factors are also considered to play an important role in determining food choices [36,37] and their relative importance is known to vary with age, population and between population subgroups [38,39].

Models of Health Behaviour

Eating and exercise behaviours are multifactorial and require a multidisciplinary approach which is grounded in a conceptual framework based on behavioural theory. Several behavioural models have been used to explain such behaviour and to guide interventions to promote behaviour change. Models of health behaviour have been used to explain behaviours as diverse as addictive behaviour and attendance at health clinics [40]. They have also been used to explore eating behaviour [41-47].

The cognitive behavioural models most commonly used to explain eating and weight loss are the Health Belief Model [32] and the Theory of Reasoned Action [34]. The original Health Belief Model suggests that the important issues which explain health behaviour are perceived susceptibility to disease and perceived severity of the disease [32]. This model was later modified to include perceived control and self-efficacy [33]. The key issue in the Theory of Reasoned Action is behavioural intention, which is then modified by the person's attitude to the action and their beliefs about how others will respond to that action [34]. The Theory of Reasoned Action was then further modified into the Theory of Planned Behavior which incorporated "perceived behavioral control" [48]. Social Learning Theory has also been used as a framework for understanding the influences of knowledge, beliefs, and psychosocial and environmental factors on food selection [35,49] and more recently Turrell and colleagues developed a conceptual framework to identify determinants of socioeconomic health inequalities [50].

The model most frequently used to describe dietary change is the Transtheoretical Model of Change (TMC) or Stages of Change Model [51,52]. This model can identify the readiness for change of an individual or group, and correctly locate different population sub-groups within the stage of change cycle, enabling a more targeted intervention. This model was initially developed in the clinical context for use with addictive behaviours [53], but it has also been used as a model of behaviour change for many health related behaviours in both the clinical and community setting, including weight control [54], eating [53-57], and exercise behaviour [54, 58, 59].

There are, however, important differences between addictive behaviour and eating behaviour [53, 60-62]. Dealing with addictive behaviour usually requires cessation of a single behaviour, which although addictive, is not necessary to sustain life (e.g. smoking). However, changing eating behaviour involves changing many behaviours whether targeting foods (e.g. increasing fruit; decreasing takeaway foods) or nutrients (e.g. increasing dietary calcium; decreasing fat intake). Moreover, unlike addictive behaviours, it is not possible to stop eating. Even the intake of fruit and vegetables which is usually assessed as a unit is more complex, as Trudeau and colleagues [63] found that intrinsic motivators (such as feeling well, controlling weight, staying healthy or preventing serious illness) were more strongly associated with fruit intake than vegetable intake.

Eating behaviour is far more complex than addictive behaviour, resulting in some limitations to the use of the TMC. For example, in its original form there were time frames for each stage, which may not be relevant to eating behaviour. Furthermore, it may be more difficult for an individual to know whether they are eating a high fibre diet or a low fat diet [53], although a single eating habit such as eating two pieces of fruit per day, is as easy to identify as not smoking cigarettes. Nevertheless the model has been used widely for eating and exercise behaviour.

The Proposed Model of Food and Weight Behaviour

A new model is proposed which can be used to both understand and change food and weight related behaviour. This model builds on the TMC and is based on: the data presented here; 15 years of clinical dietetic experience; extensive observation of food habits and lifestyle in other cultures [64]; anthropological data, which suggests that people confuse their own experience with reliable nutrition knowledge [65]; and the recognised role of cognitive dissonance (i.e. the discomfort associated with a lack of concordance between beliefs and behaviours) in aligning behaviours with beliefs [66].

There are national examples of the linkages between culture, beliefs, environment, body shape, weight, and eating habits that can serve as prototypes for interventions. These national examples indicate some potential directions for change.

The eating and activity culture of the United States of America and Australia result in high (and rising) levels of overweight and obesity [67-70], and thus provide an undesirable cultural model. The eating and activity culture of many non Anglo-Saxon countries result in lower levels of overweight and obesity, although these are also increasing [71-74]. French food culture is one of the strongest in Europe and yet the incidence of overweight and obesity of adults in France is among the lowest in Europe [74]. The levels of 32% for French women and 47% for men in France [75] compares favourably with Australian data of 52% for women and 68% for men [76] and the reported levels of overweight and obesity in the United States of America (66%) [70]. The differences in the level of obesity in these countries is even more marked: France <10% [75], Australia 19% for man and 22% for women [76] and 31% in the United States of America [70].

French culture is strongly based on food [77] and the consumption of a variety of healthful foods [78]. For example the average meal includes 3 to 5 small courses and usually contains bread, a meat (or alternative protein) dish, a vegetable or salad, a dairy product and dessert (which is often fruit). There are traditional rules relating to what a meal should contain and when it should be eaten [79]. For example, it is difficult to buy ready to eat food between meals in many regions of France, because people simply do not eat between meals. Physical activity is built into daily life more by accident than design, because of the infrastructure of European cities. However, walking for relaxation at weekends is common and the legendary extended French Sunday lunch is usually followed by a long walk, preferably in a park or the countryside.

We suggest that the important role of culture in determining eating and exercise behaviour cannot be ignored when explaining these behaviours. The proposed model builds on current models, by incorporating belief constructs and cultural concepts into the TMC [51,52]. It acknowledges that while environmental, psychosocial, physiological, personal factors and knowledge are all important in determining eating, exercise and weight loss behaviour, the relative importance of these may vary among individuals, groups, subgroups and cultures. Different issues are likely to dominate in different cultures, just as different standards of beauty are evident in different cultures [80]. A robust model, which can accommodate variety is essential in a multicultural society, such as Australia.

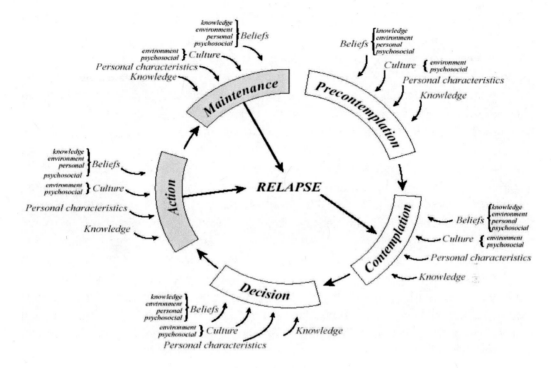

Figure 3. Model proposed for understanding and changing food and weight related behaviour. In this model the concept of relapse is based on action rather than cognition. The cognitive phase of the model is denoted by the clear boxes; the active phase of the model is denoted by the filled boxes.

Furthermore, we suggest that beliefs may be the driving force in determining eating and exercise behaviour in most Anglo-Saxon cultures. The environment, however, may be a more important influence in other cultures such as those with strong religious cultures (e.g. Buddhists, Orthodox Jews or Seventh Day Adventists) or cultures based around the table with an emphasis on fine food (e.g French, Italian or Chinese). In addition, eating behaviour is so complex that single behaviours may need to be identified before using any model to explain or change behaviour. For example, fruit and vegetables are often considered together, yet regular vegetable consumption was more common than regular fruit consumption among these adolescents.

In the suggested model (Figure 3), the classic TMC is used as a framework and to initially identify the stage of change of the individual or group, as different intervention techniques are appropriate for people at different stages of change. The model considers that when beliefs are the dominant determinants of behaviour, the personal, environmental and psychosocial factors, together with knowledge will determine the beliefs, and changing these beliefs can change behaviour. However, in strong cultures, it may be the culture, itself, which determines behaviour. The dominant features of culture in this context are the environment and psychosocial factors. Among other subgroups, knowledge, environment or personal characteristics may guide eating, exercise and weight-related behaviours.

The stages of the proposed model are those of the classic TMC: precontemplation; contemplation; decision; action and maintenance, which can be divided into two components: the cognitive component (precontemplation, contemplation and decision stages); and the active component (action and maintenance stages). In the proposed model we consider that relapse is based on action, so that at each stage of the model an individual can remain in that stage or move on to the next. In addition, in the active phase, action or maintenance, there is the potential for relapse. The route out of relapse is through the contemplation stage.

It is suggested that beliefs are the major determinants of behaviour (especially in multicultural societies such as ours, which do not have strictly defined eating or exercise patterns). Beliefs are modified by food knowledge (whether accurate or not), personal characteristics, environmental factors and psychosocial factors. Personal characteristics which have the potential to modify beliefs include: appeal of food (appearance, smell, taste, texture, familiarity, food temperature, quality, variety); demographics (age, sex, locality, education, socioeconomic level); health priorities, health status; performance (academic, fitness, sport); and physiological issues (mood, hunger, food cravings, weight).

Psychosocial factors which may modify beliefs include: advertising; body image beliefs and weight concerns; convenience; cost; fashion; family members; habit; media; mood; peers; social norms; social support; and time. Environmental issues which can affect beliefs include: accessibility; advertising; availability; culture and religion; infrastructure; media; policy (economic, health, housing, taxation, transport, welfare); role models; social norms; and weather/season. These potential influences on beliefs can also be considered as either internal or external factors.

According to this model, beliefs, culture, personal characteristics, and environment can have an impact at each stage in the change cycle. It is also possible that the issues which have an effect, may change between stages. For example: a taste preference for fatty food may decrease when dietary fat intake has been reduced for some months; beliefs about self efficacy in relation to cooking low fat meals may change with experience; and the enjoyment gained from exercise may increase with fitness.

If the hypothesis that in Anglo-Saxon societies personal beliefs are important in determining eating and exercise behaviour is correct, then a change in these behaviours is dependent, at least in part, on changing beliefs. Thus, methodology (or the manner in which information is presented) becomes extremely important. Changing beliefs is the "core business" of psychologists (and is also regularly used by advertising companies). In communities (or individuals) where beliefs determine behaviour, involvement of health psychologists in interventions to change eating, exercise and weight-related behaviour may be vital [81].

Careful attention should be paid to how dietary knowledge is presented. If it is presented in a way that is relevant to the target audience, matches their readiness to change, and has the potential to change their beliefs, it may result in change. Otherwise, no matter how good or well prepared the information might be, it will fall on deaf ears. Health professionals trying to improve the eating and exercise habits of the community will be much more effective if they employ strategies to modify the beliefs of their target audience.

Conclusion

While changing behaviour is difficult, it is more likely to be successful if interventions are designed around the perceived needs of the target group, and acknowledge the importance of beliefs, knowledge, environment and psychosocial factors which can affect behaviour and readiness to change. The model presented here may help to achieve these aims by providing a theoretical framework for interventions to alter the eating and exercise patterns of adolescents.

Appendix 1 – Methods from Section on Predictors of Weight Loss Attempts

Participants

In 1993 a questionnaire survey was conducted amongst high school students attending Grades 8, 10, 11, and 12 at four of the six non government schools in Townsville, which is an Australian tropical coastal community (latitude 19°16'S; population approximately 145,000). A total of 902 students participated with no refusals from students who were in class on the day of the study. Students in Grade 9 were not included in the sample because some of them had participated in a similar survey the previous year. Both co-educational and single sex schools, and Catholic and non-Catholic schools were included in the sample. Further details about the sample have been published previously [16]. Ethics approval was obtained from James Cook University Ethics Committee and clearance was received from Education Queensland.

Questionnaire

The standardised questionnaires (Appendix 2) were administered by teachers during a single school period and were answered anonymously. There were eight demographic questions, 15 questions relating to weight behaviour, 15 on perception of weight and body shape, and 18 on weight-related beliefs and attitudes. Demographic data included school, grade, sex, and date of birth. Information on education level of parents or socio-economic status was sought by asking the students about their parents' occupations, however, the answers received were considered too vague to be useful. Answers to questions about weight-related beliefs, attitudes, concerns and some of the body image questions were presented as a five point Likert scale with categories ranging from strongly disagree to strongly agree. Self-reports of weight and height were obtained. Height was missing for 25.4% of the students and weight was missing for 23.4%. Consequently, body mass index (BMI) could not be calculated for 35.6% of all participants. BMI was categorized into quartiles (< 18.0 kg/m^2, $18.0 - 19.9$ kg/m^2, $20.0 - 21.9$ kg/m^2, ≥ 22 kg/m^2,) and a further category containing the missing values.

Statistical Analysis

The outcome variable "tried to lose weight during the previous year" was constructed as a dichotomous variable in categories "no" or "yes". The following potentially relevant predictors of weight loss behaviour were considered: school grade; type of school (co-educational/single sex); "are you a boarder? (no/yes); "does your mother work?" (no/yes); "does your father work?" (no/yes); BMI (categories as above); the number of their body parts the students considered too fat (range: 0-12); "how do you see yourself?"(underweight/about right or don't care/overweight); "would you like to gain weight, stay the same or lose weight?" (gain weight/stay the same/lose weight); the ranking students placed on their weight among a number of issues of health and well-being (rank 1 = most important to 10 = least important); "last week how many days did you exercise or play sport continuously for 30 minutes or more?" (range: 0-7 days); and the following beliefs and behaviours: "I am happy with the way my body looks"; "other people think I am too fat"; "slim people have more friends"; "slim people are the most attractive"; "being thin is more important for a woman than a man"; "overweight women are not attractive to men"; "to be fashionable and look nice a woman must be thin"; "people who are overweight have only themselves to blame"; "most people who are fat are lazy"; "overweight people are not healthy"; "I eat more when I feel depressed"; "sometimes I eat because I am bored"; "I often eat too much and feel guilty", which were all categorised as agree and disagree or not sure.

Numerical variables were presented as mean values with standard deviations (SD) when the data were approximately normally distributed or median values with inter-quartile ranges (IQR) when they were not. Chi-square tests, t-tests, and non-parametric Wilcoxon tests were used to assess bivariate relationships between potential predictors and the outcome variable.

In preparation for CART- and logistic regression analyses, dichotomous dummy variables were created for all of the potentially influencing variables. For each potential predictor the category with the smallest probability of having "tried to lose weight during the previous year" was chosen as the baseline category of the dummy variables. Missing value categories were constructed for the following variables: BMI (n = 321; 35.6%); the number of body parts considered too fat (n = 74; 8.2%); and the ranking of the importance of weight (n = 106; 11.8%). These missing categories were included in the analyses.

CART-Analysis

For CART-analysis, associations between potential predictors and the outcome variable were assessed using bivariate chi-square test statistics. The dummy variable providing the largest statistically significant chi-square statistic was used to define the first two subgroups. This procedure was repeated within each subgroup to subdivide the data set into a tree-shaped structure. By convention a CART-analysis is considered completed when the subgroup is too small (less than the square root of the sample size) or none of the influencing variables provide a statistically significant association with the outcome variable [20]. The subgroups defined by CART-analysis were described as the proportion of students who tried to lose weight and 95%-confidence intervals (95%-CI).

Logistic Regression

Stepwise multiple logistic regression analysis (forward and backward) was used to identify independent significant predictors of weight loss attempts. Results of logistic regression analyses are presented as prevalence odds-ratios (POR) together with 95%-CI. These logistic regression models were multiplicative. Potential confounders were identified and the logistic regression models were adjusted for their effects. All possible two- and three-way interactions were investigated. Separate CART- and logistic regression analyses were performed for boys and girls, because previous analysis of the data had identified gender as the most powerful confounder [16]. Statistical analyses were performed using SPSS for Windows (release 6.1.3). Throughout the analysis p-values less than 0.05 were regarded as statistically significant.

Appendix 2 – Questionnaire

Anton Breinl Centre
Schools Nutrition Project

This is a question about the foods you eat and your opinion about food.

There are no right or wrong answers.

The questionnaire is anonymous so choose a nickname for yourself and write it down for question 1.

Q1.   Write the nickname you have chosen for yourself here

Q2.   How old are you in years?   . . . . years

Q3.   What is your date of birth? . . . . .day . . . . month . . . . year

Q4.   Which suburb do you live in?

Please Tick a Box to Answer the Following Questions

Q5.   What sex are you?   ☐ MALE   ☐   FEMALE

Q6   (a) Are you a boarder?   ☐ NO   ☐   YES

        (b) Which grade are you in?

        (c) In which grades did you do Home Economics?

        Grade 8 ☐   9 ☐   10 ☐   11 ☐   12 ☐   none ☐

(d) In which grades did you do Health and PE?

Grade 8 ☐　　　9 ☐　　　10 ☐　　　11 ☐　　　12 ☐　　　none ☐

Q7.　　Does your mother work outside the home?

NO

YES - if so what does she do?

Q8.　　Does your father work outside the home?

NO

YES - if so what does he do?

Q9.　　How many adults live in your house　　. . . . . adults

Q10.　　How many children live in your house　　. . . . . children

Q11.　　In your opinion, how important are the foods you eat to –

	Very Important	Quite Important	Not Important	I Don't Know
The way you feel generally?				
How energetic you feel?				
Your chance of getting heart disease when you are older?				
Your overall appearance?				
Your chance of getting high blood pressure when you are older?				
Your fitness?				
Your weight?				
Your chance of getting sick later in life?				
The shape of your body?				
Your chance of getting diabetes when you are older?				

Q12.   Which of the following is most important to YOU now?

Please Number Your Answers from 1 To 10, Using Number 1 for the Most Important, and 10 For the Least Important.

The way you feel generally?

How energetic you feel?

Your chance of getting heart disease when you are older?

Your overall appearance?

Your chance of getting high blood pressure when you are older?

Your fitness?

Your weight?
Your chance of getting sick later in life?

The shape of your body?

Your chance of getting diabetes when you are older?

Q13.   What kinds of foods do you eat?

How Many Days Did You Eat/Drink This Food Last Week?
Tick One Box for Each Food

	0	1	2	3	4	5	6	7
Bread								
Cereal								
Rice								
Pasta/noodles/spaghetti								
Fruit (including dried fruit)								
Fruit juice								
Green vegetables (cabbage, beans, broccoli, peas, lettuce, cauliflower, etc)								
Yellow/orange vegetables (pumpkin, corn, carrots)								

Q13.   What kinds of foods do you eat? (Continued)

	0	1	2	3	4	5	6	7
Potatoes								
Milk (plain or flavoured)								
Cheese								
3 or more glasses of water								
Yoghurt								
Icecream								
Eggs								
Chicken								
Fish (fresh or tinned)								
Meat (e.g. steak, chops, mince, roast)								
Sausages								
Cakes and biscuits								
Muesli bars								
Lollies or chocolate								
Chips or twisties								
Nuts								
Soft drink or cordial								
Wholemeal or wholegrain foods								
Low fat milk								
Eat the fat on meat								
Eat the skin on chicken								
Fried food (e.g. hot chips, fried fish, fried chicken, dim sims, chicko rolls, etc.)								
Other takeaway food (e.g. hamburgers, pizza, pies, pasties, sausage rolls, hot dogs, etc.)								
Vitamin pills								

Q14.   Last week, how many days did you:

	0	1	2	3	4	5	6	7
Add salt to your food?								
Eat breakfast?								
Eat lunch?								
Eat dinner?								
Eat between meal snacks?								
Exercise or play sport continuously for 30 minutes of more?								

Q15.   Where do you get information about food and nutrition from:

Your parents   □ NO   □ YES

Your friends   □ NO   □ YES

Classes at school   □ NO   □ YES

TV   □ NO   □ YES

Radio   □ NO   □ YES

Newspapers   □ NO   □ YES

Magazines   □ NO   □ YES

        If YES - please specify magazines

Other   □ NO   □ YES

        If YES - please specify

From where do you get the most information

Q16. What do you think about the following statements.

Please **TICK ONE BOX** for Each Statement

	Strongly Disagree	Disagree	Not Sure	Agree	Strongly Agree
The food I eat plays a role in my overall health					
Eating fried foods is bad for your health					
Eating fried foods is bad for sports performance					
Steak and eggs and a glass of Milo would be a good pre game breakfast for a young athlete					
Too much fat in the diet may lead to heart disease					
Most people need to take vitamin and mineral pills					
Skipping meals is a good way to lose weight					
Exercise is important if you want to lose weight					
Eating sugary food before exercise will improve performance					
Following a diet in a popular magazine is a good way to lose weight					
Growing kids may lose fat but would not lose weight					
Sportspeople should eat a lot of bread, rice, potatoes, and pasta					
Most takeaway foods contain a lot of fat					
Red meat is bad for you					

Q16. What do you think about the following statements. (Continued)

	Strongly Disagree	Disagree	Not Sure	Agree	Strongly Agree
Raw sugar is better for you than white sugar					
Everyone needs to add salt to their food					
Carob bars are better for you than chocolate bars					
You should not eat the fat on meat					
It is better to eat grilled fish than battered fish					

Q17. How do you feel about these statements.
TICK ONE BOX for each.

	Strongly Disagree	Disagree	Not Sure	Agree	Strongly Agree
I try to select foods that I know are good for me					
I should only worry about the food I eat if I am fat					
Sometimes I eat because I am bored					
I eat more when I feel depressed					
I feel happy with the way my body looks					
I often eat too much and feel guilty					
I often eat low fat, lite, diet or low calorie foods					
I often eat less than I want					

Q17.   How do you feel about these statements. (Continued)

	Strongly Disagree	Disagree	Not Sure	Agree	Strongly Agree
I feel guilty when I eat junk food					

Q.18   What is your opinion about the following statements.
        Please **TICK ONE BOX** for Each Statement

	Strongly Disagree	Disagree	Not Sure	Agree	Strongly Agree
Doing regular exercise is a good way to control your weight					
Slim people have more friends					
Slim people are the most attractive					
Being thin is more important for a woman than a man					
Others think I am too thin					
Overweight women are not attractive to men					
People who are overweight have only themselves to blame					
To be fashionable and look nice a woman must be thin					
Most people who are fat are lazy					
Magazines make too much of having a slim body					
Overweight people are not healthy					
Other people think I am too fat					
I feel that others pressure me to eat less					

Q19.   If you would like to make any further comments about these statements please do so on the next few lines.

....

....

....

Q20.   How often do you think about your weight?
        TICK ONE BOX

        Never or almost never

        Sometimes

        Quite often

        Most of the time

        All the time

Q21.   How often do you weigh yourself?
        TICK ONE BOX

    Every day

    Every few days

    About once a week

    About once every couple of weeks

    About once a month

    Less than once a month

    Hardly ever

Q22.   How do you see yourself?
       TICK ONE BOX

       Very underweight

       Slightly underweight

       About the right weight

       Slightly overweight

       Very overweight

       I□ve never really thought about it

Q23.   How tall are you?

       . . . . centimetres   OR   □ I don't know

Q24.   What do you weigh?

       . . . . kilograms   OR   □ I don't know

Q25.   What would you like to weigh?

       . . . . kilograms   OR   □ I don't know

Q26.   Would you like to gain weight, stay the same weight or lose weight?

       Gain weight

       Stay the same weight

       Lose weight - If you would like to lose weight, why do you want to?

       ....
       ....
       ....

Q27.   Are you trying to lose weight at the moment?

NO

YES - If so: How much weight would you like to lose

. . . . kilograms

How long do you think it will take you to lose this weight?

. . . . weeks   OR   . . . . months

Please describe what you are doing at the moment to lose weight.

....
....
....

Q28.   Have you tried to lose weight during the past year?

NO

Yes - If so how many times have you tried to lose weight

. . . . times

Please write out your diet below

....
....
....

Q29.   If the answer to Q28 was YES where did the diet come from?

Your parents

Other family members

Your friends

A doctor

A dietitian

A weight loss group

A magazine

A book

A nurse

A naturopath

A pharmacist

A teacher

Other source - please specify

Q30.   Over the past year, have you done any of these to lose weight?

Exercise for weight loss?	☐ NO	☐ YES
Taken diuretics for weight loss (to help you lose water)?	☐ NO	☐ YES
Taken laxatives for weight loss (to help you to go to the toilet)	☐ NO	☐ YES
Taken weight loss pills?	☐ NO	☐ YES
Used weight loss powders?	☐ NO	☐ YES
Vomited to help yourself lose weight?	☐ NO	☐ YES
Regularly skipped meals?	☐ NO	☐ YES
Been on a diet?	☐ NO	☐ YES
Done anything else to lose weight? ☐ NO		☐ YES

If yes - Please describe what:

....

....

....

Q31.   Over the past year, did you get any advice or information about your weight or weight loss from:

Your parents?	☐ NO	☐ YES
Other family members?	☐ NO	☐ YES
Your friends?	☐ NO	☐ YES
A doctor?	☐ NO	☐ YES
A dietitian?	☐ NO	☐ YES
A weight loss group?	☐ NO	☐ YES
A magazine?	☐ NO	☐ YES
A book?	☐ NO	☐ YES
A nurse?	☐ NO	☐ YES
A naturopath?	☐ NO	☐ YES
A pharmacist?	☐ NO	☐ YES
A teacher?	☐ NO	☐ YES
ome other source?	☐ NO	☐ YES

        If YES - please specify

Q32.   If you could change your shape, please describe what you would change. For example, would you like smaller hands, longer legs, wider shoulders, a trimmer waist etc? (If you think you are **OK**, please say so)

....

....

....

Q33.   How would you describe these different parts of your body?

Tick one Box for Each Body Part

	TOO THIN	OK	TOO FAT	DON'T KNOW
Lower legs (calves)				
Upper legs (thighs)				
Backside (buttocks)				

Q33.   How would you describe these different parts of your body? (Continued)

	TOO THIN	OK	TOO FAT	DON'T KNOW
Hips				
Waist				
Stomach				
Chest				
Lower arms				
Upper arms				
Hands				
Neck				
Shoulders				

Q34.   Imagine you wanted to gain weight. Which of the following should you do?

Tick One Box for Each Statement

Eat more bread, potatoes, rice & pasta	☐ NO ☐ YES
Use body building powders	☐ NO ☐ YES
Take vitamin pills	☐ NO ☐ YES
Take amino acid supplements	☐ NO ☐ YES
Just eat more food	☐ NO ☐ YES

Do weight training   ☐ NO   ☐ YES

Other   ☐ NO   ☐ YES - please specify

....
....
....

Q35.   Imagine you wanted to lose weight. Which of the following foods should you reduce?

Tick One Box for Each Food

Should You Reduce . . .	NO	YES	DON'T EAT NOW
Soft drinks			
Potatoes			
Pies and sausage rolls			
Bread			
Fish and chips			
Fruit			
Cakes and pastries			
Butter and cream			
Meat			
Chips and twisties			
Lollies and chocolates			
Milk and yoghurt			
The fat on meat			
Chicken			
The skin on chicken			
Breakfast cereals			
Deep fried takeaways			

Are there any other foods you would reduce?

    ☐   NO

    ☐   YES - please specify

....

....

....

Q36.   Is there a **MINIMUM** amount of food that a teenager needs to eat every day to be healthy?

    ☐ NO   ☐ YES   ☐ I DON'T KNOW

If your answer was YES then how much is the MINIMUM amount per day?

    ☐ I DON'T KNOW

OR

    . . . . slices of bread
    . . . . bowls of cereal
    . . . . pieces of fruit
    . . . . serves of vegetables
    . . . . serves of potato or rice or pasta
    . . . . glasses of milk
    . . . . serves of meat or fish or chicken or egg
    . . . . glasses of fluid

Is there anything else that a teenager needs to eat to be healthy?

    ☐ NO   ☐ YES - please specify

....

....

If you have any other comments about the foods that teenagers need to eat to be healthy please tell us here.

....

....

....

Q37.   Are you worried about the amount of the following in foods? Tick One Box for Each

Vitamins   ☐ NO   ☐ YES

Sugar   ☐ NO   ☐ YES

Additives   ☐ NO   ☐ YES

Fat   ☐ NO   ☐ YES

Pesticide   ☐ NO   ☐ YES

Salt   ☐ NO   ☐ YES

Other   ☐ NO   ☐ YES - Please specify

....

....

Q38.   What are you most concerned about in foods? **TICK ONLY ONE BOX**

☐   Vitamins

☐   Sugar

☐   Additives

☐   Fat

☐   Pesticides

☐   Salt

☐   None of them

Q.39   Do you have any specific questions about your weight or about weight loss or are there any issues about food or eating that particularly concern you?

☐   NO

☐   YES - Please write your questions or concerns here:

....

....

Thank You for Your Help

Now that you have finished please go back through the questionnaire and check that you have answered all the questions that apply to you.

Acknowledgements

The authors would like to thank: the Queensland Department of Education for permission to use questions from the NEAT project; Associate Professor David Crawford for access to unpublished questions relating to beliefs about food and weight; the principals, teachers and students of the high schools involved in the survey; and Ada Choat and Teresa Fitzgerald for data entry. This study was supported by: Queensland Health, the Parkes Bequest, and a Merit Research Grant from James Cook University. Madeleine Nowak is supported by a Research Fellowship from the Queensland Cancer Fund.

References

[1]   Kuskowska-Wolk A, Bergstrom R. Trends in body mass index and prevalence of obesity in Swedish men 1980-1989. *J Epidemiol Commun H 1993*; 47: 103-8.

[2]   Pietinen P, Vartiainen E, Mannisto S. Trends in body mass index and obesity among adults in Finland from 1972 to 1992. *Int J Obes Relat Metab Disord 1996*; 20: 114-20.

[3]   Simmons G, Jackson R, Swinburn B, Yee RL. The increasing prevalence of obesity in New Zealand: is it related to recent trends in smoking and physical activity? *New Zeal Med J 1996*; 109: 90-2.

[4]   National Health and Medical Research Council. Acting on Australia's weight: a strategy for the prevention of overweight and obesity. *Canberra: AGPS*, 1997.

[5]   Flegal KM, Carroll MD, Kuczmarski RJ, Johnson CL. Overweight and obesity in the United States: prevalence and trends, 1960-1994. *Int J Obes Relat Metab Disord 1998*; 22: 39-47.

[6]   Pi-Sunyer FX. Health implications of obesity. *Am J Clin Nutr 1991*; 53: 1595S-1603S.

[7]   Gortmaker SL, Must A, Perrin JM, Sobol AM, Dietz WH. Social and economic consequences of overweight in adolescence and young adulthood. *New Eng J Med 1993*; 329: 1008-12.

[8]   Wiseman CV, Gray JJ, Mosimann JE, Ahrens AH. Cultural expectations of thinness in women: an update. *Int J Eat Disorder 1992*; 11: 85-9.

[9]   French SA, Jeffrey RW. Consequences of dieting to lose weight: effects on physical and mental health. *Health Psychol 1994*; 13: 195-212.

[10]   Paxton SJ, Wertheim EH, Gibbons K, Szmukler GI, Hillier L, Petrovich JL. Body image satisfaction, dieting beliefs and weight loss behaviours in adolescent girls and boys. *J Youth Adolesc 1991*; 20: 361-80.

[11]   Middleman AB, Vasquez I, Durant RH. Eating patterns, physical activity and attempts to change weight among adolescents. *J Adolesc Health 1998*; 22: 37-42.

[12] Nowak M. The weight-conscious adolescent: body image, food intake, and weight-related behavior. *J Adolesc Health 1998*; 23(6): 389-98.

[13] Nowak M, Speare R, Crawford D. Gender differences in adolescent weight and shape-related beliefs and behaviours. *J Paediatr Child Health 1996*; 32: 148-52.

[14] Nowak M, Crawford D, Büttner P. A cross-sectional study of weight- and shape-related beliefs, behaviours and concerns of north Queensland adolescents. *Aust J Nutr Diet 2001*;58:174-180,185.

[15] Nowak M, Büttner P. Adolescents' food-related beliefs and behaviours: a cross-sectional study. *Nutr Diet 2002*;59:244-52.

[16] Nowak M, Crawford D. Getting the message across: adolescents' health concerns and views about the importance of food. *Aust J Nutr Diet 1998*; 55: 3-8.

[17] Morgan JN, Sonquist JA. Problems in the analysis of survey data, and a proposal. *J Am Stat Assoc 1963*; 58: 415-34.

[18] Kass GV. Significant testing in automatic interaction detection (A.I.D.) *Appl Stat 1975*; 24: 178-85.

[19] Kass GV. An exploratory technique for investigating large quantities of categorical data. *Appl Stat 1980*; 29: 119-27.

[20] Breiman L, Friedman JH, Olshen RA, Stone CJ. Classification and Regression Trees. Belmont, California; *Wadsworth International*: 1984.

[21] Segal MR, Bloch DA. A comparison of estimated proportional hazards models and regression trees. *Stat Med 1989*; 8: 539-50.

[22] Garbe C, Buettner P, Bertz J, et al. Primary cutaneous melanoma: identification of prognostic groups and estimation of individual prognosis for 5093 patients. *Cancer 1995*; 75: 2484-91.

[23] McBride WJ, Mullner H, Muller R, LaBrooy J, Wronski I. Determinants of dengue 2 infections among residents of Charters Towers, Queensland, Australia. *Am J Epidemiol 1998*; 148(11): 1111-6.

[24] Woodward DR. Teenagers and their food: The effects of physical, behavioural and socio-economic characteristics on intakes of five food categories in Tasmania. *J Food Nutr 1985;*42:7-12.

[25] Woodward DR. What influences adolescent food intakes? Human Nutr: *Appl Nutr 1986;*40;185-94.

[26] Kortt MA, Langley PC, Cox ER. A review of cost-of-illness studies on obesity. *Clin Ther 1998*; 20: 772-9.

[27] Cargill BR, Clark MM, Pera V, Niaura RS, Abrams DB. Binge eating, body image, depression, and self-efficacy in an obese clinical population. *Obes Res 1999*; 7: 379-86.

[28] Arnow B, Kenardy J, Agras WS. The Emotional Eating Scale: the development of a measure to assess coping with negative affect by eating. *Int J Eat Disorder 1995*; 18: 79-90.

[29] Davidson GC, Neale JM. *Abnormal psychology* (revised sixth edition). New York; John Wiley and Sons, Inc.: 1994.

[30] Vaughan G, Hogg M. *Introduction to social psychology*. Sydney; Prentice Hall: 1995.

[31] Nowak M, Büttner P. Relationship between adolescents' food- related beliefs and intake food intake behaviors. *Nutr Res 2003*;23:45-55.

[32] Rosenstock IM. Historical origins of the health belief model. *Health Educ Monogr 1974*;2:328-335.

[33] Rosenstock IM, Strecher VJ, Becker MH. Social learning theory and the health belief model. *Health Educ Q 1988* ;15:175-183.

[34] Fishbein M, Ajzen I. *Beliefs, attitudes, intensions and behaviour: An introduction to theory and research.* Reading MA: Addison-Wesley; 1975.

[35] Glanz K, Lewis FM, Rimer BK. *Health behavior and health education: theory, research and practice.* San Franisco: Jossey-Bass; 1997.

[36] Nestle M, Wing R, Birch L, DiSogra L, Drewnowski A, Middleton S, Sigman-Grant M, Sobal J, Winston M, Economos C. Behavioral and social influences on food choice. *Nutr Rev 1998*;56:S50-64.

[37] Birch L. Development of food preferences. *Annual Reviews of Nutrition 1999*;19:41-62.

[38] Neumark-Sztainer D, Story M, Perry C, Casey MA. Factors influencing food choices of adolescents: Findings from focus-group discussions with adolescents. *J Am Diet Assoc 1999*;99:929-934, 937.

[39] Glanz K, Basil M, Maibach E, Goldberg J, Snyder D. Why Americans eat what they do: Taste, nutrition, cost, convenience and weight control concerns as influences on food consumption. *J Am Diet Assoc 1998*;98:1118-1126.

[40] Bishop GD. *Health Psychology: integrating mind and body.* Boston: Allyn and Bacon; 1994.

[41] Rosenstock IM. The health belief model and nutrition education. *J Can Diet Assoc 1982*;43:184-192.

[42] O'Connell JK, Price JH, Roberts SM, Jurs SG, McKinley R. Utilizing the health belief model to predict dieting and exercising behavior of obese and nonobese adolescents. *Health Educ Q 1985*;12(4):343-351.

[43] Shepherd R, Stockley L. Fat consumption and attitudes towards food with a high fat content. *Human Nutr: Appl Nutr 1985*;39:431-42.

[44] Kristal AR, Bowen DJ, Curry SJ, Shattuck AL, Henry HJ. Nutrition knowledge, attitudes and perceived norms as correlates of selecting low-fat diets. *Health Educ Res, Theory and Practice 1990*;5(4):467-477.

[45] Towler G, Shepherd R. Application of Fishbein and Ajzen's expectancy-value model to understand fat intake. *Appetite 1992*;18:15-27.

[46] Schafer RB, Keith PM, Schafer E. Predicting fat in diets of marital partners using the health belief model. *J Behav Med 1995*;18:419-33.

[47] Brewer JL, Blake AJ, Rankin SA, Douglass LW. Theory of Reasoned Action predicts milk consumption in women. *J Am Diet Assoc 1999*; 99:39-44.

[48] Ajzen, I. The theory of planned behavior. *Organ Behav Hum Decis Process 1991*;50: 179-211.

[49] Harnack L, Block G, Subar A, Lane S, Brand R. Association of cancer prevention-related nutrition knowledge, beliefs, and attitudes to cancer prevention dietary behavior. *J Am Diet Assoc 1997*;97:957-65.

[50] Turrell G, Oldenberg B, McGuffog I, Dent R. Socioeconomic determinants of health: towards a national research program and a policy and intervention agenda. Queensland University of Technology, School of Public Health, Ausinfo, Canberra:1999.

[51] Prochaska JO, DiClemente CC. Transtheoretical therapy: toward a more integrative model of change. *Psychother: Theory, Res Practice 1982*;19:276-288.

[52] Prochaska JO, DiClemente CC, Norcoss JC. In search of how people change. Applications to addictive behaviors. *Am Psychol 1992*;47:1102-1114.

[53] Povey R, Conner M, Sparks P, James R, Shepherd R. A critical examination of the application of the Transtheoretical Model's stages of change to dietary behaviours. *Health Educ Res 1999*;14:641-651.

[54] Prochaska JO, Velicer WF, Rossi JS, Goldstein MG, Marcus BH, Rakowski W, Fiore C, Harlow LL, Redding CA, Rosenbloom D, Rossi SR. Stages of change and decisional balance for 12 problem behaviors. *Health Psychol 1994*;13:39-46.

[55] Glanz K, Patterson RE, Kristal AR, DiClemente CC, Heimendinger J, Linnan L, McLerran DF. Stages of change in adopting healthy diets: fat, fiber, and correlates of nutrient intake. *Health Educ Q 1994*;21:499-519.

[56] Watt RG. Stages of change for sugar and fat reduction in an adolescent sample. *Comm Dental Health 1997*;14:102-107.

[57] Greene GW, Rossi SR. Stages of change for reducing dietary fat intake over 18 months. *J Am Diet Assoc 1998*;98:529-34.

[58] Booth ML, Macaskill P, Owen N, Oldenburg B, Marcus BH, Bauman A. Population prevalence and correlates of stages of change in physical activity. *Health Educ Q 1993*;20:431-440.

[59] Marcus BH, Simkin LR. The transtheoretical model: applications to exercise behavior. *Med Sci Sports Exerc 1994*;26:1400-1404.

[60] Ni Mhurchu C, Margetts BM, Speller VM. Applying the Stages-of-Change Model to dietary change. *Nutr Rev 1997*;55:10-16.

[61] Greene GW, Rossi SR, Rossi JS, Velicer WF, Fava JL, Prochaska. Dietary applications of the Stages of Change Model. *J Am Diet Assoc 1999*;99:673-8.

[62] Kristal AR, Glanz K, Curry SJ, Patterson RE. How can stages of change be best used in dietary interventions? *J Am Diet Assoc 1999*;99:679-84.

[63] Trudeau E, Kristal A, Li S, Patterson RE. Dempographic and psychosocial predictors of fruit and vegetable intakes differ: Implications for dietary interventions. *J Am Diet Assoc 1998*;98:1412-17.

[64] Nowak M. Eat like the French and stay slim: anecdotal observations on French food culture. *Aust J Nutr Diet 1997*;52:90-92.

[65] Keane A. *Too hard to swallow? The palatability of healthy eating advice.* In: Caplan P (ed). Food Health and Identity. London: Routledge; 1997.

[66] Festinger L. *A Theory of Cognitive Dissonance.* Stanford, CA: Stanford University Press; 1957.

[67] National Health and Medical Research Council. Acting on Australia's weight: a strategy for the prevention of overweight and obesity. Canberra: Australian Government Publishing Service; 1997.

[68] Australian Institute of Health and Welfare (AIHW) 2004. Heart Stroke and Vascular Diseases- Australian Facts 2004. AIHW Cat. NO. CVD 27. Canberra: AIHW and National Heart Foundation of Australia (Cardiovascular Disease Series No. 22).

[69] Flegal KM, Carroll MD, Kuczmarski RJ, Johnson CL. Overweight and obesity in the United states: prevalence and trends, 1960-1994. *Int J Obes Rel Metab Dis 1998*;22:39-47.

[70] Hedley, AA, Ogden, CL, Johnson, CL, Carroll, MD, Curtin, LR, Flegal, KM. Overweight and obesity among US children, adolescents, and adults, 1999-2002. *J Am Med Assoc 291*:2847-50. 2004.

[71] Kuskowska-Wolk A, Bergstrom R. Trends in body mass index and prevalence of obesity in Swedish men 1980-1989. *J Epidem Comm Health 1993a*;47:103-8.

[72] Kuskowska-Wolk A, Bergstrom R. Trends in body mass index and prevalence of obesity in Swedish women 1980-1989. *J Epidem Comm Health 1993b*;47:195-9.

[73] Maillard G, Charles MA, Thibult N, Forhan A, Sermet C, Basdevant A, Eschwege E. Trends in the prevalence of obesity in the French adult population between 1980 and 1991. *Int J Obes Rel Metab Dis 1999*;23:389-394.

[74] Haftenberger M, Lahmann PH, Panico S, Gonzalez CA, Seidell JC, Boeing H, Giurdanella MC, Krogh V, Bueno-de-Mesquita HB, Peeters PH, Skeie G, Hjartaker A, Rodriguez M, Quiros JR, Berglund G, Janlert U, Khaw KT, Spencer EA, Overvad K, Tjonneland A, Clavel-Chapelon F, Tehard B, Miller AB, Klipstein-Grobusch K, Benetou V, Kiriazi G, Riboli E, Slimani N. Overweight, obesity and fat distribution in 50- to 64-year-old participants in the European Prospective Investigation into Cancer and Nutrition (EPIC). *Public Health Nutr. 2002*;5:1147-62

[75] Institut Roche de l'Ob(sit(. ObEpi 2000, le surpoids et l'ob(sit(en France: 2000. Cited in L' ob(sit(: Du d(pistage pr(coce aux traitements actuels, quelles solution? Journal N° 14 de l'URML-PACA– juin 2003. *HYPERLINK "http://www.urmlpaca.org/repertoire/journal _14complet3.html accessed 27 February 2005" http://www.urmlpaca.org/repertoire/journal _14complet3.html accessed 27 February 2005* .

[76] Cameron AJ, Welborn TA, Zimmet PZ, Dunstan DW, Owen N, Salmon J, Dalton M, Jolley D, Shaw JE. Overweight and obesity in Australia: the 1999-2000 Australian Diabetes, Obesity and Lifestyle Study (AusDiab). *Med J Aust. 2003*;178:427-32.

[77] Rozin P, Imada S, Sarubin A, Wrzesniewski A. Attitudes to food and the role of food in life in the U.S.A., Japan, Flemish Belgium and France: possible implications for the diet-health debate. *Appetite 1999*;33:163-180.

[78] Drewnowski A, Henderson SA, Shore AB, Fischler C, Preziosi P, Hercberg S. Diet quality and dietary diversity in France: implications for the French paradox. *J Am Diet Assoc 1996*;96:663-669.

[79] Mermet G. Francoscopie 1999: Comment vivent les fran(ais. Larousse, Paris: 1998.

[80] Yu DW, Shepard GH. Is beauty in the eye of the beholder? *Nature 1998*;396:321-322.

[81] Nowak M, Hawkes A. Are beliefs the missing link? *Aust J Nutr Diet 2000*;57:54.

In: Focus on Nutrition Research
Editor: Tony P. Starks, pp. 121-148

ISBN 1-59454-768-8
© 2006 Nova Science Publishers, Inc.

Chapter V

Hypothalamic Serotonin in the Control of Food Intake: Physiological Interactions and Effect of Obesity

Eliane B. Ribeiro, Mônica M. Telles, Lila M. Oyama,
Vera L.F. Silveira and Cláudia M.O. Nascimento
Federal University of São Paulo, Department of Physiology,
Division of Nutrition Physiology,
Rua Botucatu, 862, 2° andar, 04023-060,
São Paulo, SP, Brazil

Abstract

The hypothalamic serotonergic system has long been known to have an anorexigenic effect, which is likely to play a role in the control of energy homeostasis. Although the exact nature of the likely serotonergic influence on the pathogenesis of obesity remains unclear, the feeding-inhibition induced by central serotonergic stimulation has been the basis of many appetite suppressant drugs.

A complex network of hypothalamic factors has been shown to participate in the control of energy intake. This system includes anabolic effectors (which stimulate feeding), namely neuropeptide Y, orexins, melanin-concentrating hormone, and agouti-related protein, as well as catabolic effectors (which inhibit feeding), such as melanocyte-stimulating hormone, cocaine-and amphetamine-regulated transcript, corticotropin releasing hormone, and, most likely, serotonin. This system operates under the influence of peripherally borne adiposity/satiety signals, which include the adipocyte hormone leptin, the pancreatic hormone insulin, and the gastric hormone ghrelin. A large number of studies have been dedicated to elucidate the precise relationships among those multiple factors and their relevance to obesity.

This review will focus on the available data concerning the interactions of serotonin with the anabolic and catabolic hypothalamic systems as well as its putative participation as a physiological target of the adiposity signals. We also consider the status of these interactions in rodent models of hypothalamic and genetic obesity.

Introduction

The central nervous system plays an important role in the maintenance of energy balance. There is now evidence that a complex network of neuropeptides and neurotransmitters, centered at the hypothalamus, modifies energy intake and expenditure as required to keep the constancy of body weight. The adequate performance of this system, called the hypothalamic lipostat or adipostat, depends on neural, hormonal, and metabolic inputs which, generated either centrally or in the periphery, constantly inform the hypothalamus about the body energy status and necessities. Those inputs encompass not only acute signals of hunger and satiety but also, and importantly, information related to the long-term constancy of body energy stores.

It has been proposed the existence of a hypothalamic set point for body weight regulation, determined by a combination of genetic and environmental factors (Keesey and Hirvonen, 1997). Body adiposity, as stored in the white adipocyte as fat, is presently accepted as the crucial long-term parameter around which the homeostatic control system operates. The size of the adipose organ is thought to be relayed to the lipostat mainly through hormonal signals, of which leptin and insulin are the most relevant.

Besides this long-term parameter, short-term signals related to hunger and satiety also influence the system, mainly by the action of hormones of the gastrointestinal tract, such as ghrelin, CCK (cholecystokinin), and GLP-1 (glucagon-like peptide), but also through nutritional and vagal influences. Additionally, other brain centers contribute with afferent inputs concerning sensorial aspects, such as the smell, taste, and appearance of the food, as well as the hedonic component of the feeding behaviour. The integration of these multiple afferences at the hypothalamic level determine the efferent inputs which, comprising hormonal, neural, and behavioural responses, are designed to control food intake and energy expenditure.

The adiposity/satiety signals interact with several hypothalamic targets, a complex system comprising both anabolic and catabolic effectors. The anabolic effectors, which stimulate feeding and/or inhibit energy expenditure, include NPY (neuropeptide Y), orexins, MCH (melanin-concentrating hormone), and AGRP (agouti-related protein), whereas the catabolic ones, which inhibit feeding and/or stimulate energy expenditure, include α-MSH (melanocyte-stimulating hormone), CART (cocaine-and amphetamine-regulated transcript), CRH (corticotropin releasing hormone), and 5-HT (serotonin). Multiple interplays of these factors are potentially relevant to the physiological control of energy homeostasis and to the genesis of obesity. Table I lists some of those peripherally-originated (signaling) factors acting centrally as well as central effectors, whose participation in food intake control has been investigated.

Table 1. Peripheral (signaling) factors and central effectors participating in the control of energy homeostatic as catabolic (inhibit feeding and/or stimulate thermogenesis) or anabolic (stimulate feeding and/or inhibit thermogenesis) regulators.

Signaling Factors		Central Effectors	
Catabolic	Anabolic	Catabolic	Anabolic
Leptin	Ghrelin	α-MSH	NPY
Insulin		CART	AGRP
Amilin		CRH	Orexins
Adiponectin		Serotonin	MCH
CCK		CCK	Galanin
GLP-1		GLP-1	ß-Endorphin
PYY		Norepinephrine	Norepinephrine
PP		BDNF	Dopamine
IL-6		Neuromedin U	
TNF-α			

α-MSH -melanocyte-stimulating hormone, AGRP - agouti-related protein, BDNF - brain-derived neurotrophic factor, CART - cocaine-and amphetamine-regulated transcript, CCK - cholecystokinin, CRH - corticotropin-releasing hormone, GLP-1 - glucagon-like peptide, MCH - melanin-concentrating hormone, NPY - neuropeptide Y, PP - pancreatic polypeptide, PYY - peptide YY.

Leptin and Insulin as Adiposity Signals to the Hypothalamus

Leptin

Much of what is presently known about the physiological control of food intake derived from studies performed in animal models of obesity. The Ob protein or leptin (from the greek word *leptós*: thin) was identified in the obese mice of the *ob/ob* strain, as the product of the *ob* gene. A mutation at the *ob locus* leading to the production of a truncated, and hence inactive, leptin molecule, results in hyperphagia, severe early-onset obesity, and insulin resistance (Zhang et al., 1994). The rodent *ob* gene, as well as its human homologue, is expressed mainly in the white adipocyte, and leptin, a 16 kDa protein, is released to the circulation, its plasma concentration being proportional to the body adipose mass. Early experiments with recombinant leptin demonstrated that the protein reduces food intake, body mass and adiposity, and increases energy metabolism and insulin sensitivity, in both lean and obese mice, after either peripheral or intracerebroventricular administration, suggesting the existence of a central site of action (Campfield et al., 1995; Harris et al., 1998). Those effects were also observed in rodents with diet-induced obesity but were absent in obese mice of the *db/db* strain (Campfield et al., 1995). The explanation for the resistance to leptin in *db/db* mice came with the identification and cloning of the gene encoding the leptin receptor and the demonstration of its expression in the hypothalamus (Tartaglia et al., 1995; Chen et al., 1996). The *db/db* mice have a mutation of the *db* locus (Chen et al., 1996) which leads to the inactivity of the receptor protein and leptin resistance, a situation functionally similar to the leptin insufficiency of the *ob/ob* mice. These important experiments thus established that either leptin deficiency (*ob/ob* mice) or leptin resistance (*db/db* mice and Zucker *fa/fa* rats) are associated to hyperphagia and obesity.

In humans, mutations at the *ob* or *db* loci are rare, having been found only in morbidly obese subjects (O´Rahilly et al., 2003). The most frequent finding, in both animal models and obese humans, is the presence of high circulating levels of the protein, indicating that leptin resistance, rather than its deficiency, is the most common feature of obesity (Campfield et al., 1995 and 1998). This finding has led to the suggestion that, throughout evolution, leptin's physiological importance has been, more than preventing obesity, to allow accumulation of body energy for survival during periods of food scarcity in the environment (Flier and Maratos-Flier, 1998).

At least 6 isoforms of the leptin receptor (Ob-R) have been identified, generated from alternative splicing of the primary transcript of the *db* gene (Ahima and Osei, 2004). They are expressed in different intensities in various tissues, such as the coroid plexus, cerebral cortex, hypothalamus, cerebellum, lung, kidney, liver, pancreas, muscle, and white fat (Tartaglia et al.,1995; Takaya et al., 1996). Belonging to the type I citokine receptor family, the Ob-R operate through the stimulation of transcription factors of the STAT family. The long isoform of the leptin receptor (Ob-Rb) is highly expressed in the hypothalamus and acts through the JAK/STAT pathway (janus-kinase/signal transducer and activator of transcription) (Ghilardi et al., 1996). Neurons expressing Ob-Rb are present in several CNS sites, including hypothalamic nuclei involved in feeding control, as the arcuate (ARC), ventromedial (VMH), and dorsomedial (DMH) nuclei.

Leptin administration has been shown to stimulate tyrosine phosphorylation of STAT-3, inducing its translocation to the nuclear compartment, where it modulates the expression of many genes, including *c-fos* and Socs3 (suppressor of citokine signaling) (Zigman and Elmquist, 2003). Socs3 acts by feedback as a negative modulator of leptin signaling, by binding to Ob-Rb and inhibiting the tyrosine-kinase activity of JAK. There is also evidence that it can induce the degradation of Ob-Rb/JAK complexes. For these actions, Socs3 has been intensively investigated as a potential factor leading to leptin resistance in obesity. Elevated ARC Socs3 levels have been shown in response to hyperlipidic diets (Munzberg et al., 2004). Socs3-knockout mice have been shown to be more sensitive to leptin and, importantly, to not develop obesity under hyperlipidic diet (Mori et al., 2004a; Howard et al., 2004).

Besides Socs3, other negative regulators of leptin signaling have been identified, as the tyrosine-phosphatases SHP-2 (SH2-containing protein tyrosine phosphatase-2) and PTP1B (protein-tyrosine phosphatase 1B). Impairment of leptin transport into the CNS is also a potential mechanism of leptin resistance (Myers, 2004).

Insulin

The pancreatic hormone insulin also fulfills the criteria for playing a role as an afferent adiposity signal to the CNS. Its circulating levels are proportional to body adipose mass (Palaniappan et al., 2002). The hormone enters the CNS, through a saturable, facilitated transport mechanism located at endothelial cells of the blood brain barrier (Baura et al., 1993). Insulin receptors are expressed in central sites involved in the control of food intake (Havrankova et al., 1978).

The anorexigenic property of insulin, dependent on a CNS action, has long been recognized (Woods et al., 1979). Its central administration reduces food intake, whereas its deficiency, as seen in Diabetes mellitus, is associated with hyperphagia (Chavez et al., 1995; Sipols et al., 1995; Baskin et al., 1999). It has also long been known that the CNS expresses insulin receptors (IR), and that these central receptors possess tyrosine kinase activity (Havrankova et al., 1978; Rees-Jones et al., 1984; Marks et al., 1990).

Several data pointed to the physiological importance of central insulin signaling in the maintenance of energy homeostasis. Directed deletion of the neuronal IR or peri-hypothalamic administration of IR antisense oligonucleotides reportedly increased food intake and body adiposity in mice (Bruning et al., 2000; Obici et al., 2002). In rats, central administration of anti-insulin antibodies had a similar effect (McGowan et al., 1990 e 1992). These reports also found hyperinsulinemia, indicating that a state of resistance to central insulin actions may be relevant to obesity. Moreover, CNS insulin delivery has been seen to decrease after an increment in body adiposity induced by a high fat diet (Kaiyala et al., 2000). Low insulin binding to brain capillaries has been shown contribute to the hyperphagia in obese Zucker rats (Schwartz et al., 1990b).

In muscle, adipose tissue, and liver, the classical insulin target tissues, the hormone signaling pathway has been extensively studied. The binding of insulin to its receptor induces receptor autophosphorylation, activating its tyrosine kinase intrinsic activity towards the cytosolic insulin receptor substrates, the IRSs, of which IRS-1 and IRS-2 seem to be particularly relevant. These activated substrates then associate to and activate the SH2 (Src-homology 2) domain-containing proteins PI 3-K (phosphatidylinositol 3-kinase) and Grb2 (growth factor receptor binding protein 2). Distally to the activation of PI 3-K and Grb2 there is the phosphorylation of Akt (or protein kinase B, a serine/threonine kinase) and of MAPK (mitogen-activated protein kinase), respectively. While the PI 3-K pathway is particularly involved in the mediation of insulin metabolic effects, the MAPK pathway participates in the hormone actions on cell growth and gene expression (Virkamäki et al., 1999).

Recent studies indicate that, at least in its initial steps, these same pathways are responsible for insulin signaling in the hypothalamus (Carvalheira et al., 2001 and 2003; Niswender and Schwartz, 2003). For example, inhibition of PI 3-K activity (with wortmannin or LY294002) has been shown to abolish both the PKB/Akt phosphorylation and the hypophagia induced by an intracerebroventricular dose of insulin in rats (Carvalheira et al., 2003).   In mice, the knockout of the IRS-2 gene increased food ingestion and body adiposity as well as circulating levels of insulin and leptin (Burks et al., 2000). On the other hand, these responses did not follow the knockout of the IRS-1 gene (Araki et al., 1994), in agreement with the observation that IRS-2, rather than IRS-1, is the preferred substrate for the insulin receptor at the hypothalamus (Carvalheira et al., 2003).

Hunger and Satiety Signals

Ghrelin has been described as a hormone produced mainly in the stomach and, in a lesser extent, in the intestine, placenta, hypophysis and hypothalamus (De Ambrogi et al., 2003). Besides its role as a regulator of growth hormone secretion, ghrelin is an orexigenic and adipogenic hormone. In humans and rodents, systemic ghrelin administration potently stimulated food intake. Gastric ghrelin secretion is influenced by the nutritional status, decreasing during fasting and being increased in obesity (Horvath et al., 2001; Small and Bloom, 2004). For these properties, ghrelin has been pointed as a signal of energetic insufficiency to the CNS. Several brain areas express ghrelin receptors, including hypothalamic and raphe nuclei. The secreted hormone has been shown to penetrate the CNS and to interact with hypothalamic sites controlling energy homeostasis.

Amilin is produced by the pancreas and co-secreted with insulin in response to a meal. Its secretion and plasma levels have been shown to be proportional to adipose mass. It binds to central receptors and inhibits feeding, an effect not modified by vagotomy. Antagonism of the central amilin receptor increased intake and body fat content (Cancello et al., 2004).

Various other gastrointestinal hormones modulate food intake, and it has been demonstrated that, at least partially, this effect relies on central actions. This group includes cholecystokinin (CCK), pancreatic polypeptide (PP), glucagon-like peptide (GLP-1), oxyntomodulin (Oxm), peptide YY (PYY). These hormones are stimulated by the ingestion of food and inhibit feeding. The anorexigenic effect was observed after central administration and is associated with increased *c-fos* expression, specially in the arcuate nucleus of the hypothalamus (Small and Bloom, 2004). PYY levels were reportedly low in obese humans, who also failed to respond with an increase in PYY secretion after a meal (Batterham and Bloom, 2003).

Other Centrally-Acting Peripheral Factors

Besides leptin, the adipose tissue is the source of other citokine factors which reduce food intake, namely TNF-α and interleukins. It has been evidenced that hypothalamic systems, including serotonin, CRH (corticotropin-releasing hormone), NPY (neuropeptide Y), and α-MSH (melanocyte-stimulating hormone) may mediate the citokines-induced anorexia (Besedovsky and Del Rey, 1996; Langhans, 2000). In both humans and rodents, obesity has been associated with increased production of TNF-α, IL-6, and possibly other citokines, but the relevance of this to obesity genesis and maintenance has not been established (Roytblat et al., 2000; Das, 2001).

Adiponectin, also called Adipo Q and Acrp30 (adipocyte complement-related protein of 30 kDa) is an adipocyte hormone whose main effects relate to glucose and lipid metabolism, through modulation of insulin sensitivity. Its plasma levels fall in proportion to adipose mass and its cerebrospinal fluid levels have been shown to increase after systemic administration, suggesting a central mechanism of action. When injected intracerebroventricularly in mice, adiponectin reduced body mass mainly by stimulating thermogenesis, with no effect on food intake (Steppan and Lazar, 2002; Qi et al., 2004).

In summary, several hormones produced in the periphery are likely to act centrally to modulate feeding. Leptin and insulin are the most well established signaling factors of long-term body fat stores. The information on acute hunger/satiety status is mainly relayed to the hypothalamus by gastrointestinal hormones, and it is clear that the cumulative effect of these acute influences is relevant to long-term energy homeostasis.

Central Targets for the Adiposity/Satiety Signals

Once reaching the CNS, those signaling factors interact with hypothalamic neurons expressing different neuropeptides and neurotransmitters which, in turn, may be responsible for the efferent responses .

Receptors for many of the signaling hormones have been described in various hypothalamic nuclei involved in energy homeostasis. In the hypothalamus, the highest density of leptin receptors is found in the arcuate nucleus (Hakansson et al., 1998). Systemically administered leptin has been shown to penetrate the CNS and to bind mainly in the ARC (Banks et al., 1996). Following direct injection, leptin caused a more pronounced anorexia when injected at the ARC, than at the VMH and LH (Satoh et al., 1997).

At least two different ARC neuronal populations have been shown to express receptors for the adiposity/satiety signals. One such group of neurons coexpress the orexigenic factors neuropeptide Y (NPY) and agouti-related protein (AGRP). Other neurons in the ARC coexpress the anorexigenic factors proopiomelanocortin (POMC), the α-melanocyte stimulating hormone (α-MSH) precursor protein, and cocaine-and amphetamine-regulated transcript (CART). AGRP, POMC and α-MSH constitute the hypothalamic melanocortin system (Schwartz et al., 2000).

NPY is a potent stimulator of food intake whose hypothalamic levels are high in genetic and diet-induced obese mice. Its chronic central administration induces hyperphagia and obesity. Central administration of either leptin or insulin inhibits NPY expression, demonstrating that NPY neurons mediate the hypophagia induced by these hormones. However, NPY knockout mice showed a normal response to leptin, indicating that NPY neurons are not the only central target of the hormone (Erickson et al., 1996; Flier and Maratos-Flier, 1998).

CART is an anorexigenic peptide produced in ARC neurons (Calapai et al., 1999) whose expression is stimulated by leptin (Wang et al., 1999).

The hypothalamic melanocortin system is formed by the ARC proteins AGRP, POMC, and α-MSH, and also includes the MC4 melanocortin receptor, which is expressed in neurons of the PVN/VMH nuclei. The MC4R is stimulated by α-MSH, a peptide resulting from POMC cleavage by the pro-hormone convertase 1, and mediates the α-MSH-induced hypophagia. AGRP also binds to MC4R, antagonizing α-MSH, thus having an orexigenic effect. Intracerebroventricular AGRP injection has been shown to induce hyperphagia as has the deletion of MC4R, that produces hyperphagic obese mice (Spiegelman and Flier, 1996).

POMC expression is reportedly reduced in *ob/ob* mice and is stimulated by leptin treatment (Mizuno et al., 1998). On the other hand, an increased production of AGRP has been reported in these obese mice, and leptin administration decreased AGRP levels (Mizuno and Mobbs, 1998). POMC neurons also express insulin receptors and third ventricle injection of insulin has been shown to stimulate POMC expression while inhibiting feeding in rats (Benoit et al., 2002). It has also been demonstrated that POMC neurons are activated, as seen by increased Fos-like immunoreactivity, by the systemic administration of PYY (Batterham *et al.*, 2002). Central ghrelin infusion stimulated eating and also induced *c-fos* expression in ARC neurons expressing NPY and AGRP. However, these effects were abolished by vagotomy (Hewson and Dickson, 2000; Small and Bloom, 2004). Interestingly, ghrelin effects upon food intake and body adiposity were normal in NPY knockout mice (Tschop et al., 2002).

The importance of the hypothalamic melanocortin system in food intake regulation was identified in the genetically obese *agouti yellow* (A^y) mice. A mutation at the agouti locus leads to the hypothalamic expression of the agouti protein, normally expressed only in the skin, where it controls hair pigmentation through blockade of α-MSH binding to MC1R. Continuous ectopic expression of agouti in the hypothalamus causes hyperphagia and obesity due to the constant blockade of MC4R and, hence, of α-MSH inhibition of feeding. The constant blockade of MC1R leads to the yellow coat coloration of the A^y mice (Spiegelman and Flier, 1996).

In humans, mutations of melanocortin system genes are more frequent than those of the leptin system, and have been associated with morbid obesity. The most common deffect, observed in 6% of a sample of 500 morbidly obese subjects, involves the MC4R gene. Moreover, impairment of POMC processing, due to mutation of the pro-hormone convertase 1 gene, has also been detected (O´Rahilly et al., 2003).

The above data support the current concept that the ARC is a primary site of contact of the blood-borne adiposity/satiety signals with the hypothalamus. The resultant inhibition of the anabolic neurons (NPY/ AGRP) and/or stimulation of the catabolic ones (POMC/CART), would represent the initial step of the putative hypothalamic circuitries responsible for the final output, i.e. the modification of food intake. The ARC neurons are thought to relay the information to innervated sites, as the paraventricular (PVN) and ventromedial (VMH) nuclei, where MC4R and BDNF (brain-derived neurotrophic factor) are produced, as well as the lateral/perifornical area (LH/PFH), expressing the anabolic hormones MCH (melanin-concentrating hormone) and orexins (hipocretins). Additionally, other hypothalamic sites, as the VMH, LH, and PVN as well extrahypothalamic ones also contain receptors for the signaling factors, and, hence, are potential targets for the peripheral signals (Woods et al., 1998; Schwartz et al., 2000; Flier, 2004).

BDNF is an anorexigenic factor highly expressed in the VMH (Xu et al., 2003) and its haploinsufficiency caused hyperphagia in mice (Fox and Byerly, 2004). Its mRNA levels are low in the A^y yellow mouse and in mice knockout for the MC4 receptor. Accordingly, treatment with an MC4R agonist increased the number of BDNF expressing neurons in the VMH, indicating that BDNF may be a downstream factor to the activation of MC4R (Xu et al., 2003).

Orexins are also produced in LH neurons co-expressing leptin receptors (Sakurai, 1999; Funahashi et al., 2000) and orexin treatment stimulates feeding (Shiraishi et al, 2000).

MCH is a peptide produced in the lateral hypothalamus which stimulates food intake and body adiposity, and whose mRNA have been shown to increase after a high-fat diet. Hypothalamic levels of the MCH1 receptor also increased with body adiposity, showing a direct correlation with plasma leptin and insulin (Ludwig et al., 1998; Elliot et al., 2004). MCH neurons express leptin receptors (Hakansson et al., 1998) and, although leptin treatment inhibited MCH levels, MCH knockout did not abolish leptin-induced hypophagia (Shimada et al., 1998).

The number of known central mediators able to modify energy intake is still growing, as new ones are being constantly identified by the numerous studies dedicated to the subject. It has recently been shown that the enzyme AMP-activated protein kinase (AMPK) also participates in food intake control. AMPK functions as a sensor of cell energy status. It is activated when the cell needs to increase its energy production, and it acts stimulating ATP-generating metabolic pathways. Inhibition of hypothalamic AMPK has been shown after treatment with leptin, insulin, or MC4R activation. On the other hand, AGRP caused stimulation of AMPK. Absence of AMPK expression in the hypothalamus inhibited food intake whereas activation of the enzyme was orexigenic and prevented leptin-induced hypophagia (Hardie, 2003; Minokoshi et al., 2004). On the other hand, Neuromedin U (NMU) has been shown to have an anorexigenic effect independent of the leptin system, as the administration of the hormone failed to modify NMU hypothalamic levels. NMU knockout mice became obese and had low POMC levels but their response to leptin was unaffected (Hanada et al., 2004).

Serotonin

The monoaminergic neurotransmitters affect the hypothalamic mechanisms that control energy homeostasis. The role of dopamine (DA) and norepinephrine (NE) is complex and not well established. NE activity in the PVN of rats is reportedly higher at the begining of the dark period. NE had an orexigenic effect when injected in the PVN or the VMH, but its administration in the LH decreased feeding (Leibowitz et al., 1984; Hoebel et al., 1989). Activation of α-2 adrenergic receptors in the PVN stimulated whereas α-1 activation decreased intake. Inhibition of NE neuronal reuptake has been found to have a dual effect, stimulating intake in the satiated animals but lowering intake in the fasted ones. Despite these discrepancies, it is believed that at least part of the anorexigenic effect of anti-obesity drugs, such as amphetamines and phentermine, relies on their NE-releasing and α-1-stimulating properties (Wellman, 2000). Regarding dopamine, its depletion induced hypophagia in normal rats (Salamone et al., 1993) while reduced PVN levels have been associated with hyperphagia in obese mice (Oltmans, 1983). In superfused hypothalamic synaptosomes leptin failed to affect basal release of NE and DA, but reduced the depolarization-induced release of both amines (Brunetti et al., 1999).

The hypothalamic serotonergic system has long been known to have an anorexigenic effect and serotonergic drugs have been widely used clinically to treat obesity (Glazer, 2001; Gerozissis, 2004). The hypothalamus is richly innervated by serotonergic projections from the raphe nuclei, the main source of brain 5-HT (Jacobs and Azmitia, 1992). At least 14 distinct receptor sub-types for 5-HT have been identified, with $5-HT_{1A}$ auto-receptor and the $5-HT_{1B}$ and $5-HT_{2C}$ sub-types having been more directly associated with the hypophagic effect, although other sub-types, such as the $5-HT_{2B}$ and $5-HT_6$, have recently been implicated (Barnes and Sharp, 1999; Vickers and Dourish, 2004). Pharmacological activation of the system (by inhibition of neuronal reuptake or stimulation of neurotransmitter release) induces anorexia in both animals and humans (Nielsen et al., 1992; Ward et al., 1999), while serotonergic inhibition (with $5-HT_{1A}$ auto receptor agonists or $5-HT_{1B}/5-HT_{2C}$ receptor antagonists) stimulates feeding (Leibowitz and Alexander, 1998; Voigt et al., 2000).

The reduction in energy intake following serotonergic activation has been associated with a selective inhibition of carbohydrate consumption (Wurtman and Wurtman, 1996) but it has later been suggested that fat and protein intakes may be preferentially reduced by serotonergic drugs (Heisler et al., 1999). A modification of the structure of feeding behavior, with reduction of meal size and eating rate, has been proposed to account for the feeding inhibition and to explain a serotonergic modulation of the processes of acute satiation and post-absortive satiety (Halford, 2001). The hypophagic effect of 5-HT has been specially associated with medial hypothalamic sites (Leibowitz and Alexander, 1998) but the involvement of the ARC (Heisler et al., 2003) and the lateral hypothalamus (LH) (Bernardis and Bellinger, 1996; Meguid et al., 2000) has also been evidenced.

Serotonin, Food Intake and Glucocorticoids

Several lines of evidence point to a physiological role of serotonin on the mechanisms responsible for food intake regulation. Deletion of the $5-HT_{2C}$ receptor gene in mice resulted in hyperphagia and increased body weight (Tecott et al., 1995; Nonogaki et al., 1998). Classical microdialysis experiments have indicated that the eating of a palatable meal (a mash of chow and condensed milk) elicited an increase in the serotonin levels recovered in microdialysate samples of the lateral and the medial hypothalamus of normal rats. This serotonergic stimulation was seen both during light-phase and dark-phase eating (Schwartz et al., 1989 and 1990a). In our laboratory, we demostrated that the day-time intake of a balanced mash (standard powdered chow and water) also stimulated serotonin release in the lateral hypothalamus of normal rats, as measured by microdialysis (Mori et al., 1999). In the absence of an increased palatability of the food, we used an overnight fast as the stimulus eliciting food intake. Those data indicate that the normal hypothalamic response to feeding includes the stimulation of serotonergic activity, as part of the mechanisms modulating satiety.

The mechanisms coupling the intake of food and the observed serotonergic activation are probably numerous. It is known that the nucleus tractus solitarius (NTS) receives vagal afferences about the amount and composition of the food eaten. Since efferent NTS projections to the raphe nuclei and the hypothalamus itself have been described (Jean, 1991; Herbert and Saper, 1992), this is a likely mechanism through which food could modify serotonergic neurotransmission, either at the terminal level or at the cell bodies of serotonergic neurons. Feeding also stimulates the release of intestinal peptides, such as cholecystokinin (CCK) and glucagon-like peptide 1 (GLP-1), whose central actions play important roles in satiety, through vagally mediated and direct mechanisms (Schwartz et al., 2000; Meier et al., 2002). Both these peptides have been shown to induce serotonergic activation in the hypothalamus (Voigt et al., 1998; Owji et al., 2002) and there is evidence that serotonergic receptors are involved in CCK-induced anorexia (Hayes et al., 2004).

The serotonergic system has been shown to also respond to insulin (Orosco et al., 1991; Dunbar et al., 1995), a hormone whose hypothalamic levels increase after feeding (Gerozissis et al., 1998). Insulin deficient diabetic rats had a reduced turnover of 5-HT (Martin et al., 1995) and insulin increased 5-HT release in the medial hypothalamus (Orosco et al., 2000). Systemic infusion of glucose elevated cerebral levels of 5-HT (Vahabzadeh et al., 1995) and ingestion of a glucose solution or an amino acid mixture increased hypothalamic serotonin metabolism (Yamauchi et al., 1995).

Increased glucocorticoid levels have also been described after food intake (Merali et al., 1998, Guimarães et al., 2002) and these hormones have been shown to affect the 5-HT system. Dorsal raphe neurons express glucocorticoid receptors (Joels and Vreugdenhil, 1998) whose activation inhibited 5-HT1A auto-receptors, thus stimulating 5-HT neurons (Laaris et al., 1995). Moreover, adrenalectomy has been shown to reduce 5-HT synthesis and turnover rates in rats (Van Loon et al., 1981; Dinan, 1996), and corticosterone supplementation reversed these effects (De Kloet et al., 1982). On the other hand, acute administration of high doses of corticosterone has been shown to reduce 5-HT metabolism (Inoue and Koyama, 1996).

We performed brain microdialysis in adrenalectomized rats to address the question of whether glucocorticoid hormones are relevant to the food-induced stimulation of LH 5-HT release. We observed that the LH serotonergic response to feeding was completely abolished in the adrenalectomized animals (Guimarães et al., 2002).

This could be due to the absence of a permissive effect of glucocorticoids, since such an effect has been described for the stress-induced serotonergic stimulation (Meijer and De Kloet, 1998) and tryptophan hydroxylase activity (Chaouloff, 1993). The high levels of CRH (corticotropin-releasing hormone) induced by the withdrawal of glucocorticoids may also have been important. The raphe nuclei are innervated by CRH neurons and express CRH receptors. Intracerebroventricular or intra-raphe CRH inhibited raphe neurons and 5-HT release at innervated sites (Chalmers et al., 1995; Kirby et al., 2000; Price and Lucki, 2001). CRH receptors have also been described in the LH (Chalmers et al., 1995).

The existence of a bi-directional relationship between the serotonergic and the CRHergic systems has been indicated. Serotonin and serotonergic drugs stimulated CRH release and gene expression (Kageyama et al., 1998) and CRH has been hypothesized to mediate the weight-reducing effects of serotonergic drugs (Appel et al., 1991).

Although the existence of a serotonergic component contributing to the feeding disturbance of obesity is widely accepted, the precise nature of the defect is still controversial. In obese humans, 5-HT turnover has been found to be reduced (Ashley et al., 1985) or elevated (Lambert et al., 1999). In rats, there are reports of low 5-HIAA levels in the VMH and PVN of obese Zuckers (Koulu et al., 1990). A low activity level was also indicated by the finding of diminished 5-HT turnover in the hypothalamus of the genetically obese Zucker rat (Routh et al., 1994). On the other hand, we and others have found indications of an exacerbated 5-HT response to food intake in the VMH and in the LH of obese Zucker rats (Orosco et al., 1995; Mori et al., 1999; De Fanti et al., 2001;) suggesting that an impairment of the physiological actions of the released neurotransmitter may also contribute to the impaired energy balance. This proposition is in agreement with the observation of a blunted hypophagic response to central serotonin administration in genetically obese mice (Currie, 1993). On the other hand, a normal response to the systemic administration of a $5-HT_{1B}$ agonist has been reported in the Zucker obesity (Koulu et al., 1990).

A low 5-HT content in the VMH has also been described in animals with hypothalamic obesity of the hyperphagic type (Silva and Hernandez, 1989). A non-hyperphagic obesity syndrome is produced by the neonatal treatment with monosodium glutamate (MSG). This excitotoxin induces hypothalamic lesions, specially at the arcuate nucleus, and several neuroendocrine disturbances, with reduction of metabolic rate, disrupted fat metabolism and consequent excess energy deposition as fat (Tokuyama and Himms-Hagen, 1989; Nascimento et al., 1991; Ribeiro et al., 1997; Morris et al., 1998). Hypothalamic 5-HT turnover has been reported not to be altered in this hypometabolic obesity model (Dawson, 1986; Lorden and Caudle, 1986; Caputo et al., 1996), as was the response to fenfluramine, a serotonin releaser and reuptake blocker (Leigh et al., 1992). Accordingly, the food-induced release of 5-HT in the LH was similar to that of normal rats (Mori et al., 1999).

A common feature of many obesity syndromes, including animal models and central obesity in men, is the presence of high corticosteroid secretion rates and/or circulating levels. The MSG obesity shows increased serum corticosterone levels and blunted circadian rhythm (Magarinos et al., 1988) and adrenalectomy has been shown to prevent the development of the MSG obesity (Tokuyama and Himms-Hagen, 1989). High glucocorticoid levels are thought to play a role in hyperphagic obesity models, partly due to the induction of feeding, which has been shown to involve increased expression of arcuate nucleus NPY (Larsen et al., 1994). In the MSG obesity this mechanism is probably not operative, due to the neurotoxin-induced destruction of the arcuate nucleus (Stricker-Krongrad et al., 1996a). We demonstrated that, unlike normal rats, MSG-obese rats showed a sharp decrease of circulating corticosterone during feeding. However, they had a similar response to adrenalectomy as the normal rats, i.e., abolition the feeding-induced release of serotonin in the LH (Guimarães et al., 2002).

Serotonin and NPY Interactions

A functional interaction of the NPYergic and the serotonergic systems has been indicated. NPY neurons express 5-HT receptors (Makarenko et al., 2002). Hypothalamic NPY levels were elevated by 5-HT antagonists or synthesis inhibitors, while they were decreased after chronic administration of 5-hydroxy-tryptophan (Dryden et al., 1995; Kakigi and Maeda, 1992). NPY-induced hyperphagia was attenuated by serotonergic activation in some studies (Grignaschi et al., 1996; Currie et al., 2002) but in others it failed to change (Brown and Coscina, 1995). These discrepancies have been associated to the nucleus of injection of the serotonergic agonists, with the PVN but not the PFH or the VMH being an effective site (Currie and Coscina, 1997; Currie et al., 1999). Contrarily, other authors found that serotonergic receptors outside the PVN mediate the inhibition of NPY hyperphagia induced by 5-HT agonists (Grignaschi et al., 1996). The above data indicate that inhibition of NPY neurons may play a role in serotonin-induced hypophagia.

The hypothalamic NPY system is a physiological inducer of feeding and its levels increase during fasting (Beck et al., 1990; Kalra and Kalra, 2004). The effect of NPY-induced feeding on hypothalamic serotonin release was evaluated by some authors. Push-pull experiments found that local 5-HT levels either increased or remained unchanged when NPY was perfused in the preoptic area (Myers et al., 1996). NPY stimulated intake when perfused directly in the PFH, but failed to modify local 5-HT efflux (Myers et al., 1992). 5-HT levels in PVN microdialysates were unaffected when intake was induced by an intracerebroventricular injection of NPY (Matos et al., 1996). In protocols in which the animals were not allowed to eat after the NPY treatment, it was possible to observe a decrease in serotonin release in the VMH and the LH (Shimizu and Bray, 1989; Yeung and Castonguay, 2000).

We have recently been able to demonstrate that the presence or absence of a 5-HT stimulation in response to NPY-induced eating is dependent on the amount of peptide administered. We tested three different NPY doses, which were given intracerebroventricularly to satiated rats. Only after the lowest dose, of 1.0 µg NPY, there was a significant stimulation of 5-HT release in the lateral hypothalamus, as measured by microdialysis (Mori et al., 2004b). Interestingly, the amount of food eaten by these animals closely resembled the intake stimulated by an overnight fast, as we had previously shown (Mori et al., 1999). This observation supports the suggestion that the NPY treatment felt into the physiological range, leading to hypothalamic levels closer to the ones endogenously achieved in situations of increased NPY stimulation, as overnight fasting. A different pattern was observed after the administration of higher doses of NPY, as serotonin release was not significantly affected during feeding evoked by either 2.0 µ or 5.0 µg of the peptide. These results indicate that, when feeding is stimulated by NPY, serotonergic inhibition is not always observed. On the contrary, the intake physiologically stimulated by enhanced endogenous NPY activity is probably followed by the serotonergic stimulation aimed at modulating satiety. A high NPY dose, more in the pharmacological range, is necessary to inhibit the normal serotonergic response to food.

Serotonin and Leptin Interactions

A serotonin effect upon leptin secretion has been investigated by a few studies, with contradictory results. Indeed, increasing 5-HT synthesis, by the systemic administration of the precursor 5-hydroxytryptophan, has been shown to either increase (Yamada et al., 2003) or decrease leptin circulating levels (Choi et al., 2003). The leptin and the serotonin systems have even been suggested not to interact at all in the control of feeding (Halford and Blundell, 2000).

However, based on available data, a role for hypothalamic serotonin as one catabolic system targeted by leptin signaling can not be ruled out. Serotonin neurons of the mesencephalic raphe nuclei, the major source of brain serotonergic innervation, have been found to express leptin receptors (Finn et al., 2001; Hay-Schmidt et al., 2001; Elmquist et al., 1998). Leptin administration has been shown to activate the signal transduction pathway mediated by the Ob-Rb receptor in the brainstem and also in the LH (Hakansson and Meister, 1998; Hosoi et al., 2002). Chronic i.c.v. leptin decreased serotonin transporter binding sites in the frontal cortex but not in the raphe nuclei (Charnay et al., 2000). The anorexia induced by i.c.v. leptin has been shown to involve activation of the 5-HT_{2C} receptor (von Meyenburg et al., 2003).

Contrarily, down regulation of dorsal raphe serotonin transporter expression has been associated with leptin deficiency (Collin et al., 2000). Studies on leptin´s acute effect on serotonin release *in vitro* found that both basal and potassium-stimulated serotonin overflow were unaltered by the addition of leptin to synaptosomes or superfusion preparations of rat hypothalami (Orlando et al., 2001; Hastings et al., 2002). Moreover, mice knockout for the 5-HT_{2C} receptor gene responded normally to leptin (Nonogaki et al., 1998).

In vivo effects of leptin have been examined in few studies, which performed indirect estimations of serotonergic activity. A daily intraperitoneal injection of leptin for 7 days increased serotonin metabolism, as evaluated in homogenates of hypothalamic tissue, in obese (*ob/ob*) but not in normal mice (Harris et al., 1998). Other authors were able to see an increase in serotonin turnover in normal mice, after 5 daily i.p. or i.c.v. leptin injections, and also reported an acute stimulatory effect of leptin on hypothalamic serotonin turnover, 3 hours after a single i.c.v. administration (Calapai et al., 1999).

Using microdialysis we have directly assessed the acute effect of a single intracerebroventricular leptin injection on 5-HT release in the lateral hypothalamus of normal rats. In the absence of food, leptin failed to affect serotonin levels in LH microdialysates. However, when food was available, leptin significantly accentuated the food-induced serotonergic activation, while it decreased intake. This indicates that leptin probably intensifyed the serotonergic-stimulating mechanisms elicited by food intake. The additional serotonergic activation induced by leptin may be significant for the hormone effects on energy balance (Telles et al., 2003).

Figure 1 summarizes our microdialysis results on the alterations of serotonin release in the lateral hypothalamus (LH) of normal rats. Serotonin release is stimulated when the rats eat after an overnight fasting period, likely representing a physiological response towards satiety (Mori et al., 1999). Concomitantly, glucocorticoid circulating levels increase, and these levels are important for the serotonergic stimulation, since this activation is abolished in adrenalectomized rats (Guimarães et al., 2002). The intake induced by the intracerebroventricular injection of NPY in fed rats has a dual effect on LH serotonin release. When a dose of NPY is able to elicit a similar intake as the one evoked by short fasting, the modulatory serotonergic stimulation is maintained. Contrarily, higher NPY doses promote a more pronounced intake while inhibiting the serotonergic activation (Mori et al., 2004b).

When a single leptin injection is given i.c.v. to overnight-fasted rats, it decreases intake and the level of LH serotonin stimulation is higher (Telles et al., 2003).

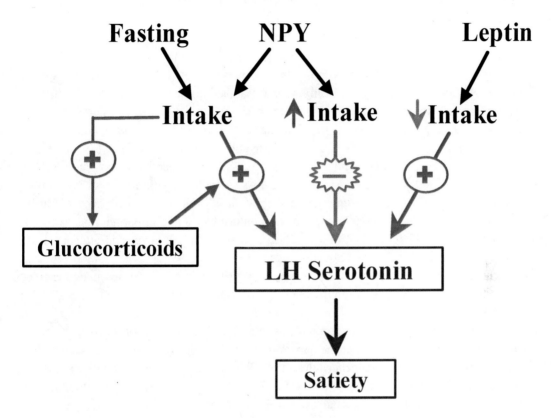

Figure 1. Summary of the effects of food intake, as evoked by fasting, NPY, or leptin, on the serotonin release in the lateral hypothalamus (LH). For details, see text.

More Serotonin Interactions: POMC, Orexins, CART, Inflammatory Citokines, Nitric Oxide

Recently, the hypothalamic melanocortin system has emerged as an important dowstream mediator of serotonin hypophagia. It has been shown that the anorexia induced by the serotonergic drug dexfenfluramine was attenuated by the blockade of the MC3 and MC4 receptors. Moreover, POMC neurons in the arcuate nucleus have been shown to be activated by serotonergic drugs, an effect mediated by 5-HT_{2C} receptors (Heisler et al., 2002 and 2003).

It has also been reported that 5-HT caused hyperpolarization of orexin neurons in the lateral hypothalamus, indicating that inhibition of this orexigenic system may play a role in serotonin-induced hypophagia (Muraki et al., 2004). Conversely, CART mRNA levels reportedly decreased after a sub-chronic systemic treatment with 5-hydroxytryptophan (Choi et al., 2003). The depolarization-stimulated serotonin release from rat hypothalamic synaptosomes was inhibited by orexins while CART had no effect on 5-HT release (Orlando et al., 2001).

As already mentioned, the proinflammatory citokines also have been shown to influence feeding and body weight (Banks, 2001). Interleukin 1ß (IL-1ß) dose-dependently inhibited food intake when i.c.v. injected in normal rats (Yang et al., 1994, Plata-Salamán et al., 1996; Sonti et al., 1997) and stimulated 5-HT in various hypothalamic sites (Shintani et al., 1993; Linthorst et al., 1996; Brebner et al., 2000). The 5-HT$_{2C}$ receptor has been shown to mediate IL-1ß anorexia (von Meyenburg et al., 2003).

Additionally, the nitric oxide (NO) system has been pointed as a factor stimulating food intake, as NOS inhibitors reduced feeding in both lean and obese mice and rats (Squadrito et al., 1994a and 1994b; Hui et al., 1995; Stricker-Krongrad et al., 1996b). The participation of a high NO tonus in the pathogenesis of obesity has been proposed, from the demonstration of increased levels of NOS and NOS mRNA in the hypothalamus of *ob/ob* mice (Morley et al., 1995). However, decreased hypothalamic NOS expression has been shown in obese Zucker rats (Kim et al., 2000). The administration of the NO precursor L-arginine or of NO donors increased 5-HT levels in the pre-optic area and striatum (Lorrain and Hull, 1993). Contrarily, L-arginine abolished the serotonergic stimulation induced by leptin in normal mice (Calapai et al., 1999) and NOS inhibition increased diencephalic 5-HT turnover and attenuated the hyperphagia of obese Zucker rats (Squadrito et al., 1994a and 1994b). Other authors reported that, although NOS inhibition attenuated the hyperphagia elicited by a serotonin autoreceptor agonist, this was not related to modification of 5-HT metabolism (Sugimoto et al., 1999; Yamada et al., 2000).

We have recently used brain microdialysis to address the question of whether the 5-HT system in the VMH participates in the anorexia induced by IL-1ß in obese Zucker rats, and whether the NO system affects this interaction. We found that 5-HT release was highly stimulated by a single i.c.v. injection of IL-1ß, which also significantly inhibited food intake. The pre-treatment with the NO precursor L-arginine abolished both the hypophagia and the serotonergic stimulation induced by the cytokine (Iuras et al., 2005).

All the above evidence demonstrate that the hypothalamic serotonergic system is an integrant component of the intricate central nervous system mechanism responsible for controlling food intake and energy homeostasis. Given the complexity of such mechanism, which involves numerous mediators and their multiple interactions, much is still unknown regarding the precise nature of the serotonergic participation, the specific pathways involved, as well as the relevance of serotonergic disturbances to the pathogenesis of obesity. The understanding of these aspects is highly relevant, since serotonergic agents are still largely employed as anti-obesity drugs, in spite of several limiting factors, such as treatment inefficacy, undesired side effects, and development of tolerance.

References

Ahima RS, Osei SY. Leptin Signaling. *Physiol Behav 81*: 223-41, 2004.

Appel, N. M.; Owens, M. J.; Culp, S.; Zaczek, R.; Contera, J. F.; Bissette, G.; Nemeroff, C. B.; De Souza, E.B. Role of brain corticotropin-releasing factor in the weight reducing effects of chronic fenfluramine treatment in rats. *Endocrinology 128*: 3237-3246; 1991

Araki E, Lipes MA, Patti ME, Bruning JC, Haag B, Johnson RS, Kahn CR. Alternative pathway of insulin signaling in mice with targeted disruption of the IRS-1 gene. *Nature 372*: 186-90, 1994.

Ashley DV, Fleury MO, Golay A, Maeder E, Leathwood PD. Evidence for diminished 5-hydroxytryptamine biosynthesis in obese diabetic and non-diabetic humans. *Am J Clin Nutr 42*: 1240-5, 1985.

Banks WA, Kastin AJ, Huang W, Jaspan JB, Maness LM. Leptin enters the brain by a saturable system independent of insulin. *Peptides 17* (2): 305-11, 1996.

Banks WA. Anorectic effects of circulating citokines: role of the vascular blood-brain barrier. *Nutrition 17*: 434-7, 2001.

Barnes NM, Sharp T. A review of central 5-HT receptors and their function. *Neuropharmacology 38*: 1083-1152, 1999.

Baskin DG, Lattermann DF, Seeley RJ, Woods SC, Porte Jr D, Schwartz MW. Insulin and leptin: dual adiposity signals to the brain for the regulation of food intake and body weight. *Brain Res 848*: 114-23, 1999.

Batterham RL, Bloom SR. The gut hormone Peptide YY regulates appetite. *Ann N Y Acad Sci 994:* 162-8, 2003.

Batterham RL, Cowley MA, Small CJ, Herzog H, Cohen MA, Dakin CL, Wren AM, Brynes AE, Low MJ, Ghatei MA, Cone RD, Bloom SR. Gut hormone PYY (3-36) physiologically inhibits food intake. *Nature 418* (6898): 650-4, 2002.

Baura GD, Foster DM, Porte Jr D, Kahn SE, Bergman RN, Cobelli C, Schwartz MW. Saturable transport of insulin from plasma into the central nervous system of dogs in vivo. A mechanism for regulated insulin delivery to the brain. *J Clin Invest 92*: 1824-30, 1993.

Beck B, Jhanwar-Uniyal M, Burlet A, Chapleur-Chateau M, Leibowitz SF, Burlet C. Rapid and localized alterations of neuropeptide Y (NPY) in the discrete hypothalamic nuclei with feeding status. *Brain Res 528*: 245-9, 1990.

Benoit SC, Air EL, Coolen LM, Strauss R, Jackman A, Clegg DJ, Seeley RJ, Woods SC. The catabolic action of insulin in the brain is mediated by melanocortins. *J Neurosci 22* (20): 9048-52, 2002.

Bernardis LL, Bellinger LL. The lateral hypothalamic area revisited: ingestive behavior. *Neurosci Biobehav Rev 20* (2): 189-287, 1996.

Besedovsky HO, Del Rey A. Immune-neuro-endocrine interactions: facts and hypotheses. *Endocr Rev 17* (1): 64-102, 1996.

Brebner K, Hayley S, Zacharko R, Merali Z, Anisman H. Sinergystic effects of interleukin-1(, interleukin-6, and tumor necrosis factor-(: central monoamine, corticosterone, and behavioral variations. *Neuropsychopharmacology 22*: 566-80, 2000.

Brown CM, Coscina DV. Ineffectiveness of hypothalamic serotonin to block neuropeptide Y-induced feeding. *Pharmacol Biochem Behav 51*: 641-6, 1995.

Brunetti, L.; Michelotto, B.; Orlando, G.; Vacca, M. - Leptin inhibits norepinephrine and dopamine release from rat hypothalamic neuronal endings. *Eur J Pharmacol 372*: 237-40, 1999.

Bruning JC, Gautam D, Burks DJ, Gillette J, Schubert M, Orban PC, Klein R, Krone W, Muller-Wieland D, Kahn CR. Role of brain insulin receptor in control of body weight and reproduction. *Science 289*: 2122-5, 2000.

Burks DJ, de Mora JF, Schubert M, Withers DJ, Myers MG, Towery HH, Altamuro SL, Flint CL, White MF. IRS-2 pathways integrate female reproduction and energy homeostasis. *Nature 407*: 377-82, 2000.

Calapai G, Corica F, Corsonello A, Sautebin L, Di Rosa M, Campo JM, Bruemi M, Mauro VN, Caputi AP. Leptin increases serotonin turnover by inhibition of nitric oxide synthesis. *J Clin Invest 104*: 975-82, 1999.

Campfield L, Smith FJ, Guisez Y, Devos R, Burn P. Recombinant mouse OB protein: evidence for a peripheral signal linking adiposity and central neural networks. *Science 269*: 546-9, 1995.

Campfield LA, Smith FJ, Burn P. Strategies and potential molecular targets for obesity treatment. *Science 280* (5368): 1383-7, 1998.

Cancello R, Tounian A, Poitou C, Clément K. Adiposity signals, genetic and body weight regulation in humans. *Diabetes Metab 30* (3): 215-27, 2004.

Caputo FA, Ali SF, Guisez Y, Devos R, Burn P. Neonatal MSG reduces hypothalamic DA, beta-endorphin, and delays weight gain in genetically obese (A viable yellow/alpha) mice. *Pharmacol Biochem Behav 53* (2): 425-32, 1996.

Carvalheira JBC, Ribeiro EB, Telles MM, Gontijo JAR, Velloso LA, Saad MJA. Selective impairment of insulin signaling in the hypothalamus of obese Zucker rats. *Diabetologia 46* (12): 1629-40, 2003.

Carvalheira JBC, Siloto RMP, Ignacchitti I, Brenelli SL, Carvalho CRO, Leite A, Velloso LA, Gontijo JA, Saad MJA. Insulin modulates leptin-induced STAT3 activation in rat hypothalamus. *FEBS Lett 500*: 119-24, 2001.

Chalmers DT, Lovenberg TW, De Souza EB. Localization of novel corticotropin-releasing factor receptor (CRF2) mRNA expression to specific subcortical nuclei in rat brain: comparison with CRF1 receptor mRNA expression. *J Neurosci 15* (10): 6340-50, 1995.

Chaouloff F. Physiopharmacological interactions between stress hormones and central serotonergic systems. *Brain Res Rev 8*: 1-32, 1993.

Charnay Y, Cusin I, Vallet PG, Muzzin P, Rohner-Jeanrenaud F, Bouras C. Intracerebroventricular infusion of leptin decreases serotonin transporter binding sites in the frontal cortex of the rat. *Neurosci Letters 283*: 89-92, 2000.

Chavez M, Kaiyala K, Madden LJ. Intraventricular insulin and level of maintained body weight in rats. *Behav Neurosci 109* (3): 528-31, 1995.

Chen H, Charlat O, Tartaglia LA, Woolf EA, Weng X, Ellis SJ, Lakey ND, Culpepper J, Moore KJ, Breitbart RE, Duky GM, Tepper RI, Morgenstern JP. Evidence that the diabetes gene encodes the leptin receptor: identification of a mutant in the leptin receptor gene in *db/db* mice. *Cell 84*: 491-5, 1996.

Choi SH, Kwon BS, Lee S, Houpt TA, Lee HT, Kim DG, Jahng JW. Systemic 5-hydroxy-L-tryptophan down-regulates the arcuate CART mRNA level in rats. *Regul Pept 115*: 73-80, 2003.

Collin M, Håkansson-Ovesjö M, Misane I, Ögren SO, Meister B. Decreased 5-HT transporter mRNA in neurons of the dorsal raphe nucleus and behavioral depression in the obese leptin-deficient *ob/ob* mouse. *Mol Brain Res 81*: 51-61, 2000.

Currie PJ, Coiro CD, Niyomchai AL, Lira A, Farahmand F. Hypothalamic paraventricular 5-hydroxytryptamine: receptor-specific inhibition of NPY-stimulated eating and energy metabolism. *Pharmacol Biochem Behav 71*: 709-16, 2002.

Currie PJ, Coscina DV. Stimulation of 5-HT 2A/2C receptors within specific hypothalamic nuclei differentially antagonize NPY-induced feeding. *Neuroreport 8*: 3759-62, 1997.

Currie PJ, Saxena N, Tu AY. 5-HT2A/2C receptor antagonists in the paraventricular nucleus attenuate the action of DOI on NPY-stimulated eating. *Neuroreport 10*: 3033-6, 1999.

Currie PJ. Differential effects of NE, CLON, and 5-HT on feeding and macronutrient selection in genetically obese (ob/ob) and lean mice. Brain Res Bull 32: 133-42, 1993.

Das UN. Is obesity an inflammatory condition? *Nutrition 17*: 953-66, 2001.

Dawson R Jr. Developmental and sex-specific effects of low dose neonatal monosodium glutamate administration on mediobasal hypothalamic chemistry. *Neuroendocrinology 42*: 158-66, 1986.

De Ambrogi M, Volpe S, Tamanini C. Ghrelin: central and peripheral effects of a novel peptydil hormone. *Med Sci Monit 9* (9): RA217-24, 2003.

De Fanti BA, Hamilton JS, Horwitz BA. Meal-induced changes in extracellular 5-HT in medial hypothalamus of lean (Fa/Fa) and obese (fa/fa) Zucker rats. *Brain Res 902* (2): 164-70, 2001.

De Kloet ER, Kovács GL, Szabó G, Telegdy G, Bohus B, Versteg DHG. Decreased serotonin turnover in the dorsal hippocampus of rat brain shortly after adrenalectomy: selective normalization after corticosterone substitution. *Brain Res 239*: 659-63, 1982.

Dinan TG. Serotonin and the regulation of hypothalamic-pituitary-adrenal axis function. *Life Sci 58* (20): 1683-94, 1996.

Dryden S, Wang Q, Frankish HM, Pickavance L, Williams, G. The serotonin (5-HT) antagonist methisergide increases neuropeptide Y (NPY) synthesis and secretion in the hypothalamus of the rat. *Brain Res 699*: 8-12, 1995.

Dunbar JC, Clough-Helfman C, Barraco RA, Anderson GF. Effect of insulin and clonidine on the evoked release of norepinephrine and serotonin from de nucleus tractus solitarius of the diabetic rat. *Pharmacology 51*: 370-80, 1995.

Elliott JC, Harrold JA, Brodin P, Enquist K, Backman A, Bystrom M, Lindgren K, King P, Williams G. Increases in melanin-concentrating hormone and MCH receptor levels in the hypothalamus of dietary-obese rats. *Mol Brain Res. 128* (2): 150-9, 2004.

Elmquist JK, Bjørbæk C, Ahima RS, Flier JS, Saper CB. Distributions of leptin receptor mRNA isoforms in the rat brain. *J Comp Neurol 395*: 535-47, 1998.

Erickson JC, Clegg KE, Palmiter RD. Sensitivity to leptin and susceptibility to seizures of mice lacking neuropeptide Y. *Nature 381*: 415-21, 1996.

Finn PD, Cunningham MJ, Rickard DG, Clifton DK, Steiner RA. Serotonergic neurons are targets for leptin in the monkey. *J Clin Endocrinol Metab 86*: 422-6, 2001.

Flier JS, Maratos-Flier E. Obesity and the hypothalamus: novel peptides for new pathways. *Cell 92*: 437-40, 1998.

Flier JS. Obesity wars: molecular progress confronts an expanding epidemic. *Cell* *116*(2):337-50, 2004.

Fox EA, Byerly MS. A mechanism underlying mature-onset obesity: evidence from the hyperphagic phenotype of brain-derived neurotrophic factor mutants. *Am J Physiol 286* (6): R994-1004, 2004.

Funahashi H, Hori T, Shimoda Y, Mizushima H, Ryushi T, Katoh S, Shioda S. Morphological evidence for neural interactions between leptin and orexin in the hypothalamus. *Regul Pept 92* (1-3): 31-5, 2000.

Gerozissis K, Rouch C, Nicolaïdis S, Orosco M. Brain insulin response to feeding in the rat is both macronutrient and area specific. *Physiol Behav 65*: 271-5, 1998.

Gerozissis K. Brain insulin and feeding: a bi-directional communication. *Eur J Pharmacol 490* (1-3): 59-70, 2004.

Ghilardi C, Ziegler S, Wiestner A, Stoffel R, Heim MH, Skoda RC. Defective STAT signaling by the leptin receptor in diabetic mice. *Proc Natl Acad Sci 93*: 6231-5, 1996.

Glazer G. Long-term pharmacotherapy of obesity 2000: a review of efficacy and safety. *Arch Intern Med 161*: 1814-24, 2001.

Grignaschi G, Sironi F, Samanin R. Stimulation of 5-HT2A receptors in the paraventricular hypothalamus attenuates neuropeptide Y-induced hyperphagia. *Brain Res 708*: 173-6, 1996.

Guimarães RB, Telles MM, Coelho VBO, Mori RCT, Nascimento CMO, Ribeiro EB. Adrenalectomy abolishes the food-induced hypothalamic serotonin release in both normal and monosodium glutamate-obese rats. *Brain Res Bull 58* (4): 363-9, 2002.

Hakansson ML, Brown H, Ghilardi N, Skoda RC, Meister B. Leptin receptor immunoreactivity in chemically defined target neurons of the hypothalamus. *J Neurosci. 18* (1): 559-72, 1998.

Hakansson M-L, Meister B. Transcription factor STAT3 in leptin target neurons of the rat hypothalamus. *Neuroendocrinology 68*: 420-7, 1998.

Halford JC, Blundell JE. Pharmacology of appetite suppression. *Prog Drug Res 54*: 25-58, 2000.

Halford JC. Pharmacology of appetite suppression: implication for the treatment of obesity. *Curr Drug Targets 2* (4): 353-70, 2001.

Hanada R, Teranishi H, Pearson JT, Kurokawa M, Hosoda H, Fukushima N, Fukue Y, Serino R, Fujihara H, Ueta Y, Ikawa M, Okabe M, Murakami N, Shirai M, Yoshimatsu H, Kangawa K, Kojima M. Neuromedin U has a novel anorexigenic effect independent of the leptin signaling pathway. *Nat Med 10* (10): 1067-73, 2004.

Hardie DG. Minireview: The AMP-activated protein kinase cascade: the key sensor of cellular energy status. *Endocrinology 144* (12): 5179-83, 2003.

Harris RBS, Zhou J, Redmann Jr SM, Smagin GN, Smith SR, Rogers E, Zachwieja JJ. A leptin dose-response study in obese (*ob/ob*) and lean (+/?) mice. *Endocrinology 139* (1): 8-19, 1998.

Hastings JA, Wiesner G, Lambert G, Morris MJ, Head G, Esler M. Influence of leptin on neurotransmitter overflow from the rat brain in vitro. *Regul Pept 103*: 67-74, 2002.

Havrankova J, Roth J, Browntein M. Insulin receptors are widely distributed in the central nervous system of the rat. *Nature 272*: 827-9, 1978.

Hayes MR, Savastano DM, Covasa M. Cholecystokinin-induced satiety is mediated through interdependent cooperation of CCK-A and 5-HT3 receptors. *Physiol Behav 82*: 663-9, 2004.

Hay-Schmidt A, Helboe L, Larsen PJ. Leptin receptor immunoreactivity is present in ascending serotonergic and catecholaminergic neurons of the rat. *Neuroendocrinology 73* (4): 215-26, 2001.

Heisler LK, Cowley MA, Kishl T, Tecott LH, Fan W, Low MJ, Smart JL, Rubinstein M, Tatro JB, Zigman JM, Cone RD, Elmquist JK. Central serotonin and melanocortin pathways regulating energy homeosthasis. *Ann N Y Acad Sci 994*: 169-74, 2003.

Heisler LK, Cowley MA, Tecott LH, Fan W, Low MJ, Smart JL, Rubinstein M, Tatro JB, Marcus JN, Holstege H, Lee CE, Cone RD, Elmquist JK. Activation of central melanocortin pathways by fenfluramine. *Science 297*: 609-11, 2002.

Heisler LK, Kanarek RB, Homoleski B. Reduction of fat and protein intakes but not carbohydrate intake following acute and chronic fluoxetine in female rats. *Pharmacol Biochem Behav 63* (3): 377-85, 1999.

Herbert H, Saper CB. Organization of medullary adrenergic and noradrenergic projections to the periaquedutal gray matter in the rat. *J Comp Neurol 315* (1): 34-52, 1992.

Hewson AK, Dickson SL. Systemic administration of ghrelin induces Fos and Egr-1 proteins in the hypothalamic arcuate nucleus of fasted and fed rats. *J Neuroendocrinol 12*: 1047-9, 2000.

Hoebel BG, Hernandez L, Schwartz DH, Mark GP, Hunter GA. Microdialysis studies of brain norepinephrine, serotonin and dopamine during ingestive behavior. Theoretical and clinical implications. *Ann N Y Acad Sci 575*: 171-91, 1989.

Horvath TL, Diano S, Sotonyi P, Heiman M, Tschop M. Minireview: ghrelin and the regulation of energy balance - a hypothalamic perspective. *Endocrinology 142*: 4163-9, 2001.

Hosoi T, Kawagishi T, Okuma Y, Tanaka J, Nomura Y. Brain stem is a direct target for leptin's action in the central nervous system. *Endocrinology 143* (9): 3498-504, 2002.

Howard JK, Cave BJ, Oksanen LJ, tzameli I, Bjorbaek C, Flier JS. Enhanced leptin sensitivity and attenuation of diet-induced obesity in mice with haploinsufficiency of Socs3. *Nature Med 10*: 734-8, 2004.

Hui SC, Chan TY. Mechanisms mediating NG-nitro-L-arginine methyl ester-induced hypophagia in mice. *Eur J Pharmacol 283*: 141-50, 1995.

Inoue T, Koyama T. Effects of acute and chronic administration of high-dose corticosterone and dexamethasone on regional brain dopamine and serotonin metabolism in rats. *Prog Neuropsychopharmacol Psychiatr 20:*147-56, 1996.

Iuras A, Telles MM, Bertoncini CRA, Ko GM, Andrade IS, Silveira VLF, Ribeiro EB. Central administration of a nitric oxide precursor abolishes both the hypothalamic serotonin release and the hypophagia induced by interleukin 1ß in obese Zucker rats. *Regul Pept 124* (1-3): 145-50, 2005.

Jacobs BL, Azmitia EC. Struture and function of the brain serotonin system. *Physiol Rev 72*: 165-229, 1992.

Jean, A. The nucleus tractus solitarius: neuroanatomic, neurochemical and functional aspects. *Arch Int Physiol Biochim Biophys 99* (5): A3-52, 1991.

Joels M, Vreugdenhil E. Corticosteroids in the brain - Cellular and molecular actions. *Mol Neurobiol 17* (1-3): 87-108, 1998.

Kageyama K, Tozawa F, Horiba N, Watanobe H, Suda, T. Serotonin stimulates corticotropin-releasing factor gene expression in the hypothalamic paraventricular nucleus of conscious rats. *Neurosci Lett 243*: 17-20, 1998.

Kaiyala KJ, Prigeon RL, Kahn SE, Woods SC, Schwartz MW. Obesity induced by a high-fat diet is associated with reduced brain insulin transport in dogs. *Diabetes 49* (9):1525-33, 2000.

Kakigi T, Maeda K. Effect of serotonergic agents on regional concentrations of somatostatin and neuropeptide Y-like immunorreactivities in the brain. *Brain Res 599*: 45-50, 1992.

Kalra SP, Kalra PS. NPY- an endearing journey in search of a neurochemical on/off switch of appetite, sex and reproduction. *Peptides 25*: 465-71, 2004.

Keesey RE, Hirvonen MD. Body weight set-points: determination and adjustment. *J Nutr 127*: 1875S-83S, 1997.

Kim MJ, Kim Y, Kun B, Choe BK, Kim SA, Lee HJ, Kim J-W, Huh Y, Kim C, Chung J-H. Differential expression of nicotinamide adenine dinucleotide phosphate-diaphorase in hypothalamic areas of obese Zucker rats. *Neurosci Lett 292*: 60-2, 2000.

Kirby LG, Rice KG, Valentino RJ. Effects of corticotropin-releasing factor on neuronal activity in the serotonergic dorsal raphe nucleus. *Neuropsychopharmacology 22*: 148-61, 2000.

Koulu M, Huuponen R, Hanninen H, Personen U, Rouru J, Seppala T. Hypothalamic neurochemistry and feeding behavioral responses to clonidine, an alpha-2 agonist, and to trifluoromethillphenilpiperazine, a putative 5-hidroxytriptamine 1-B agonist, in genetically obese Zucker rats. *Neuroendocrinology 52*: 503-10, 1990.

Laaris N. Haj-Dahmane S, Hamon M, Lanfumey L. Glucocorticoid receptor-mediated inhibition by corticosterone of 5 HT_{1A} autoreceptor functioning in the rat dorsal raphe nucleus. *Neuropharmacology 34*: 1201-10, 1995.

Lambert GW, Vaz M, Cox HS, Turner AG, Kaye DM, Jennings GL, Esler MD. Human obesity is associated with a chronic elevation in brain 5-hydroxytryptamine turnover. *Clin Sci 96* (2): 191-7, 1999.

Langhans W. Anorexia of infection: current prospects. *Nutrition 16*: 996-1005, 2000.

Larsen PJ, Jessop DS, Chowdrey HS, Lightman SL, Mikkelsen JD. Chronic administration of glucocorticoids directly upregulates prepro-neuropeptide Y and Y1-receptor mRNA levels in the arcuate nucleus of the rat. *J Neuroendocrinol l6*: 153-9, 1994.

Leibowitz SF, Alexander JT. Hypothalamic serotonin in control of eating behavior, meal size and body weight. *Biol Psychiatry 44*: 851-64, 1998.

Leibowitz SF, Roossin P, Rosenn M. Chronic norepinephrine injection into the hypothalamic paraventricular nucleus produces hyperphagia and increased body weight in rats. *Pharmacol Biochem Behav 21*: 801-8, 1984.

Leigh FS, Kaufman LN, Young JB. Diminished epinephrine excretion in genetically obese (ob/ob) mice and monosodium glutamate-treated rats. *Int J Obes Relat Metab Disord 16* (8): 597-604, 1992.

Linthorst ACE, Flachskamm C, Holsbor F, Reul JM. Activation of serotonergic and noradrenergic neurotrasmission in the rat hippocampus after peripheral administration of bacterial endotoxin: envolvement of the cyclo-oxygenase pathway. *Neuroscience 72*: 989-97, 1996.

Lorden JF, Caudle A. Behavioral and endocrinological effects of single injections of monosodium glutamate in the mouse. Neurobehav Toxicol Teratol 8 (5): 509-19, 1986.

Lorrain DS, Hull EM. Nitric oxide increases dopamine and serotonin release in the medial preoptic area. *Neuroreport 5*: 87-9, 1993.

Ludwig DS, Mountjoy KG, Tatro JB, Gillette JA, Frederich RC, Flier JS, Marathos-Flier E. Melanocortin-concentrating hormone a functional melanocortin antagonist in the hypothalamus. *Am J Physiol 274 (Endocrinol Metab 37)*: E627-33, 1998.

Magarinos AM, Estivariz F, Morado MI, De Nicola AF. Regulation of the central nervous system-pituitary-adrenal axis in rats after neonatal treatment with monosodium glutamate. *Neuroendocrinology 48* (2): 105-111, 1988.

Makarenko IG, Meguid MM, Ugrumov MV. Distribution of serotonin 5-hydroxytriptamine 1B (5-HT(1B)) receptors in the normal rat hypothalamus. *Neurosci Lett 328*: 155–9, 2002.

Marks JL, Porte D, Stahl WL, Baskin DG. Localization of insulin receptor mRNA in rat brain by in situ hybridization. *Endocrinology 127*: 3234-6, 1990.

Martin FJ, Miguez JM, Aldegunde M, Atienza G. Effect of streptozotocin-induced diabetes mellitus on serotonin measures of peripheral tissues in rats. *Life Sci 56*: 51-9, 1995.

Matos FF, Guss V, Korpinen C. Effects of neuropeptide Y (NPY) and [D-Trp^{32}] on monoamine and metabolite levels in dialysates from rat hypothalamus during feeding behavior. *Neuropeptides 30*: 391-8, 1996.

McGowan MK, Andrews KM, Grossman SP. Chronic intrahypothalamic infusions of insulin or insulin antibodies alter body weight and food intake in the rat. *Physiol Behav 51*: 753-66, 1992.

McGowan MK, Andrews KM, Kelly J, Grossman SP. Effects of chronic intrahypothalamic infusion of insulin on food intake and diurnal meal patterning in the rat. *Behav Neurosci 104*: 373-85, 1990.

Meguid MM, Fetissov SO, Varma MV, Sato T, Zhang L, Laviano A, Rossi-Fanelli F. Hypothalamic dopamine and serotonin in the regulation of food intake. *Nutrition 16*: 843-57, 2000.

Meier JJ, Gallwitz B, Schmidt WE, Nauck MA. Glucagon-like peptide 1 as a regulator of food intake and body weight: therapeutic perspectives. *Eur J Pharmacol 440* (2-3): 269-79, 2002.

Meijer OC, De Kloet ER. Corticosterone and serotonergic neurotransmission in the hippocampus: functional implications of central corticosteroid receptor diversity. *Crit Rev Neurobiol 12* (1-2): 1-20, 1998.

Merali Z, Mcintosh J, Kent P, Michaud D, Anisman H. Aversive and appetitive events evoke the release of corticotropin-releasing hormone and bombesin-like peptides at the central nucleus of the amygdala. *J Neurosci 18* (12): 4758-66, 1998.

Minokoshi Y, Alquier T, Furukawa N, Kim YB, Lee A, Xue B, Mu J, Foufelle F, Ferre P, Birnbaum MJ, Stuck BJ, Kahn BB. AMP-kinase regulates food intake by responding to hormonal and nutrient signals in the hypothalamus. *Nature 428*: 569-74, 2004.

Mizuno TM, Kleopoulos SP, Bergen HT, Roberts JL, Priest CA, Mobbs CV. Hypothalamic pro-opiomelanocortin mRNA is reduced by fasting and [corrected] in ob/ob and db/db mice, but is stimulated by leptin. *Diabetes 47* (2): 294-7, 1998.

Mizuno TM, Mobbs CV. Hypothalamic agouti-related protein mesenger ribonucleic acid is inhibited by leptin and stimulated by fasting. *Endocrinology 140*: 814-7, 1998.

Mori H, Hanada R, Hanada T, Aki D, Mashima R, Nishinakamura H, Torisu T, Chien KR, Yasukawa H, Yoshimura A. Socs3 deficiency in the brain elevates leptin sensitivity and confers resistance to diet-induced obesity. *Nature Med 10*: 739-43, 2004a.

Mori RCT, Guimarães RB, Nascimento CMO, Ribeiro EB. Lateral hypothalamic serotonergic responsiveness to food intake in rat obesity as measured by microdialysis. *Can J Physiol Pharmacol 77*: 286-92, 1999.

Mori RCT, Telles MM, Guimarães RB, Nascimento CMO, Ribeiro EB. Effect of neuropeptide Y-induced feeding on the release of serotonin in the lateral hypothalamus of normal rats, as measured by microdialysis. *Nutr Neurosci 7* (4): 235-9, 2004b.

Morley JE, Kumar VB, Mattamal M, Villareal DT. Measurement of nitric oxide synthase and its mRNA in genetically obese (ob/ob) mice. *Life Sci 57*: 1327-31, 1995.

Morley JE, Mattammal MB. Nitric oxide synthase levels in obese Zucker rats. *Neurosci Lett 209*: 137-9, 1996.

Morris MJ, Tortelli CF, Filippis A, Proietto J. Reduced BAT function as a mechanism for obesity in the hypophagic, neuropeptide Y deficient monosodium glutamate-treated rat. *Regul Pept 75-6*: 441-7, 1998.

Munzberg H, Flier JS, Bjorbaek C. Region-specific leptin resistance within the hypothalamus of diet-induced-obese mice. *Endocrinology 145* (11): 4880-9, 2004.

Muraki Y, yamanaka A, Tsujino N, Kilduff TS, Goto K, Sakurai T. Serotonergic regulation of the orexin/hypocretin neurons through the 5-HT1A receptor. *J Neurosci 24* (32): 7159-66, 2004.

Myers MG Jr. Leptin receptor signaling and the regulation of mammalian physiology. *Recent Prog Horm Res 59*: 287-304, 2004.

Myers RD, Lankford MF, Paez X. Norepinephrine, dopamine, and 5-HT release from perfused hypothalamus of the rat during feeding induced by neuropeptide Y. *Neurochem Res 17*: 1123-32, 1992.

Myers RD, Lankford MF, Roscoe AK. Neuropeptide Y perfused in the preoptic area of rats shifts extracellular eflux of dopamine, norepinephrine, and serotonin during hypothermia and feeding. *Neurochem Res 21*: 637-48, 1996.

Nascimento CMOC, Marmo MR, Egami M, Ribeiro EB, Andrade IS, Dolnikoff MS. Effect of monosodium glutamate treatment during neonatal development on lipogenesis rate and LPL activity. *Biochem Int 24* (5): 927-35, 1991.

Nielsen JA, Chapin DS, Johnson Jr JL, Torgensen LK. Sertraline, a serotonin-uptake inhibitor, reduces food intake and body weight in lean rats and genetically obese mice. *Am J Clin Nutr 55 (Suppl 1)*: 185S-9S, 1992.

Niswender KD, Schwartz MW. Insulin and leptin revisited: adiposity signals with overlapping physiological and intracellular signaling capabilities. *Front Neuroendocrinol 24*: 1-10, 2003.

Nonogaki, K.; Strack, A.; Dallman, M.; Tecott, L. - Leptin-independent hyperphagia and type 2 diabetes in mice with a mutated serotonin 5-HT$_{2C}$ receptor gene. *Nature Med 4*: 1152-6, 1998.

O´Rahilly S, Farooqi S, Yeo GSH, Challis BG. Minireview: Human obesity - lessons from monogenic disorders. *Endocrinology 144*: 3757-64, 2003.

Obici S, Feng Z, Karkanias G, Baskin DG, Rosseti L. Decreasing hypothalamic insulin receptors causes hyperphagia and insulin resistance in rats. Nat Neuroci 5: 566-72, 2002.

Oltmans G. Norepinephrine and dopamine levels in hypothalamic nuclei of genetically obese mouse (ob/ob). *Brain Res 273*: 369-73, 1983.

Orlando G, Brunetti L, Chiara DN, Michelotto B, Recinella L, Ciabattoni G, Vacca M. Effects of cocaine- and amphetamine-regulated transcript peptide, leptin and orexins on hypothalamic serotonin release. *Eur J Pharmacol 430*: 269-72, 2001

Orosco M, Rouch C, Gerozissis K. Activation of hypothalamic insulin by serotonin is the primary event of the insulin-serotonin interaction involved in the control of feeding. *Brain Res 872*: 64-70, 2000.

Orosco M, Rouch C, Gripois D, Blouquit MF, Roffi J, Jacquot C, Cohen Y. Effects of insulin on brain monoamine metabolism in the Zucker rat: influence of genotype and age. *Psychoneuroendocrinology 16*: 537-46, 1991.

Orosco M, Rouch C, Meile MJ, Nicolaidis S. Spontaneous feeding related changes in rostromedial hypothalamus of the obese Zucker rat: a microdialysis study. *Physiol Behav 57* (6): 1103-6, 1995.

Owji AA, Khoshdel Z, Sanea F, Panjehshahin MR, Fard MS, Smith DM, Coppock HA, Ghatei MA, Bloom SR. Effects of intracerebroventricular injection of glucagon-like peptide-1 and its related peptides on serotonin metabolism and on levels of amino acids in the rat hypothalamus. *Brain Res 929* (1): 70-5, 2002.

Palaniappan LP, Carnethon MR, Fortmann SP. Heterogeneity in the relationship between ethnicity, BMI, and fasting insulin. *Diabetes Care 25* (8): 1351-7, 2002.

Plata-Salamán CR, Sonti G, Borkoski JP, Wilson CD, French-Mullen JM. Anorexia induced by chronic central administration of cytokines at estimated pathophysiological concentrations. *Physiol Behav 60*: 867-75, 1996.

Price ML, Lucki I. Regulation of serotonin release in the lateral septum and striatum by corticotropin-releasing factor. *J Neurosci 21* (8): 2833-41, 2001.

Qi Y, Takahashi N, Hileman S, Patel HR, Berg AH, Pajvani UB, Scherer PE, Ahima RS. Adiponectin acts in the brain to decrease body weight. *Nat Med 10* (5): 5249, 2004.

Rees-Jones RW, Hendricks SA, Quarum M, Roth J. The insulin receptor of rat brain is coupled to tyrosine kinase activity. *J Clin Invest 259*: 3470-4, 1984.

Ribeiro EB, Nascimento CMO, Andrade IS, Hirata AE, Dolnikoff MS. Hormonal and metabolic adaptations to fasting in monosodium glutamate-obese rats. *J Comp Physiol B 167*: 430-7, 1997.

Routh VH, Stern JS, Horwitz BA. Serotonergic activity is depressed in the ventromedial hypothalamic nucleus of 12-day-old obese Zucker rats. *Am J Physiol 267*: 12-19, 1994.

Roytblat L, Rachinsky M, Fisher A, Greemberg L, Shapira Y, Douvdevani A, Gelman S. Raised interleukin-6 levels in obese patients. *Obes Res 8*: 673-75, 2000.

Sakurai T. Orexins and orexin receptors: implication in feeding behavior. *Regul Pept 85* (1): 25-30, 1999.

Salamone J, Mahan K, Rogers S. Ventrolateral striatal dopamine depletions impair feeding and food handling in rats. *Pharmacol Biochem Behav 44*: 605-10, 1993.

Satoh N, Ogawa Y, Katsuura G, Hayase M, Tsuji T, Imagawa K, Yoshimasa Y, Nishi S, Hosoda K, Nakao K. The arcuate nucleus as a primary site of satiety effect of leptin in rats. *Neurosci Lett 224* (3): 149-52, 1997.

Schwartz DH, Hernandez L, Hoebel B. Serotonin release in lateral and medial hypothalamus during feeding and its anticipation. *Brain Res Bull 25*: 797-802, 1990a.

Schwartz DH, Mcclane S, Hernandez L, Hoebel BG. Feeding increases extracellular serotonin in the lateral hypothalamus of the rat as measured by microdyalisis. *Brain Res 479*: 349-54, 1989.

Schwartz MW, Figlewicz DF, Kahn SE, Baskin DG, Greenwood MR, Porte D Jr. Insulin binding to brain capillaries is reduced in genetically obese, hyperinsulinemic Zucker rats. *Peptides 11*: 467-72, 1990b.

Schwartz MW, Woods SC, Porte D, Seeley RJ, Baskin DG. Central nervous system control of food intake. *Nature 404*: 661-71, 2000.

Shimada M, Tritos NA, Lowell BB, Flier JS, Maratos-Flier E. Mice lacking melanin-concentrating hormone are hypophagic and lean. *Nature 396* (6712): 670-4, 1998.

Shimizu H, Bray GA. Effects of neuropeptide Y on norepinephrine and serotonin metabolism in rat hypothalamus in vivo. *Brain Res Bull 22*: 945-50, 1989.

Shintani F, Kanba S, Nakaki T, Nibuya M, Kinoshita N, Suzuki E, Yagi G, Kato R, Asai M. Interleukin-1 beta augments release of norepinephrina, dopamine, and serotonin in the rat anterior hypothalamus. *J Neurosci 13*: 3574-81, 1993.

Shiraishi T, Oomura Y, Sasaki K, Wayner MJ. Effects of leptin and orexin-A on food intake and feeding related hypothalamic neurons. *Physiol Behav 71* (3-4): 251-61, 2000.

Silva E, Hernandez L. Goldthioglucose causes brain norepinephrine and serotonin depletion correlated with increased body weight. *Brain Res 490*: 192-5, 1989.

Sipols AJ, Baskin DG, Schwartz MW. Effect of intracerebroventricular insulin infusion on diabetic hyperphagia and hypothalamic neuropeptide gene expression. *Diabetes 44*: 147-51, 1995.

Small CJ, Bloom SR. Gut hormones and the control of appetite. *Trends Endocrinol Metab 15* (6): 259-63, 2004.

Sonti G, Flynn MC, Plata-Salamán CR. Interleukin (IL-1) receptor type I mediates anorexia but not adipsia induced by centrally admistered IL-1(. Physiol Behav 62: 1179-83, 1997.

Spiegelman BM, Flier JS. Adipogenesis and obesity: rounding out the big picture. *Cell 87*: 377-89, 1996.

Squadrito F Calapai G, Altavilla D, Cuccinota D, Zingarelli B, Arcoraci V, Campo GM, Caputi AP. Central serotoninergic system involvement in the anorexia induced by NG-nitro-L-arginin, an inhibitor of nitric oxide synthase. *Eur J Pharmacol 255*: 51-5, 1994a.

Squadrito F, Calapai G, Altavilla D, Cucinotta D, Zingarelli B, Campo GM, Arcoraci V, Sautebin L, Mazzaglia G, Caputi AP. Food deprivation increases brain nitric oxide synthase and depresses brain serotonin levels in rats. *Neuropharmacology 33*: 83-6, 1994b.

Steppan CM, Lazar MA. Resistin and obesity-associated insulin resistance. *Trends Endocrinol Metab 13* (1): 18-23, 2002.

Stricker-Krongrad A, Beck B, Burlet C. Enhanced feeding response to neuropeptide Y in hypothalamic neuropeptide Y-depleted rats. *Eur J Phamacol 295* (1): 27-34, 1996a.

Stricker-Krongrad A, Beck B, Burlet C. Nitric oxide mediates hyperphagia of obese Zucker rats: Relation to specific changes in the microstructure of feeding behavior. *Life Sci 58*: 9-15, 1996b.

Sugimoto Y, Yamada J, Yoshikawa T. A neuronal nitric oxide synthase inhibitor 7-nitroindazole reduces the 5-HT1A receptor agonist 8-OH-DPAT-elicited hyperphagia in rats. *Eur J Pharmacol 376*: 1-5, 1999.

Takaya K, Ogawa Y, Isse N, Okazaki T, Satoh N, Masuzaki H, Mori K, Tamura N, Hosoda K, Nakao K. Molecular cloning of rat leptin receptor isoform complementary DNAs - Identification of a missense mutation in Zucker fatty (fa/fa) rats. *Biochem Biophys Res Commun 225*: 75-83, 1996.

Tartaglia LA, Dembrski M, Weng X, Deng N, Culpepper J, Devos R, Richards GJ, Camplifield LA, Clark FT, Deeds J, Muir C, Sanker S, Moriarty A, Moore KJ, Smutko JS, Mays GG, Woolf EA, Monroe CA, Tepper RI. Identification and expression cloning of a leptin receptor, OB-R. *Cell 83:* 1263-71, 1995.

Tecott LH, Sun LM, Akana, SF, Strack AM, Lowenstein DH, Dallman M, Julius D. Eating disorder and epilepsy in mice lacking 5-HT2C serotonin receptors. *Nature 374*: 542-6, 1995.

Telles MM, Guimarães RB, Ribeiro EB. Effect of leptin on the acute feeding-induced hypothalamic serotonergic stimulation in normal rats. *Regul Pept 115*: 11-18, 2003.

Tokuyama K, Himms-Hagen J. Adrenalectomy prevents obesity in glutamate-treated mice. *Am J Physiol 257*: E139-44, 1989.

Tschop M, Statnick MA, Suter TM, Heiman ML. GH-releasing peptide-2 increases fat mass in mice lacking NPY: indication for a crucial mediating role of hypothalamic agouti-related protein. *Endocrinology 143*: 558-68, 2002.

Vahabzadeh A, Boutelle MG, Fillenz M. Effects of changes in rat brain glucose on serotonergic and noradrenergic neurons. *Eur J Neurosci 7*:175-9, 1995.

Van Loon GR, Shum A, Sole MJ. Decreased brain serotonin turnover after short term (two-hour) adrenalectomy in rats: A comparison of four turnover methods. *Endocrinology 108*: 1392-402, 1981.

Vickers SP, Dourish CT, Serotonin receptor ligands and the treatment of obesity. *Curr Opin Investig Drugs 5* (4): 377-88, 2004.

Virkamäki A, Ueki K, Kahn RC. Protein-protein interaction in insulin signaling and the molecular mechanisms of insulin resistance. *J Clin Invest 103* (7): 931-43, 1999.

Voigt J, Kienzle F, Sohr R, Rex A, Fink H. Feeding and 8-OHDPAT-related release of serotonin in the rat lateral hypothalamus. *Pharmacol Biochem Behav 65* (1): 183-9, 2000.

Voigt J-P, Sohr R, Fink H. CCK-8S facilitates 5-HT release in rat hypothalamus. *Pharmacol Biochem Behav 59* (1): 179-82, 1998.

von Meyenburg C, Langhans W, Hrupka BJ. Evidence for a role of 5-HT2C receptor in central lipopolysaccharide-, interleukin-1ß-, and leptin-induced anorexia. *Pharmacol Biochem Behav 74*: 1025-31, 2003.

Wang ZW, Zhou YT, Kakuma T, Lee Y, Higa M, Kalra SP, Dube MG, Kalra PS, Unger RH. Comparing the hypothalamic and extrahypothalamic actions of endogenous hyperleptinemia. *Proc Natl Acad Sci USA 96* (18): 10373-8, 1999.

Ward AS, Comer SD, Haney M, Fischman MW, Foltin RW. Fluoxetine-maintained obese humans: Effect on food intake and body weight. *Physiol Behav 66* (5): 815-21, 1999.

Wellman PJ. Norepinephrine and control of food intake. *Nutrition 16*: 837-42, 2000.

Woods SC, Lotter EC, McKay LD, Porte D. Chronic intracerebroventricular infusion of insulin reduces food intake and body weight of baboons. *Nature 282*: 503-5, 1979.

Woods SC, Seeley RJ, Porte Jr D, Schwartz MW. Signals that regulate food intake and energy homeostasis. *Science 280*: 1378-83, 1998.

Wurtman RJ, Wurtman JJ. Brain serotonin, carbohydrate craving, obesity and depression. *Adv Exp Med Biol 398*: 35-41, 1996.

Xu B, Goulding, Zang K, Cepoi D, Cone RD, Jones KR, Tecott LH, Reichardt LF. Brain-derived neurotrophic factor regulates energy balance downstream of melanocortin-4 receptor. *Nat Neurosci 6* (7): 736-42, 2003.

Yamada J, Sugimoto Y, Kunitomo M. A nitric oxide synthase inhibitor reduces hyperphagia induced in rats by the 5-HT1A receptor agonist, 8-OH-DPAT, independently of hypothalamic serotonin metabolism. *Eur J Pharmacol 402*: 247-50, 2000.

Yamada J, Sugimoto Y, Ujikawa M, Goko H, Yagura T. Hyperleptinemia elicited by the 5-HT precursor, 5-hydroxytryptophan in mice: involvement of insulin. *Life Sci 73*: 2335-44, 2003.

Yamauchi A, Shizuka F, Yamamoto T, Nikawa T, Kido Y, Rokutan K, Kishi K. Amino acids and glucose differently increased extracellular 5-hydroyindolacetic acid in the rat brain. *J Nutr Sci Vitaminol 41* (3): 325-40, 1995.

Yang ZJ, Koseki M, Meguid MM, Gleason JR, Debonis D. Sinergistic effect of rhTNF-(and rhIL-1(in inducing anorexia in rats. *Am J Physiol 267*: 1056-64, 1994.

Yeung SK, Castonguay TW. The effect of neuropeptide Y on hypothalamic serotonin overflow. *Nutr Neurosci 3*, 373-81, 2000.

Zhang Y, Proença P, Maffei M, Barone M, Leopold L, Friedman JM. Positional cloning of the mouse obese gene and its human homologue. *Nature 372*: 425-32, 1994.

Zigman JM, Elmquist JK. Minireview: from anorexia to obesity - the yin and yang of body weight control. *Endocrinology 144*: 3749-3756, 2003.

In: Focus on Nutrition Research
Editor: Tony P. Starks, pp. 149-163

ISBN 1-59454-768-8
© 2006 Nova Science Publishers, Inc.

Chapter VI

Hypovitaminosis D in Elderly People Living in an Overpopulated City: Buenos Aires, Argentina

L. Plantalech[1], A. Bagur[2], J. Fassi[1], H. Salerni[3], M.J. Pozzo[4],
M. Ercolano[5], M. Ladizesky[2], C. Casco[2], S.N. Zeni[2*],*
*J. Somoza[2**] and B. Oliveri[2*]*

Research Committee of the Asociación Argentina de Osteología y Metabolismo Mineral
(AAOMM).
[1] Sección Osteopatías Médicas, División Endocrinología, Hospital Italiano, Buenos Aires,
[2] Sección Osteopatías Médicas, Hospital de Clínicas, Universidad de Buenos Aires,
[3] Sección Osteopatías Médicas, Hospital Durand, Buenos Aires,
[4] Division de Endocrinología, Hospital Alemán, Buenos Aires and
[5] Unidad de Osteopatías Médicas, División Endocrinología, Hospital Ramos Mejía,
Buenos Aires.
*Researcher of the National Council for Scientific and Technological Research
(CONICET)
**Technician of the National Council for Scientific and Technological Research
(CONICET)

Abstract

Background: Elderly people are susceptible to hypovitaminosis D. Bone loss and fractures have been associated with Vitamin D deficiency. Urban populations are prone to suffering Hypovitaminosis D due to the type of housing (large apartment buildings),

---

[1] Correspondence and reprint requests: Luisa Plantalech –Sección Osteopatías Médicas- Servicio de Endocrinología, Hospital Italiano, Gascon 450 (C11814ACH) Ciudad de Buenos Aires, Argentina. Email: luisa.plantalech@hospitalitaliano.org.ar

lack of green spaces, and indoor lifestyle. In addition, low-income elderly subjects have been reported to be a risk population. The aim of this study was to determine winter 25OHD serum levels of the non-institutionalized elderly population of a large overpopulated city, and to analyze their determining factors.

Population and Methods: A population of healthy people aged 71.5 ± 5.4 years (x±se) (113 women and 56 men) living in the city of Buenos Aires (34° SL), was studied at the end of winter. None of the subjects were receiving treatment with Vitamin D supplements. Exposure to sunlight, housing, type of clothing worn in summer, Vitamin D rich food (D food) intake and socioeconomic status, were assessed using specific questionnaires. Calcium, Parathyroid hormone (PTH), bone turn-over markers and 25OHD were measured.

Results: Mean 25OHD circulating levels were 17.9 ± 0.64 ng/ml. Only 51 % of subjects had sunlight exposure; 63 % consumed D food. 25OHD levels were higher in men (19.8 ± 0.2 vs 17.0 ± 0.1ng/ml p < 0.04) and in subjects who had more than 3.5 hrs /week of sun exposure (21.4 ± 1.5 vs 16.6 ± 0.6 ng/ml; p < 0.0001), ate D food three times /week or more (21.6 ± 0.2 vs 16.4 ± 0.1ng/ml; p < 0.0001), lived in a house (19.5 ± 0.1 vs 17.1 ± 0.1 ng/ml; p < 0.018), and wore light clothes in summer (20.9 ± 2.3 vs 18.0 ± 2.7 ng/ml; p< 0.006).

A multivariable regression linear model showed that gender, {Beta coefficient 2.44, CI 95% (0.25-5.15), p<0.076} sunlight exposure {Beta coefficient 0.96, CI 95% (0.45-1.46),p<0.0001} and D food intake (Beta coefficient 5.03, CI 95% (2.0-8.1), p<0.001), with adjusted R squared 0.22; p<0.0001, were predictors of 25OHD serum levels. Subjects with low income were found to have less time/week of sunlight exposure (Low: 1.9 ± 05 Middle: 2.9 ±0.6, High Income: 5.8 ±1.6 hours /week; p< 0.004), and poor D food intake (60%, 22.9% and 18.8% respectively; p< 0.002). Low-income subjects also showed increased PTH levels and bone turn over. 25OHD serum levels were similar in all three socioeconomic levels, although high-income subjects tended to have better Vitamin D status.

Conclusions: Hypovitaminosis D is common in elderly people living in a big city, as is the case of Buenos Aires, during winter; it is related to low sunlight exposure and poor intake of Vitamin D rich foods, which counteract seasonal changes in Vitamin D synthesis. Subjects with low income are most vulnerable.

Key Words: Hypovitaminosis D, elderly, urban population, sun exposure, vitamin D-rich foods.

Introduction

Hypovitaminosis D in the elderly is a major worldwide public health problem. Bone loss and fractures have been linked with vitamin D deficiency [1,2]. Restricted sunlight exposure, decreased skin synthesis of vitamin D and low vitamin D intake are the main etiologic factors in elderly people [3].

Photo-conversion of pre-vitamin D_3 to cholecalciferol in human skin is the major source of vitamin D [4]. During winter, photo-conversion is either lacking or limited. Consumption of vitamin D rich-food and dietary enriched nutrients counteract the deficiency caused by seasonal changes, geographic latitude and the time spent indoors [3].

Vitamin D status has been typed as follows: vitamin D deficiency which leads to osteomalacia, with the ensuing histomorphometric changes [1], vitamin D insufficiency which affects calcium homeostasis decreasing calcium absorption and 1, 25(OH)2D levels, and leads to secondary hyperparathyroidism [5], and vitamin D sufficiency which does not affect calcium homeostasis. The threshold of serum 25OHD that establishes the difference between vitamin D sufficiency and insufficiency is generally defined by its biological effect, primarily by the increase in serum parathyroid hormone (PTH). According to the literature, the levels of serum 25OHD below which PTH begins to rise are between 12 and 20 ng/ml [6-9]. More recent reports have established higher levels of 25OHD as limits of insufficiency: 25 , 31 or 44ng/ml [11-12]. A new category of desirable levels has been proposed, based on the levels of 25OHD required to decrease hip fractures [2,9] or those required to improve intestinal calcium absorption [13].

It must be pointed out however, that the aforementioned reports used different techniques to measure 25OHD, i.e. radioimmunoassay, competitive protein binding assay and immunoradiometric assay. This may account for the variation in results. Another possible intervening factor that would explain the different findings is the association between calcium intake and vitamin D status, since calcium intake varied among the studied populations [9].

The type of housing (apartment buildings), lack of green spaces, pollution, and indoor lifestyle, render the urban population prone to suffering hypovitaminosis D. The low income, elderly population is also at risk of suffering vitamin D deficiency. Harris et al [14] observed hypovitaminosis D in low class elderly Caucasian and African-Americans living in Boston.

Buenos Aires (34° SL) is an overpopulated city. Several research studies have reported hypovitaminosis D in the elderly, mainly in institutionalized subjects [15-17]. However, environmental causes have not been fully evaluated to date. The aim of this study was to assess the vitamin D status of healthy non-institutionalized elderly people living in Buenos Aires and to evaluate its association with exposure to sunlight, dietary intake, and socioeconomic status.

Population and Methods

Population

One hundred and sixty nine subjects over 65 years of age recruited at hospitals and medical centers in Buenos Aires agreed to participate. The subjects were on the preventive programs of the hospitals or centers, were relatives of patients admitted to the program/hospital or were on the hospital staff. The subjects had no history of organ failure, malignancy, malabsorptive syndromes, osteoporotic fractures or metabolic bone disease. None of the subjects were receiving vitamin D or any medication affecting mineral metabolism. Based on biochemical determinations, two women who presented primary hyperparathyroidism and eight subjects with high serum creatinine levels (> 1.4 mg%) were excluded from the study. The study population comprised 157 subjects (102 women and 55 men). The study was carried out at the end of the winter and beginning of spring (August 15-October 15/2000).

All subjects gave informed consent prior to the onset of the study. The study protocol was approved by the Research Committee of each Hospital and Institution and by the Asociación Argentina de Osteología y Metabolismo Mineral.

Methods

1-Questionnaires
The subjects were asked to complete three different questionnaires.

A. Information regarding sunlight exposure in winter was measured in total hours/week (hours during sunny periods). Subjects were asked about the time spent outdoors (-10am to 4pm-, -8 to 10am and 4-6pm–and after 6pm-). In order to evaluate indirect sunshine exposure during summer, type of clothing was recorded - long / short sleeves, light clothes, and so forth -and a score was used to assess covered/uncovered skin (0 to 3). Housing, i.e., house or apartment, was also recorded.

B. Calcium and vitamin D-rich food intake (eggs, fish, mushrooms, chicken liver) was assessed by means of a checklist administered by a trained physician. The score was calculated according to times/week (0 to 7) of vitamin D-rich foods intake. Dairy calcium intake was calculated from dairy products consumption and expressed in mg/day.Questions under a and b were adapted from the EURONUT-SENECA study [18].

C. Socioeconomic status was evaluated according to a test provided by the Argentine Marketing Association [19]. Three socio-economic levels were defined according to income, cultural level, property owned, automobiles and furniture:

1. High socioeconomic level (score ≥ 64)
2. Middle socioeconomic level (score 64-34)
3. Low socioeconomic level (score < 34)

One hundred and forty five subjects completed the socioeconomic questionnaire.

2-The Following Serum Biochemical Measurements were Performed
Calcium (atomic absorptiometry spectrophotometry), creatinine (colorimetric), bone alkaline phosphatase (BAP) (wheat lectin precipitation), 25 hydroxyvitamin D (25OHD) (RIA-IDS) and mid-molecular parathormone (PTH) (RIA, employing the antiserum that recognizes intact hormone, such as mid molecular and carboxyterminal fragments).

All biochemical determinations were performed at the laboratory of the Hospital de Clínicas using methods described elsewhere [20-22].

Serum levels of 25OHD vitamin D expressed vitamin D status and were typed as desirable: > 30 ng/ml, hypovitaminosis D: < 30ng/ml; vitamin D insufficiency: < 20ng/ml; vitamin D deficiency: < 10ng/ml.

Statistical analysis was performed using the Stata 8 statistical software package. Continuous variables were analyzed using the Kruskall Wallis test, Wilcoxon sum rank test and and/or multiple linear regression analysis, as needed. A value of $p < 0.05$ was considered to indicate statistical significance.

Results

Mean age of the population (X ±SE) was 71.5 ± 5.4 years, nutritional status, expressed by albumin (4.1 mg/ml) was normal and mean serum 25OHD was 17.9±0.64 ng/ml, indicating vitamin D insufficiency. The women had slightly yet significantly lower levels of 25OHD vitamin D.

Table 1. 25 OH Vitamin D levels (X ± SE) in the elderly population of Buenos Aires according to gender, duration and quality of solar exposure during the winter, summer clothing, housing and vitamin D- intake.

		25OHD ng/ml n p
Hours of solar exposure		
≥ 3.5 hs/week	21.4+1.5	45
≥ ≥ 3.5 hs/week	16.6+0.6112	0.0001
Period of sunlight exposure		
10 am-4 pm	21.3+0.2	49
Other hours	18.8+0.2	32
No exposure	15.2+0.876	0.0006
Summer clothes		
Full cover	18.0+2.7	10
Half cover	16.8+0.7	112
Light cover	20.9+/-2.335	0.006
Housing		
Apartment	17.1+0.1	103
House	19.5+0.151	0.018
Vitamin D-rich foods intake	16.4+0.1	112
< 3 (times/week)	21.6+0.245	0.0001
≥ 3 (times/week)		
Dairy Vitamin D intake		
<100 IU/day	17.6 ± 0.8 109	
>100 IU/day	18.8 ± 1.8 59 ns	

Only 52% of subjects spent time outdoors during the day. The mean number of hours per week spent outdoors was 3.46 ± 0.44, nearly thirty minutes/day. Less than 12.4% of the population stayed indoors (less than half an hour per week spent outdoors). Sixty eight percent of subjects lived in an apartment. Vitamin D-rich foods were consumed 1.84 times a week. Vitamin D intake in dairy products was 117 ±15 IU/day. Calcium intake was very low in the overall population (x 473.73 ± 23.78 mg/day). When associated diseases were assessed, 69% of subjects presented co-morbidities related to their age (Table 1).

Subjects exposed to more than 3.5 hours of sun per week had better levels of 25OHD, as well as those who spent time outdoors during maximal sunshine or sunny days. Subjects that wore light clothes during the summer and lived in a house, had higher levels of 25OHD than those who wore regular clothes and lived in an apartment. A similar finding was observed in subjects who ate vitamin D- rich foods more than three times a week (Table 1).

To assess the independent effect of each characteristic, all these variables were included in a multivariate regression linear model. Independent predictors for levels of 25OHD vitamin D were sunlight exposure between 10 am and 4 pm {B coefficient 0.96, CI 95% (0.45-1.46), $p<0.0001$}, gender {B coefficient 2.44, CI 95% (0.25-5.15), $p<0.076$} and intake of vitamin D-rich foods {B coefficient 5.03, CI 95% (2.0-8.1), $p<0.001$}, with adjusted R-squared =0.22, $p<0.0001$.

Based on international classifications of acceptable 25OHD levels, levels above 30 ng/ml were considered appropriate. As regards circulating levels of 25OHD vitamin D, subjects presenting 25OHD vitamin D above 30 ng/ml were young, had greater exposure to sunlight, high calcium intake and ate natural vitamin D rich foods more than three times/week (Table 2).

Table 2. Age, intake of calcium and vitamin D rich foods, and sunlight exposure according to 25OHD serum levels (X+SE).

	<10 ng /ml (18)	10 - <20 ng /ml (79)	20 - >30 ng /ml (47)	> 30 ng /ml (15)
Age (years)	71.8 ± 1.2	72.1 ± 0.7	72.7 ± 0.8	68.3 ± 0.7 *
Calcium intake gr/day	345.7 ± 46.9	437.1 ± 32.8	553.4 ± 45.8	573.6 ± 98.1*
Vitamin D-food intake (time/week)	1.3 ± 0.2	1.8 ± 0.1	2.0 ± 0.2	2.4 ± 0.3*
Sunlight exposure (hr/week)	1.4 ± 0.6	2.6 ± 0.6	3.7 ± 0.8	8.9 ± 2.5**
Sunlight exposure 10 am-4pm hr/week	0.7 ± 0.4	1.0 ± 0.3	1.8 ± 0.4	4.2 ± 1.4***

Anova * $p < 0.05$; ** $p= 0.0001$; ***$p= 0.002$; **(n)**

Analysis of the socioeconomic questionnaire showed that 15.2% , 37.3% and 47.5 % of the population belonged to the high, middle and low socioeconomic level. Low socioeconomic subjects presented more co-morbidities associated with age, less exposure to sunlight during the hours of highest solar radiation (average: 34 minutes per week), with a total daily exposure of 16 minutes at different hours; in contrast, 60% of weekly exposure of high socioeconomic level subjects occurred during the peak hours of solar radiation, and the overall daily average was approximately 50 minutes (30 minutes between 10 am and 4 pm). Near thirty two percent of high-income subjects, 38.9% of middle-income subjects and

62.3% of low-income subjects had no sunlight exposure (x^2 p<0.001). No variations in calcium intake or vitamin D intake in dairy products were observed among social levels. However, consumption of vitamin D-rich foods varied significantly, and weekly consumption was highest in high-income subjects (Table 3). Low-income subjects showed lower 25OHD levels, associated with an increase in parathyroid hormone and bone turnover, as confirmed by the finding of higher levels of bone alkaline phosphatase (Table 4). 25OHD levels were below 20 ng/ml in 68.1% of low – income subjects, but were ≥ 20 ng/ml in 59.1% of high-income subjects.

Table 3. Evaluation of parameters determining circulating levels of 25OH vitamin D, according to socioeconomic level. (X+SE)

Parameter	High class	Middle class	Low class	p
N	20	47 68		
Age (years)	70.4 ± 0.9	71.0 ± 0.8	72.8± 0.6	Ns
Gender F/M	9/13	36/18	56/13	-
Co-morbidity	45 %	62 %	80% 0.0001	
House/Apartment	18 %	33 %	34 %	ns
Calcium intake gr /day	461.6 ± 13.7	466.5 ± 6.3	471.9 ± 4.5	ns
Vit D rich food intake	60 %	22.9 %	19 % 0.002	
(>3 times/week) Vit D intake from dairy food (IU/day)	121.7 ± 21.9	104.1 ± 19.1	123.7 ± 16.3	ns
Exposure to sunlight				
10 am-4 pm (hr/week)	3.9 ± 1.2	1.4 ± 0.3	0.6±0.2 0.001	
Total exposure (hr/week)	5.8 +1.6	2.9 + 0.6	1.9±0.5 0.004	

Table 4. Serum Levels of 25OHD. (X+SE) and Parameters of Mineral and Bone metabolism, according to socioeconomic level.

Parameters	High class (20)	Middle class (47)	Low class (68)
Calcemia mg%	9.4 ± 0.1	9.5 ± 0.1	9.5 ± 0.1
25OHD ng/ml	21.2 ± 2.1	18.4 ± 1.3	16.4 ± 0.8
PTH pg/ml	43.5 ± 0.8	50.3 ± 0.4	61.3 ± 0.5*
BAP IU/ml	53.4 ± 0.7	59.5 ± 0.4	64.9 ± 0.3**

* p=0.06 **p=0.04 , (n)

Discussion

The importance of housing and its relation to hypovitaminosis D was first described in the XVIIth century. The advent of industrialization and urban development has brought about new bone diseases in children and adults, associated to environmental pollution, overcrowded living conditions and lack of exposure to direct sunlight. In the XIXth century, it was shown that exposure to sunlight could cure such diseases, which were later known as rickets and osteomalacia [23]. Hypovitaminosis D causes bone loss and osteoporosis, as observed in recent decades [24]. Elderly adults are one of the populations at risk, and hip fracture is the most feared consequence [1]. Thus, the population of a large city is potentially at risk of developing this disorder.

Buenos Aires is a large densely populated city. (2 776 138 inhabitants) [25]. It is located at 34° SL, and has four well-defined seasons. Urban lifestyle is prevalent, with most people living in apartment buildings. Although vitamin D supplementation of food products is not mandatory, more than 80% of dairy products are vitamin D enriched.

Based on modern criteria defining optimal vitamin D values (25OHD > 30 ng /ml), a high percentage of our city population over 65 years of age was found to present hypovitaminosis D. Our results are in agreement with previous studies reporting similar values in the adult and elderly population and a marked deficiency in institutionalized elderly subjects during winter [26,27]. Buenos Aires is located in a temperate climate region; this explains the higher circulating levels of 25OHD detected in our study as compared to the average values of populations living at higher latitudes in the country [26]. 25OHD levels were found to be similar to those reported in the EPIDOS [27] study performed in France, and higher than the average value reported for the European population of elderly outpatients studied in the Euronut-Seneca study.

Solar radiation, accumulation of vitamin D deposited during summer, and intake of vitamin D-rich foods or supplements, contribute to maintaining circulating levels of 25OHD during winter [28-30]. In the present study, the average time spent outdoors was found to be 30 minutes. Only 21% of subjects were exposed to sunlight during the hours of high solar radiation. Average 25OHD values of subjects exposed to sunlight more than 3.5 hours/week were above 20 ng /ml, and those who were outdoors an average 9 hours per week, with exposure to peak solar radiation during 4.14 hours a week, had 25OHD levels above 30 ng/ml. This is equivalent to more than 1 hour/day of exposure at any time during sunlight hours and 35 minutes/day of exposure during the hours of maximum UV radiation. The hours of exposure observed herein are similar to those observed by Webb et al. at the end of autumn in a study using polysulphone badges to measure UV radiation [28]. Winters in Buenos Aires are less harsh than at other latitudes and photo-conversion of pro vitamin D3 to cholecalciferol is preserved even during the winter months since people can be outdoors a great deal during winter [31]. Hence, in contrast to the study by Webb et al., the number of patients with 25OHD levels below 15 ng/ml in our study was 48% vs 55% in the population of Boston.

Housing also contributes to improved circulating levels of vitamin D; in fact, people who live in houses with patios or gardens exhibit 25OHD levels above those of people who live in apartment buildings. It is well documented that the city per se entails a risk of hypovitaminosis D as compared to rural areas, due to the lack of green spaces, environmental pollution, and city lifestyle which encourages people to stay indoors. All these factors hinder the effects of UV radiation on the skin and the synthesis of vitamin D. Previous studies assessed the differences between young populations living in urban and rural areas in countries with adequate solar radiation [32].

A number of studies have evaluated the effect of summer indirectly in areas of harsh winters. The lack of vacation periods (i.e., spending the summer in sunny regions) greatly contributes to the risk of suffering hypovitaminosis D (odds ratio: 3.9) [33]. Studies performed in the U.S. confirmed better 25OHD levels in subjects who spent more than 3 months in sunny regions of the southern states [29]. In our study, vitamin D synthesis during the summer was assessed indirectly and showed that people who wore light clothes during the summer had higher winter levels of 25OHD. These findings are in agreement with the Euronut-Séneca study [18]. However, the values reported herein are higher (20.9 ng/ml vs 16.4 ng /ml) and may be associated to the latitude and the mild weather of Buenos Aires, which allows engaging in outdoor activities. Clothing issues related to vitamin D levels were assessed in young Jordanians, Jewish orthodox, and Muslims, whose deficit in 25OHD in spite of living in countries receiving adequate solar radiation, was attributed to the fact that they keep their body completely covered [34-36]. Holick also investigated this issue after 24-hour exposure of the whole body in subjects wearing summer, autumn, or no clothing, and arrived at a similar conclusion [4].

Consumption of foods that are naturally rich in vitamin D, supplemented foods, and pharmacological supplements contribute to maintaining circulating levels of 25OHD during winter. In our country, vitamin D enriched milk and yogurt contain 40 and 30 IU per 100 ml of vitamin D respectively. Although supplementation is not mandatory, almost all the products on the market are vitamin D enriched. Our results showed that subjects who ate vitamin D-enriched foods more than three times a week had 25OHD levels above 20 ng /ml. Subjects with sufficient levels of 25OHD consumed foods that are naturally rich in vitamin D more than twice a week. The results obtained with our qualitative and semi-quantitative assessment are in keeping with the quantitative findings reported in the Euronut-Seneca study [18]. However, other studies disagree on the importance of the exclusive contribution of dietary intake of vitamin D. Webb et al reported that dietary intake of vitamin D was 24 IU/day, whereas Omdhall et al [37] found it to be 81–100 IU/day in men and women. Burnand et al.[33] posited that meat and fish intake is a poor predictor of 25OHD levels (odds ratio: 0.9). Similar conclusions can be drawn from the study by Salamone [30], who found that the population that only consumed non-enriched foods exhibited average levels of 25OOHD equivalent to 16 ng/ml. Intake of vitamin D-rich foods, associated with the low solar radiation at high latitudes and harsh weather, which hinders people from leaving their homes, explain the differences observed in comparison with our experience.

Intake of vitamin D in enriched foods (milk and yogurt) is low (117 IU /day) compared to the daily intake requirements recommended by international agencies (400 IU/day) for this population. Given that sun radiation in South America is high, recommended dietary intake is 200 IU/day (Mercosur Agency) in the belief that solar radiation alone is sufficient to ensure adequate levels of vitamin D. However, the results obtained in this study, which was performed during winter, seem to indicate that this measure should be reconsidered. Webb

[28] showed that intake of vitamin D from enriched foods is in the range of 52 to 352 IU/day. Our results showed it to be between 0 and 460 IU /day; 14.5 % of subjects did not eat dairy products and hence did not receive this source of vitamin D. People whose calcium intake was over 500 mg/day had 25OHD levels above 20 ng/ml. Several studies have reported a direct correlation between calcium intake and 25OHD levels [29,30,37,38]. In agreement with other reports, our results showed that calcium intake was low [39]. The increase in calcium intake and hence, in vitamin D, entails an increase in intake of enriched dairy products. In addition, low calcium intake leads to secondary hyperparathyroidism, an increase in calcitriol synthesis and a decrease in the substrate, i.e. 25OHD [40].

Vitamin D supplementation prevents hypovitaminosis D and is frequently used in the U.S. A study by Krall et al [38] reported that daily supplements greater than 316 IU/day correlated with 25OHD levels above 30 ng/ml; subjects who consumed less than 220 IU /day exhibited a greater rise in PTH at the end of winter and in spring. Additionally, the Framingham [29] study showed that an intake below 200 IU /day increased the odds ratio for hypovitaminosis D in a population of elderly people. Subjects receiving supplementation were excluded from the present study since our aim was to evaluate environmental factors. Our results, as well as previous studies carried out in Buenos Aires, show that 61% of subjects exhibited 25OHD levels below 20 ng/ml in winter; reaching 28.6 ng/ml in summer. Only 14.7% of subjects clearly exhibited hypovitaminosis D [16]. Nevertheless, subjects over the age of 80 failed to reach satisfactory levels of vitamin D during summer [15]. Based on our results, it can be inferred that the population of older adults should receive vitamin D supplementation during winter. This would not apply to subjects who are exposed to sunlight more than 30 minutes a day during the hours of maximum radiation, and consume vitamin D enriched dairy products and vitamin D-rich foods more than 3 times a week. It would seem appropriate to prescribe permanent vitamin D supplementation to the very elderly (more than 80 years of age).

As regards the characteristics of subjects who reached optimal 25OHD levels without supplementation, they account for 9% of the population, were younger, spent more time outdoors, and had higher calcium and vitamin D intake due to consumption of enriched dairy products and foods that are naturally rich in vitamin D. No socioeconomic differences were observed compared to the remaining subjects. Linear and multi-step regression analysis showed the following to be predictive factors of 25OHD levels in our study population: sunlight exposure during the hours of bright sunshine, vitamin D intake in foods that are naturally rich in vitamin D, and gender. Other authors have confirmed similar independent predictive factors: parameters of sunlight exposure such as the season of the year, winter time, lack of a recent vacation, time spent daily outdoors, gender, age, vitamin D intake, low milk intake and body mass index [11,28,29,33,37,38]. As regards gender, it is well documented that women have lower circulating levels of vitamin D, probably due to the fact that they have a larger amount of adipose tissue than men [41].

Although few studies have related 25OH D levels in the elderly to their socioeconomic status, a recent study performed in Britain shows that the low-income population over the age of 75 years is at high risk of suffering hypovitaminosis D, among other dietary deficiencies [42]. Several research studies have been performed in low-income populations [15,30,43,44]. Moreover, socioeconomic stratification and its association with 25OH D levels was assessed in a group of young women from Bangladesh [45], showing a greater percentage of hypovitaminosis D in the lower-income population. Our results show that low-income subjects are more prone to hypovitaminosis D: 25OHD levels were below 10 ng/ml in 23% of low-socioeconomic level subjects and in only 5% of high-socioeconomic level subjects. Scarce exposure to sunlight (60% of subjects is not exposed to direct sunlight) and low intake of foods that are naturally rich in vitamin D are likely causes of this difference. The high rate of co-morbidities (excluding serious diseases) observed in this socioeconomic group is also related to the aforementioned factors. Such co-morbidities interfere with the well being during every-day life and leisure time spent outside the home, while favoring indoor life. Several research works addressing these issues strongly suggest that hypovitominosis D and disability to perform every-day activities are associated [18,29,46-48]. This relation can be clearly observed in hospitalized subjects [49-52]. Although we observed no differences between low socioeconomic level subjects and middle and high-socioeconomic level subjects as regards intake of vitamin D and calcium in dairy products, their daily intake from this source is low. Contribution of vitamin D by other sources, such as vitamin D containing foods, is limited since these foods are high priced and are too often beyond the people's purchasing power.

Our results evidence a marked trend toward hypovitaminosis D in the middle as well as the low-income subjects. In the latter it was associated with higher levels of parthormone and an increase in bone turnover, as shown by bone alkaline phosphatase. Although the mean age of this socioeconomic group does not differ significantly from that of the other two groups, the population is in fact older and this would also contribute to the lower circulating levels of 25OHD. Our results strongly suggest that the environmental factors addressed in this study contribute to lowering 25OHD levels. Age, a decrease in glomerular filtration rate, and co-morbidities may also explain the increase in parathyroid hormone. The latter would also contribute to a rise in bone alkaline phosphatase. The immobilization caused by various co-morbidities increases bone turnover [53]. Other authors [29] have confirmed that vitamin D levels are higher in people who are more active.

We can conclude that hypovitaminosis D is a common finding in the non-institutionalized elderly population of Buenos Aires city. Contributing environmental factors include poor sunlight exposure during winter and summer, and low intake of vitamin D rich foods and enriched dairy products. This condition is more prevalent in low socioeconomic subjects. It would seem advisable to recommend vitamin D supplementation during the winter to the elderly living in densely populated built-up districts of the city and to the low-income elderly population.

References

[1]   Parfitt, MA; Gallagher, JC; Heaney, RP; Johnston, CC; Neer,R; Whedon, GD. Vitamin D and bone health in the elderly. *Am J Clin Nutr 1982*; 36: 1014-31.

[2]   Chapuy, MC; Arlot, M; Dubeof, F; Brun, ; Crouzet, B; Arnaud, S; Delmas, P; Meunier, P. Vitamin D_3 and calcium to prevent hip fractures in elderly women. *N Engl J Med 1992*; 327: 1637-42.

[3]   Chapuy C.M. and Meunier P. *Vitamin D insufficiency in adults and the elderly.* Feldman D. ed .In Vitamin D, Academic Press, San Diego: 1997; 679-694.

[4]   Holick, MF. MacCollum .Award lecture, 1994: Vitamin D-new horizons for the 21st century. *Am J Clin Nutr1994*; 60: 619-30.

[5]   Peacock M, Selby PL, Francis RM, Brown WB, Horden L: *Vitamin D deficiency, insufficiency and intoxication: What do they mean?* In Norman AW, Schaefer K, Grigoleit HG, Herrat D editors. Vitamin D: Chemical, biochemical and Clinical update: Berlin Walter de Gruiter 1985;569-70

[6]   Bouillon RA, Aurweerch MD, Lissens WD, Pelemans WK: Vitamin D status in the elderly, seasonal substrate deficiency causes 1,25(OH) cholecalciferol defficiency. *Am J Clin Nutr 1987*; 45:755-63.

[7]   Gloth FM, Gunberg CM, Hollis BW, Haddad JG, Tobin JD. Vitamin D deficiency in homebound elderly persons. *JAMA 1995*; 274 : 1683-1686.

[8]   Ooms ME, Lips P , Roos JC, van der Vijgh WJF, Popp.Snijders C, Bezemer D, Bouter LM. Vitamin D status and sex hormone binding globulin: determinants of bone turnover and bone mineral density in elderly women. *J Bone Miner Res 1995*;10:1177-1184.

[9]   Malachi J, Mc Kenna MJ and Freaney R. *Defining hypovitaminosis D in the elderly.* In Nutritional Aspects of Osteoporosis. Burckardt P, Dawson-Hughes B and Heaney RP eds. Springer-Verlag New York. 1998:268-277

[10]   Chapuy MC, Preziosi P, Maamer M, Arnaud S, Galan P, Hereberg S and Meunier PJ. Prevalence of vitamin D deficiency in an adult normal population. *Osteoporosis Int 7.* 439-443, 1997

[11]   Dawson-Hughes B, Harris A, Dallal G. Plasma calcidiol, season and PTH concentration in healthy elderly men and women. *Am J Clin Nutr 65*: 67-71,1997.

[12]   Haden ST, Fuleihan GEH, Angell JE, Cotran NM, LeBoff MS. Calcidiol and PTH levels in women attending an osteoporosis Program. *Calcif Tissue Int 64*:275-279,1999.

[13]   Heaney RP, Dowell M, Hale C, Bendich A: Calcium absorption varies within the reference range for serum 25-hydroxivitamin D. *J Am Coll Nutr 2003*:22:142-146

[14]   Harris, SS; Soteriades, E; Coolidge, JA; Mudgal, S; Dawson–Hudges, B. Vitamin D insufficiency in low income, multiracial, elderly population. *J Clin Endocrinol Metab 2000*; 85: 4125-30.

[15]   Fradinger, E; Zanchetta, J. Niveles de Vitamina D en mujeres de la ciudad de Buenos Aires. *Medicina (Buenos Aires)1999*; 59: 449-52.

[16]   Fassi, J; Russo Picasso, MF; Furci, A; Sorroche, P; Jauregui, JR; Plantalech, L. Seasonal variations in 25-hydroxyvitamin D in young and elderly population in Buenos Aires City. *Medicina (Buenos Aires) 2003*; 63: 215-220.

[17]   Plantalech, L; Knoblovits, P; Cambiazzo, E; et al. Hipovitaminosis D en ancianos institucionalizados de Buenos Aires. *Medicina (Buenos Aires)1997*; 57: 29-35.

[18]   Van der Wielen, R; Lowik, M; Van der Berg, H; et al. Serum vitamin D concentrations among elderly people in Europe. *Lancet 1995*; 346:207-10.

[19]   Comisión de Investigación de Mercado. Indice de Nivel Socioeconómico Argentino. *Asociación Argentina de Marketing. Buenos Aires. 1998*; 43-72.

[20] Oliveri MB, Ladizesky M, Mautalen C, Alonso A, Martinez L. Seasonal variations of 25 hydroxyvitaminD, 1,25 dihydroxyvitaminD and parathyroid hormone in Ushuaia (Argentina) the southernmost city of the world. *Bone and Mineral 20*:99-108, 1993.

[21] Casco, C; Bagur, A; Mautalen, C. Determinación de parathormona con un suero polivalente. Su utilidad en el diagnóstico y en la estimación de la severidad del hiperparatiroidismo primario. *Revista Argentina de Endocrinología 1988*; 25:3-8.

[22] Zeni S, Wittich A, Di Gregorio S, Casco C, Oviedo A, Somoza J, Gómez Acotto C, Bagur A, González D, Portela M, Mautalen CA. Utilidad Clínica de los Marcadores de Formación y Resorción Osea. Acta Bioquím. *Clin. 2001*: 35, 3-36

[23] Rajakumar, K. Vitamin D, cod liver, sunlight and rickets: a historical perspective. *Pediatrics 2003*; 112: 132-35.

[24] Mc Kenna, MJ; Freaney, R. Secondary hyperparathyroidism in the elderly: means to defining hypovitaminosis D. *Osteop Int 1998*; Suppl. 8: S3-6.

[25] Censo Nacional Poblacional 2001 de la República Argentina. Instituto Nacional de Estadísticas y Censo de la República Argentina (INDEC).www.indec.gov.ar.

[26] Oliveri, B; Plantalech, L; Bagur, A et al. High prevalence of vitamin D insufficiency in healthy elderly people living at home in Argentina. *Eur J Clin Nutr 2004*; 58: 337-42.

[27] Chapuy, M; Schott, A; Garnero, P, et al. Healthy elderly French people women living at home have secondary hyperparathyroidism and high bone turnover in winter. *J Clin Endocrinol Metab 1996*; 81:1129-33.

[28] Webb, AR; Pilbeam, C; Hanafin, N and Holick, M F. An evaluation of the relative contributions of exposure to sunlight and of diet to the circulating concentrations of 25-hydroxyvitamin D in an elderly nursing home population in Boston. *Am J Clin Nutr 1990*; 51:1075-81.

[29] Jacques, PF; Felson, DT; Tucker, KL; Mahnken, B; Wilson, PWF; Rosenbeg, IH; Rush, D. Plasma 25-hydroxyvitamin D and its determinants in an elderly population sample. *Am J Clin Nutr 1997*; 66: 929-36.

[30] Salamome, L; Dallal, GE; Zantos, D; Makraner, F; Dawson–Hudges, B. Contribution of Vitamin D intake and seasonal sunlight exposure to plasma 25-hydroxyvitamin D circulation in elderly women. *Am J Clin Nutr 1993*; 58:80-6.

[31] Ladizesky,M; Lu, Z; Oliveri, B; San Román, N; Díaz, S; Holick, MF; Mautalen, C. Solar utraviolet B radiation and photoproduction of Vitamin D_3 in central and southern areas of Argentina. *J Bone Min Res 1995*; 10:545-49.

[32] Gannagé-Yared, MH; Chemali, R; Yaacoub, N; Halaby,G. Hypovitaminosis D in a sunny country: Relation to lifestyle and bone markers. *J Bone Miner Res 2000*; 15: 1856-62.

[33] Burnard, B; Sloutskis, F; Gianoli, F; et al. Serum 25 hydroxyvitamin D: distribution and determinants in the Swiss population. *Am J Clin Nutr 1992*; 56:537-42.

[34] Mishal, AA. Effects of different dress styles on vitamin D levels in healthy young Jordanian women. *Osteoporosis Int 2001*; 12: 931-5

[35] Mukamel, MN; Weisman, Y; Somech, R; Eisenberg, Z; Landman, J; Shapira, M; Spirer, Z, Jurgenson U. Vitamin D deficiency and insufficiency in Orthodox and non Ortodox Jewish mothers in Israel. *Isr Med Assoc 2001*; 3: 419-21.

[36] Diamond, TH; Levy, S; Smith, A; Day, P. High bone turnover in Muslim women with vitamin D deficiency. *Med J Aust 2002*; 177:139-41.

[37] Omdhall, JL; Garry, PJ; Hunsareck, LA; Hunt, WC; Goodwin, JS. Nutritional status in a healthy elderly population: Vitamin D. *Am J Clin Nutr 1982*;36:1225-33.

[38] Krall, E; Sahyoun, N; Tannenbaum, S; Dalla, G; Dawson – Hughes, B. Effect of Vitamin D intake on seasonal variations in parathyroid hormone secretion in postmenopausal women. *N Eng J Med 1989*; 321:1777-83.

[39] Ercolano, M; Drnovsek, M; Moran, M; Salerni, H; Guadagna M; Rubin, Z; et al. Encuesta sobre ingesta de calcio en mujeres de Capital federal y Gran Buenos Aires. *Revista Argentina de Endocrinología. 2001*; 36: Suppl: S 91-93.

[40] Clements, MR; Johnson, L; Frase, DR. A new mechanism for induced vitamin D deficiency in calcium deprivation. *Nature 1987*; 325:62-65.

[41] Arunabh, S; Pollack, S; Yeh, J; Aloia, JF. Body fat content and 25-hydroxyvitamin D levels in healthy women. *J Clin Endocrinol Metab 2003*; 88:157-161.

[42] McNeill, G; Vyvyan, J; Peace, H; Mckie, L; Seymour, G; Hendry, J; Mac Pherson, I. Predictors of micronutrient status in men and women over 75 years old living in the community. *Br J Nutr 2004* ;88: 555-561.

[43] Delvin, E; Imbach, A; Copi, M. Vitamin D nutritional status and related biochemical indices in an autonomous elderly population. *Am J Clin Nutr 1988*; 48: 373-8.

[44] Gonzalez-Clemente, JM; Martinez-Osaba, MJ; Minarro, A; Delgado, MP; Mauricio,D; Ribera, F. Hipovitaminosis D: its high prevalence in elderly outpatients in Barcelona. Associated factors. *Med Clin (Barcelona) 1999*; 113: 641-45.

[45] Islam, MZ; Lamberg-Allardt, C; Karkkainen, M; Outila, T; Salamatullah, Q; Shamim, AA. Vitamin D deficiency: a concern in pre-menopausal Bangladeshi women of two socioeconomic groups in rural and urban region. *Eur J Clin Nutr 2002*; 56:51-6.

[46] Semba, RD; Garret, E; Johnson, BA; Garalnik, JM; Freíd, LP. Vitamin D deficiency among older women with and without disability. *Am J Clin Nutr 2000*;72:1529-34

[47] Nashimoto, M; Nakamura, K; Matsuyama, S; Hatakeyama, M; Yamamoto, M. Hypovitaminosis D and hyperparathyroidism in physically inactive elderly Japanese living in nursing homes: relationship with age, sunlight exposure and activities of daily living. *Aging Clin Exp Res 2002*;14: 5-12.

[48] Zamboni, M; Zoico, E; Tosoni, P; Zivelonghi, A; Bortolani, A; Maggi, S; Di Francesco,V; Bosello, O. Relation between vitamin D; physical performance and disability in elderly persons. *J Gerontol A Biol Sci Med Sci. 2002*; 57: M7-11.

[49] Thomas, MK; Lloyd-Jones, DM; Thadhani, RI; Shaw, AC; Deraska, DJ; Kitch, BT; Vamvakas, EC; Dick, IM; Prince, RL; Finkelstein, JS. Hypovitaminosis D in medical in patients. *N Engl J Med 1998*; 338: 777-83.

[50] Hochwald, O; Harman-Boehm, I; Castel, H. Hypovitaminosis D among in-patients in a sunny country. *Isr Med Assoc J 2004*; 6:82-87.

[51] Kauppinen-Makelin, R; Tahtela, R; Loyttyniemi, E; Karkkainen, J; Valimaki, MJ. A high prevalence of hypovitaminosis D in Finnish medical in- and outpatients. *J Intern Med 2001*; 249:559-63.

[52] Warodowichit, D; Leelawattana, R; Luanseng, N; Thammakumpee, N. Hypovitaminosis D in long stay hospitalized patients in Songklanarind. *J Med Assoc Thai. 2002*; 85:990-7.

[53] Theiler, R; Stähelin, HB; Kränzlin, M; Somorjai, G; Singer-Lindpaintner, L; Conzelmann, M; Geusens, P; Bischoff, HA. Influence of physical mobility and season on 25-hydroxyvitamin D-parathyroid hormone interaction and bone remodeling in the elderly. *Eur J Endocrinol 2000*; 143: 673-79.

In: Focus on Nutrition Research   ISBN 1-59454-768-8
Editor: Tony P. Starks, pp. 165-186   © 2006 Nova Science Publishers, Inc.

Chapter VII

The Intestinal Transportation of Zinc Sulfate and Zinc Methionine and Their Effects on Growth in Mice

Y. U. Ze-Peng, Shi Yong-Hui, L. E. Guo-Wei[1] and L. I. Lu-Mu

Laboratory of Nutrition and Biotechnology, School of Food Science
and Technology, Southern Yangtze University,
Wuxi, Jiangsu Province, 214036,
People's Republic of China

Abstract

Objective: This experiment was conducted to investigate the effect of zinc sulfate ($ZnSO_4$) and zinc methionine (Zn-Met) on growth and the expression of growth-related genes in mice; the further purpose was to study the transportation regulation of different zinc forms in the intestine of mice.

Material and Methods: Ninety male KM mice were randomly divided into three treatments. The control was fed on basal diet. The $ZnSO_4$ group and Zn-Met group were fed on the diets supplemented with $ZnSO_4$ or Zn-Met. The mice were offered the test diets for 10 days. Weight gains were measured, zinc contents in liver and serum were determined using atomic absorption spectrophotometry (AAS); growth hormone (GH) was determined by radioimmunoassay (RIA), the levels of growth hormone receptor (GHR), insulin-like growth factor I (IGF-I), ZnT1 (zinc transporter), ZnT4, DCT1 (divalent cation transporter) and MT-1 (metallothionein) mRNAs were determined using semi-quantification reverse transcript polymerase chain reaction (RT-PCR).

Results: The weight gain of the mice was enhanced by both $ZnSO_4$ and Zn-Met. The both forms of zinc had no effect on the concentration of plasma GH and the expression of GHR mRNA, but they up-regulated the expression of IGF-I mRNA. As compared to $ZnSO_4$, Zn-Met enhanced the weight gain and the level of IGF-I mRNA significantly.

[1] Corresponding author; Fax: +86-510-5869236; E-mail: lgw@sytu.edu.cn.YU Ze-peng, currently works for Anui Agriculture University, P. R. China; E-mail: yuzepeng@mail.hf.ah.cn.

Both $ZnSO_4$ and Zn-Met significantly decreased the expression of ZnT1 mRNA, ZnT4 mRNA and DCT1 mRNA in intestine, while they significantly increased MT-1 mRNAs expression in liver and intestine. The expressions of ZnT1 and DCT1 mRNAs were down-regulated significantly by Zn-Met as compared to $ZnSO_4$; there were no difference between the two zinc sources on ZnT4 mRNA expression. The MT-1 mRNA expression was up-regulated markedly by Zn-Met comparing to $ZnSO_4$.

Conclusions: Zn-Met could improve the weight gain efficiently by up-regulating the expression of IGF-I mRNA. It was deduced that there might be different transportation ways in organic and inorganic zinc base on their different effects on the expression of ZnTs, DCT1 and MT-1 gene.

Key words: zinc sulfate, zinc methionine, growth, zinc transporter, divalent cation transporter, transportation

1. Introduction

Zinc is an essential ion for cells with a vital role to play in controlling the cellular processes of the cell, such as growth, development and differentiation. It is essential to cell growth and is a cofactor for more than 300 enzymes, representing over 50 different enzyme classes [Urani, C., 2003]. Zinc is involved in protein, nucleic acid, carbohydrate and lipid metabolism, as well as in the control of gene transcription and the coordination of other biological processes controlled by proteins containing DNA-binding zinc finger motifs, RING fingers and LIM domains.

Zinc is an essential trace-element required for growth. Growth retardation is a principal sign of zinc deficiency in humans and animals [Hambidge, K.M., 1986], but the underlying mechanisms remain to be elucidated.

The classic function of growth hormone (GH) is the regulation of the growth and differentiation of various cell types and the control of anabolism and metabolism in organs and tissues. The insulin-like growth factors (IGF-I and IGF-II) are major metabolic and mitogenic factors involved in body growth. The production of IGF-I and IGF-II depends on the actions of GH and insulin. IGF-I produced by the liver and other tissues is considered to be the prime effector of growth hormone actions on growth and development. The ability of IGF-I to stimulate growth in GH-deficient humans and animals has been well documented [Froesch, E. R., 1990; Jones, J. I., 1995].

IGF, as a major downstream target of GH, is essential for regulating growth and body size both prenatally (IGF-I and IGF-II) and postnatally (IGF-I) [Nakae, J., 2001; Efstratiadis, A.,1998; Herington, AC.,1991; Sara, V, 1990; Wang, HS, 1999]. IGF-I stimulates both proliferation and differentiation of target cells [Florini, JR, 1991], whereas IGF-II seems to be primarily involved in the regulation of prenatal growth [Froesch, E.R.,1985] via paracrine, autocrine and endocrine signaling [Lackey, B. R., 1999]. Regulation of plasma IGF-I concentration is mainly through nutrients and hormones and concentrations depend on stage of development [Cohick, W, 1993; Cordanoa, P., 2000].

Extensive studies of mammalian insulin/IGF biology have shown that the insulin/IGF system is split into two complementary and interacting subsystems that govern growth, metabolism, reproduction and longevity [Nakae, J., 2001; Efstratiadis, A, 1998; Saltiel, A.R., 2001]. Insulin, secreted from the pancreatic b cells in response to elevated glucose and amino acid levels, primarily regulates anabolic metabolism in the classical insulin-responsive tissues such as adipose, muscle and liver [Saltiel, A.R., 2001]. Insulin, IGF-I and IGF-II, all possibly act through the insulin receptor (IR) [Nakae, J., 2001].

IGF-I mRNA abundance indicated that IGF-I synthesis takes place in most organs. The liver is considered to be the major source of circulating IGF-I. IGF-I actions are therefore due to locally and hepatically produced IGF-I. Hepatic IGF-I gene expression is modified by GH, insulin and other hormones and is dependent on energy and protein intakes [Lackey, B. R., 1999]. Hepatic GH and insulin effects are mediated by GH and insulin receptors (GHR and IR, respectively). Plasmatic IGF-I circulates mainly bound to six binding proteins (IGFBPs), which are synthesized by various tissues. IGFBPs modulate the IGF-I activity, whose actions of IGF-I are mainly mediated by the type-1 IGF receptor (IGF-IR).

In order for zinc to have a varied role in cells, and because it is a small hydrophilic charged species, which cannot cross biological membranes by passive diffusion, it has to be transported into the intracellular compartments of a cell where it is required for these zinc-dependent processes. A group of proteins called zinc transporters is dedicated to this transport of zinc across cell membranes [Eide, D., 1997; Reyes, J.G., 1996].

The understanding of mechanisms controlling zinc absorption and metabolism at the molecular level has advanced recently. The accumulation of Zn in the cell is a sum of influx and efflux processes via Zn transporter proteins, like the divalent cation transporter 1 (DCT1) and the zinc transporters, and of storage processes bound to metallothionein (MT) [Bhatnagar, S., 2001; Choi, D.W., 1998; Cousins, R. J., 2000]. Zinc-associated genetic disorders like acrodermatitis enteropathica, familial hypozincemia in humans have been thought possibly due to defects in zinc transport systems.

Kinetics of zinc transport have been investigated for many years, but only recently have genes coding for proteins thought to be involved in the transport process been cloned. Four putative zinc transporters, known as ZnT-1 through ZnT-4, have now been well described [Mcmahon, R. J., 1998].

Among these, ZnT-1, the first zinc transporter to be cloned, localized in mouse and rat at the plasma membrane with six membrane spanning domains, is important for eliminating potentially toxic levels of zinc. Although its expression is not ubiquitous in animal cells, it is believed to be involved in zinc homeostasis [Cousins, R.J., 2000; Langmade, S. J., 2000]. ZnT-4 is believed to be involved in either zinc efflux or compartmentalization and is abundant in mammary epithelia and brain, and is found in lesser amounts in a variety of tissues, such as the liver, heart, and spleen. A nonsense mutation in the ZnT-4 gene is responsible for the condition in mice known as lethal milk, in which decreased zinc transport into the mammary glands of mutant mothers causes zinc deficiency and death in nursing pups. ZnT-1 and ZnT-4 are involved in the efflux of zinc in intestine, kidney tubules, mammary epithelium and synaptic vesicles. ZnT-2 and ZnT-3 have been shown to be involved in the translocation of zinc from the cytosol to endosomal/lysosomal vesicles in the intestine, kidney, testis and brain [Palmiter, R. D., 1995, 1996; Wang, Z. Y., 2003; Lopantsev, V., 2003].

These transporters genes predict putative proteins with multiple membrane spanning domains and all have histidine rich intracellular loop. They are organ specific and are involved in the specialized function of zinc transport [Palmiter, R. D., 1995, 1996; Lopantsev, V., 2003]. However, the mechanism of transport for these transporters is poorly understood, although they show specificity for zinc. None of the known zinc transporters are believed to be responsible for uptake of zinc into cells via its transport across the plasma membrane at present [Clifford, K. S., 2000].

A type of metal ion transporter has been cloned from rat intestine and is termed DCT1 (divalent cation transporter) [Gunshin, H., 1997]. This transporter is quite different from the ZnT family and is highly expressed in the proximal duodenum, kidney, thymus, and brain. It is a much larger protein with 12 putative membrane spanning domains. It has an unusually broad substrate range that includes Fe^{2+}, Zn^{2+}, Mn^{2+}, Co^{2+}, Cd^{2+}, Cu^{2+}, Ni^{2+} and Pb^{2+}. So, DCT1 was proposed to act as a common entry pathway for a number of divalent metals including zinc [Yamaji, S., 2001]. Recent cloning strategies have greatly improved our knowledge concerning the mechanisms by which iron crosses the intestinal barrier from the diet into the blood. At the apical membrane, the divalent metal transporter DCT1 takes iron into enterocytes via a pH-dependent mechanism. The situation for zinc, however, is not so clear.

Some studies showed that DCT1 is predominantly an iron transporter, with lower affinity for other metals. Several studies have shown that increasing dietary iron down-regulates DCT1. Interestingly, some studies indicated that zinc up-regulates DCT1 protein and mRNA expression [Yamaji, S., 2001].

Zinc is a component of hormones and part of the active site of numerous metalloenzymes, especially metallothionein, which acts as an intracellular pool of zinc. Excess zinc can also be toxic to cells and aberrant levels of zinc have been linked to various disease states thereby making it vital that the level of intracellular zinc is tightly controlled. MTs are ubiquitous in eukaryotes and highly conserved, cysteine-rich, low molecular weight proteins; they have unique structural characteristics that give potent metal-binding. The most widely expressed in mammals, MT is rapidly induced in the liver by a wide range of metals, drugs and inflammatory mediators. Although MT is thought to play a crucial role in the metabolism, transport, homeostasis and toxicity or detoxication of certain metals, an unequivocally established function is still lacking [Davis, S. R., 2000; Coyle, P., 2002]. The relationship between recently-cloned mammalian zinc transporters and previously measured zinc fluxes in intact animal zinc homeostasis is unclear at present.

Zinc is an essential element that serves structural and catalytic roles in enzymes and transcription factors [Lipscomb, W. L., 1996]. The enzyme activity and gene expression of proteins influenced by zinc affect reproduction, growth, milk production and the immune system of the animals [Chesters, J. K., 1997]. Zinc may affect these physiological functions by its influence on feed intake, mitogenic hormones, signal transduction, gene transcription and RNA synthesis [MacDonald, R.S., 2000].

Zinc sources of greater bioavailability or high dietary levels of zinc [Kincaid, R. L., 1976, 1997] can improve the growth of animal and increase the concentration of zinc in tissues. Zinc methionine (Zn-Met) has been shown to have greater bioavailability than traditional zinc sources in some situations [Wedekind, K.J., 1992; Cao, J., 2000]. The aim of our study was to evaluate the effect of zinc sulfate and zinc methionine on growth, plasma GH concentration, and the expression of GHR, IGF-I mRNAs in weanling mice. In this report we also investigated the regulation of the expression of ZnT-1, ZnT-4, DCT1 and MT-1 mRNAs in rat intestine and/or liver by dietary zinc, the goal was to provide much needed new information on the mechanism of zinc ion influx and efflux across the small intestine and the regulation mechanism.

2. Material and Methods

2.1. Animal and Diets

Ninety male KM weanling mice of 21d old were purchased and assigned by weight to 3 treatments with 30 mice each. Mice in the control were fed on a semi-purified basal diet containing 11.67mg/kg zinc, described in table 1. Mice treated with $ZnSO_4$ and Zn-Met were fed on one of two additional diets prepared by adding 30mg/kg of $ZnSO_4$ ($ZnSO_4 \cdot 7H_2O$, AR) or Zn-Met (prepared by our lab with Microwave Method, Patent No.:01138045.4; purity: 97.5%). Test diets of treatments $ZnSO_4$ and Zn-Met contained 40.05, 40.75mg/kg of zinc respectively (measured by atomic absorption spectrophotometry). All mice had free access to food and deionized water. Test diets were offered to the mice for ten days according to our previous works. Body weights were measured at the beginning and the end of the experiment.

Table 1. Composition of basal diet.

Ingredient	Ratio
Corn starch	63
Casein	20
Corn oil	8
Cellulose	3
Minerals mixture	5
Vitamins mixture	1

1. Minerals mixture (g/kg): $CaHPO_4$ 500, NaCl 74, $K_3C_6H_5O_7 \cdot 12H_2O$ 220, K_2SO_4 52, $MnCO_3$ 3.5, K_2SO_4 52, KIO_3 0.3, $Na_2SeO_3 \cdot 5H_2O$ 0.01, $CrK(SO_4)_2 \cdot 12H_2O$ 0.55, $CuCO_3$ 0.3, Ferric Ditrate 15-16, can sugar to 1000g.
2. Vitamins mixture (per kg): VA 400000IU, VD_3 100000IU, VE 5000IU, VB_1 600mg, VB_2 600mg, VB_6 700mg, Folic acid 200mg, D-Biotin 20mg, Niacin 3g, VB_3 1.6g, VK 5mg , can sugar to 1000g.

2.2. Blood and Tissue Sampling

Blood samples were taken before animals were slaughtered. Tubes containing heparin sodium were used to collect blood for the determination of plasma GH concentrations. Blood samples were centrifuged at 1000g for 20 min; the supernatants (serum or plasma) were stored at –80°C until analyzed. Liver and intestine samples were taken immediately after slaughter from the right large lobe, frozen in liquid nitrogen, and then stored at –80°C until analyzed.

Zinc concentrations in all samples were measured by atomic absorption spectrophotometry (SpectrAA220, VARIAN, America). Approximately 0.5g of each tissue and debris pellet was digested with nitric acid (80%) and perchloric acid (20%).

Serum GH concentrations were determined using a double-antibody radioimmunoassay (RIA); the iodine labeled (I^{125}) GH concentration detection kit was bought from Beijing Northern Biotechnology Research Institute.

Serum alkaline phosphatase (AKP) activity was measured with AKP activity detection kit (bought from Nanjing Jiancheng Biotechnology Research Institute).

2.3. Semi-Quantitive RT-PCR

2.3.1. Genes and Primers

The sequences of GHR, IGF-I, ZnT1, ZnT4, DCT1, MT-1 and beta actin mRNAs were obtained from NCBI; the primers were designed with Oligo 6.67, the results were shown in table 2.

Table 2. Information of genes and primers.

Gene		Primer	Size of Product
β-actin	Forward	5'CTGGCACCACACCTTCTACAAT3'	635 bp
	Reverse	5'TGTTGGCATAGAGGTCTTTACGG3'	
GHR	Forward	5' AGGGAAAGCCAACGACAAG3'	498bp
	Reverse	5' GACTTCGCTGAACTCGCTGTA3'	
IGF-I	Forward	5'GCTCTTCAGTTCGTGTGTGG3'	212bp
	Reverse	5'TTGGGCATGTCAGTGTGG3'	
ZnT-1	Forward	5'CTGACAATCTGGAAGCGGAAGAC3'	476bp
	Reverse	5'TATGTGGGCAGTGGCGATGAT3'	
ZnT-4	Forward	5'AATGACACCAGCGCCTTCGACT3'	590bp
	Reverse	5'ATGAGCATGACATCGCCGTTT3'	
DCT1	Forward	5' AGG TGT CTC CAG TCT CTA CC 3'	201bp
	Reverse	5' GATCCTTGA ACTTACTGGCTG 3'	
MT-1	Forward	5'AGTACCTTCTCCTCACTTA3'	306bp
	Reverse	5'TGGAACTGTATAGGAAGACG3'	

2.3.2. Isolation of RNA

Total RNA of the liver was extracted using Trizol™ Reagent (Gibco, BRL) according to the manufacturer's instructions. RNA was resuspended in ribonuclease (RNase)-free water, treated with diethylpyrocarbonate (DEPC, Sigma). The amount of total RNA was measured spectrophotometrically at 260 nm.

2.3.3. Synthesis of cDNA

Ten micrograms of the total RNA added with 2μl 0.5μg/μl Oligo d(T)16mer was incubated at 70°C for 5min; then added with 5×RT buffer 5μl, dNTPs (10mmol each) 1μl, M-MLV reverse transcriptase 300U, RNasin 0.5μl; incubated at 42°C for 65min; and then, at 95°C for 5min to denature the enzyme. The cDNA samples were kept at -20°C.

2.3.4. Polymerase Chain Reaction (PCR)

A reaction volume of 50μl contained 2.5U AmpliTaq of DNA polymerase, 10×PCR buffer, 1μM of each particular oligonucleotide of primer and 2μl of cDNA. The samples were denatured for 5 min at 94°C and subjected to 26-30 cycles of amplification in automated Thermal Cycler. The cycling conditions were as follows, 30-second denaturation at 94°C, 40-second anneal at 57°C, 1-min prolongation at 72°C and final 8 min step at 72°C. The reaction was performed in DNA Thermal Cycler (Hybaid, UK).

2.3.5. Semi-Quantization of GHR And IGF-I mRNA Abundance

The RT-PCR products were analyzed by electrophoresis on 1.5% agarose gel; the amounts of the products amplified by RT-PCR were quantified by comparing to the relative intensities of the amplified beta actin using a Gel-Pro 4.5 imaging analyzer.

2.4. Statistic Analysis

Results were presented as mean ± S.D. and the data had been analyzed with SAS 8.1 using analysis of variance (ANOVA) and Dancan's multiple rang test. A value of $P<0.05$ was considered statistically significant.

3. Results

3.1. Effect of Different Forms of Zinc on Weight Gain, Zinc Contents in Tissues and Serum AKP Activity

Weight gains of mice treated $ZnSO_4$ and Zn-Met were higher than the control ($P<0.05$ for Zn-Met; shown in Table 3.). This indicated that both forms of zinc could improve the growth of mice; Zn-Met did more efficiently than $ZnSO_4$ ($P<0.05$). Zinc supplementing markedly enhanced the food intake of mice ($P<0.05$); the food intake of mice treated with Zn-Met was significantly higher than those treated with $ZnSO_4$ ($P<0.05$). As compared to the control, both $ZnSO_4$ and Zn-Met enhanced zinc content in liver and serum obviously ($P<0.05$ for Zn-Met). Zinc contents in liver and serum of mice treated with Zn-Met were higher than those treated with $ZnSO_4$.

Activity of AKP in group $ZnSO_4$ and Zn-Met was markedly higher than the control ($P<0.05$); it did not differ between the two zinc sources ($P>0.05$). This means zinc deficiency reduced the activity of AKP.

Table 3. Effect of different forms of zinc on growth and biological index of the mice

Treatment	Weight Gain (g)	Total Food Intake (g)	Liver zinc content (mg/kg)	Serum zinc content (μg/ml)	AKP activity (u/ml)
Control	10.86±1.26[B]	31.53±2.10[C]	24.69±1.17[B]	1.46±0.38[B]	5.44±0.76[B]
ZnSO4	11.99±1.00[B]	33.68±2.31[B]	26.15±0.68[AB]	1.86±0.24[AB]	6.35±0.71[A]
Zn-Met	15.21±1.45[A]	37.13±1.94[A]	27.75±1.23[A]	1.96±0.24[A]	6.26±0.55[A]

Values in the same column not sharing common superscript small letter were significantly different from Zn-Met at $P<0.05$. Values are means± S.D

3.2. Effect of Different Forms of Zinc on Plasma GH Concentration of Mice

Plasma GH concentration did not differ among the three treatments ($P>0.05$; Table 4). Zinc supplementing tended to enhance the GH concentration slightly. There was no significant difference between the two treatments of ZnSO4 and Zn-Met.

Table 4. Effect of different forms of zinc on plasma GH concentration

Treatment	GH (ng/ml)
Control	2.62±0.94 A
ZnSO4	2.79±1.20 A
Zn-Met	2.83±0.74 A

Values in the same column sharing common superscript small letter showed no significant difference among the treatments ($P>0.05$). Values are means± S.D.

3.3. Effect of Different Forms of Zinc on the Expression of GHR mRNA

There was no significant difference among the three treatments ($P>0.05$; shown in figure 1); this indicated that zinc supplementing had no effect on GHR gene expression. The parallelism of the amplification between the target and beta actin was tested during the exponential and the plateau phase of the PCR. The same PCR reaction on cDNA was run in seven separated tubes, and one tube after the other was taken away from the PCR machine after 24, 26, 28, 30, 32, 34, and 36 cycles. The RT-PCR products were then quantified in a 1.5% agarose gel. Between cycle number 26 to 30 there was an exponential increase in the amount of both products (target and beta actin), followed by the plateau phase.

3.4. Effect of Different Forms of Zinc on the Expression IGF-I mRNA

As compared to the control, $ZnSO_4$ and Zn-Met enhanced the abundance of IGF-I mRNA significantly (P<0.05; shown in figure 2). The effect of Zn-Met was markedly different from $ZnSO_4$ (P<0.05).

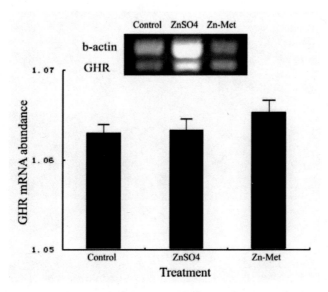

Figure 1. GHR mRNA abundance The RT-PCR products of GHR were analyzed by electrophoresis on 1.5% agarose gel, and stained with ethidium bromide. There was no significant difference among the three treatments (P>0.05).

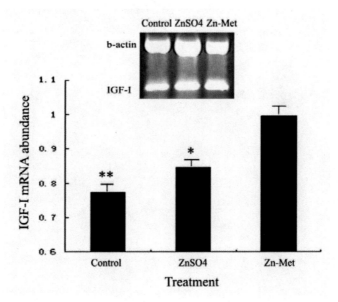

Figure 2. IGF-I mRNA abundance. The RT-PCR products of IGF-I were analyzed by electrophoresis on 1.5% agarose gel, and stained with ethidium bromide. As compared to the control, ZnSO4 and Zn-Met enhanced the abundance of IGF-I mRNA significantly (P<0.05). The effect of Zn-Met was markedly different from ZnSO4 (P<0.05).

3.5. Effect of Different Forms of Zinc on the Expression of ZnT-1 And ZnT-4 mRNAs

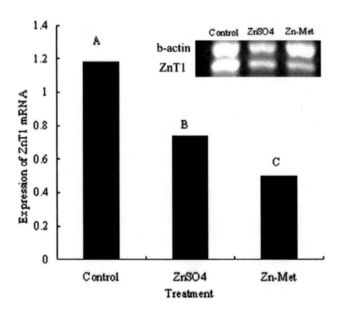

Figure 3. ZnT-1 mRNA abundance.The RT-PCR products of ZnT-1 were analyzed by electrophoresis on 1.5% agarose gel, and stained with ethidium bromide. ZnSO4 and Zn-Met decreased the expression of ZnT-1 mRNA by 37.68%, 57.98% respectively as compared to the control. Zn-Met decreased the level of mRNA more efficiently than ZnSO4. Values not sharing common capital letter were significantly different at $P<0.05$.

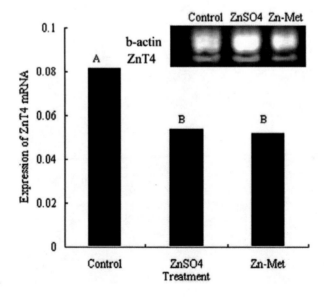

Figure 4. ZnT-4 mRNA abundance.The RT-PCR products of ZnT-4 were analyzed by electrophoresis on 1.5% agarose gel, and stained with ethidium bromide. Both ZnSO4 and Zn-Me decreased the expression of ZnT4 mRNA comparing to the control. There was no significant difference between ZnSO4 and Zn-Met. Values not sharing common capital letter were significantly different at $P<0.05$.

The expression of ZnT-1 mRNA differed among the three treatments ($P<0.05$, shown in figure 3); $ZnSO_4$ and Zn-Met decreased the level of ZnT-1 mRNA expression by 37.68%, 57.98% respectively. Zn-Met decreased the level of mRNA expression more efficiently as compared to $ZnSO_4$ ($P<0.05$).

The expression of ZnT-4 mRNA in the control was markedly higher than those supplemented with ZnSO4 or Zn-Met ($P<0.05$, shown in figure 4), $ZnSO_4$ and Zn-Met decreased the level of mRNA expression by 33.96%, 36.12% respectively ($P<0.05$) comparing to the control. There was no significant difference between $ZnSO_4$ and Zn-Met ($P>0.05$).

3.6. Effect of Different Forms of Zinc on the Expression of DCT1 mRNA

$ZnSO_4$ and Zn-Met decreased the expression of DCT-1 mRNA significantly ($P<0.05$, shown in figure 5), Zn-Met inhibited the expression more efficiently than $ZnSO_4$ ($P<0.05$).

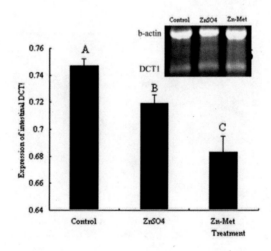

Figure 5. DCT1 mRNA abundance. The RT-PCR products of DCT1 were analyzed by electrophoresis on 1.5% agarose gel, and stained with ethidium bromide. ZnSO4 and Zn-Met decreased the expression of DCT-1 mRNA significantly; Zn-Met inhibited the expression more efficiently than ZnSO4. Values not sharing common capital letter were significantly different at P<0.05.

3.7. Effect of Different Forms of Zinc on the Expression of MT-1 mRNA

Zinc supplementation increased intestine and liver MT-1 expression markedly ($P<0.05$, shown in figure 6 and 7). $ZnSO_4$ and Zn-Met increased the level of MT-1 mRNA by 29.74%, 45.48% respectively in the intestine while they were 66.77% and 268.89% in the liver. The expression of MT-1 mRNA in both intestine and liver of mice treated with Zn-Met was higher than those treated with $ZnSO_4$ ($P<0.05$).

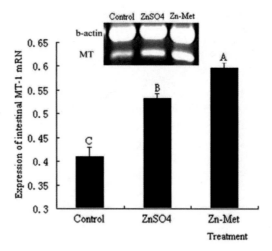

Figure 6. Intestine MT-1 mRNA abundance.The RT-PCR products of MT-1 were analyzed by electrophoresis on 1.5% agarose gel, and stained with ethidium bromide. Zinc supplementation increased intestine MT-1 expression markedly. The expression of MT-1 mRNA treated with Zn-Met was higher than those treated with ZnSO4. Values not sharing common capital letter were significantly different at P<0.05.

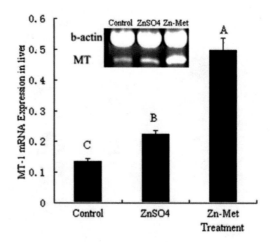

Figure 7. Liver MT-1 mRNA abundance.The RT-PCR products of MT-1 were analyzed by electrophoresis on 1.5% agarose gel, and stained with ethidium bromide. Zinc supplementation increased liver MT-1 expression significantly. The expression of MT-1 mRNA in liver of mice treated with Zn-Met was higher than those treated with ZnSO4.Values not sharing common capital letter were significantly different at P<0.05.

4. Discussion

4.1. Effect of Different Forms of Zinc on Growth, Tissue Zinc Contents and Activity of Serum AKP

In our present experiment, the basal diet containing 11.67mg/kg zinc retarded the growth of mice; zinc supplementing with ZnSO$_4$ and Zn-Met containing 40.05, 40.75 mg/kg of zinc respectively which were equal to commercially diet, improved growth retard, enhanced food intake, and increased zinc contents in tissues and the activity of serum AKP.

Slow growth is dominant feature in zinc deficient animals. Studies showed that growth ceases and anorexia develops after feeding a low zinc diets containing less than 1mg/kg zinc for a few days (less than one week) in young rats [Chesters, J. K., 1970, 1997]. Zinc content in the control diet in present experiment was somewhat higher than other studies which used the diets contained zinc ranging from 0 to 5mg/kg; but the same conclusion could still be drawn.

Reduction in growth is correlated with cell proliferation and DNA synthesis in zinc deficient animals. Zinc plays an important role in growth; two mechanisms could be responsible for the dramatic effects of zinc deficiency on growth. One possibility is that zinc itself is not available for the normal cellular activity. It has a recognized action of zinc on more than 300 enzymes by participating in their structure or in their catalytic and regulatory actions, such as thymidine kinase and DNA polymerases, which are essential for cell proliferation. It is also a structural ion of biological membranes and closely related to protein synthesis. Furthermore, zinc finger transcription factors such as Gli proteins, TFIIIA, retinoic acid receptors, vitamin D receptors all require zinc for maintaining three-dimension structure [Campbell, G. L., 2000].

Increasing evidence shows that labile intracellular zinc is metabolically important. Depletion of labile intracellular zinc using chelators suppresses DNA synthesis. Labile intracellular zinc could be modulated *via* varying zinc nutrition. 3T3 cells are the most frequently used model for understanding the influence of zinc on growth. When 3T3 cells was cultured in zinc-depleted medium using diethylenetrinitrilopenta acetate (DTPA), an extracellular divalent cation chelator, labile intracellular zinc was diminished along with a suppressed DNA synthesis and cell proliferation. In contrast, supplementation of zinc to the medium increased the labile intracellular zinc and promoted DNA synthesis and cell proliferation [Vanhaesebroeck, B., 2001]. Furthermore, growth factor-dependent stimulation of DNA synthesis and cell proliferation was also accompanied by increased labile intracellular zinc. These suggested that labile intracellular zinc could be an important cellular link between zinc nutrition and growth [Paski, S. C., 2001].

It is interesting to note that while DNA synthesis was suppressed by DTPA, total cell zinc concentration determined using atomic absorption spectrophotometer, remained unchanged [Vanhaesebroeck, B.2001]. There are some other studies indicated that, in rats, severe zinc deficiency retards growth while tissue zinc concentration often remains unaffected [Hammermueller, J. D., 1987; Taylor, C. G., 1988]. Therefore, it is possible that the effect of zinc deprivation, whether induced by dietary zinc deficiency or by chelators, on growth are mediated *via* a change in intracellular zinc and this change is too small to be detected by conventional determination of total zinc concentration [MacDonald, R. S., 1998].

In our present experiment, Zn-Met showed more effectively than $ZnSO_4$ in promoting the growth of mice. Zn-Met has been shown to have greater bioavailability, such as higher absorption rate in animal intestine, than traditional zinc sources [Wedekind, K.J., 1992; Cao, J., 2000]. Wedekind (1992) reported that the bioavailability of zinc from zinc methionine (Zn-Met) in poultry was greater than that of zinc sulfate and the difference in bioavailability increased as complexity of the diet increased. The bioavailability of Zn-Met relative to that of zinc sulfate was 117% in a crystalline amino acid purified diet and 206% in a complex corn-soybean diet [Wedekind, K.J., 1992]. Spears (1989) found that zinc from Zn-Met and zinc oxide were absorbed similarly in lambs, but that zinc retention was higher in animals fed on Zn-Met. He interpreted this to indicate that zinc from the two sources was utilized differently after absorption [Spears, J. W., 1989]. However, the metabolic pathway of Zn-Met is not clear at present.

AKP is a zinc-containing enzyme, zinc is essential to maintain its activity. Zinc deficiency reduced its activity significantly in present study; there was no significant difference between Zn-Met and $ZnSO_4$. This may mainly due to the both forms of zinc provided sufficient zinc for the enzyme to maintain its normal activity in the body.

4.2. Effect of Different Forms of Zinc on Plasma GH Concentration and GHR, IGF-I mRNA Abundance

An alternative mechanism could be responsible for the effect of zinc on the growth of mice is that zinc deficiency could indirectly affect the growth through changing hormones or peptide growth factors.

Our present study showed that zinc supplementing had no obvious effect on plasma GH concentration and the expression of GHR mRNA, but enhanced IGF-I gene expression significantly. Some other studies using primary culture of rat hepatocytes and culture of rat pituitary tumor cells have showed that zinc deficiency reduced serum GH and IGF-I levels [Lefebvre, D., 1998; Sciaudone, M. P., 2000]. The latter was associated with decreased IGF-I expression in liver. These findings raised the possibility that zinc deficiency affects growth through the GH-IGF axis [Browning, J. D., 1998].

Growth hormone (GH) production is stimulated and inhibited by the hypothalamic hormone, growth hormone releasing hormone and somatostatin, respectively. GH stimulates somatostatin synthesis and secretion by the periventricular nucleus [Lackey, B. R., 1999]. GH exerts pleiotrophic action on many biological systems, including the reproductive and immune. GH increases hepatic production of IGF-I and IGFBP-3 and also acts at other tissues to stimulate autocrine/paracrine release of IGF. It acts as a primary stimulator of IGF. However, GH and IGF concentrations are not always correlated [Lackey, B. R., 1999]. In addition, infusion of GH and IGF-I could not reverse the effects of zinc deficiency [Campbell, G. L., 2000; Browning, J. D., 1998]. Thus, the changes in circulating GH and IGF-I may not be fully responsible for the defects of the zinc deficient state.

IGFs are polypeptides that regulate growth, differentiation and survival in a multitude of cells and tissues. It is an important growth factor which mediates most of the postnatal. Growth-promoting actions of GH, insulin and nutrition are the main regulators of circulating IGF-I [Mathews, L. S., 1986; Thissen, J. P., 1994]. The impaired growth induced by zinc deficiency in rats is associated with reduced plasma IGF-I, hepatic GHR and serum GH binding protein (GHBP) levels, together with a decrease of their hepatic mRNAs [Ninh, N. X., 1995]. GH infusion in zinc deficient rats normalized liver GHR but failed to restore normal plasma IGF-I and growth [Ninh, N. X., 1998]. These results suggested that zinc deficiency causes GH resistance at a post-receptor level. Our present study approved both

$ZnSO_4$ and Zn-Met modulated the growth of mice at the downstream of GHR via GH-IGF axis.

Despite the variations of IGF-I gene expression induced by zinc supplementation, our results showed that neither $ZnSO_4$ nor Zn-Met supplementation affected plasma GH concentration and the expression of GHR. These observations suggested that the transduction pathways stimulated IGF-I gene transcription are affected by zinc availability. In our experiment, zinc deficiency induced a state of GH insensitivity. It is therefore possible that more chronic zinc deficiency or lower zinc level is required to alter the GH and GHR mRNA expression. In present experiment, the basal diet contained 11.67mg/kg zinc; it was perhaps enough for GH to be synthesized and secreted in the body under this condition.

The mechanisms by which zinc regulates IGF-I gene expression are still unknown. One can postulate the existence of direct mechanisms such as those occurring for the metallothionein gene by which extracellular zinc availability is directly responsible for the gene regulation [Dunn, M. A., 1987]. But some studies showed that, exposition of cells to the zinc chelator DTPA did not decrease IGF-I while zinc excess decreased IGF-I and GHR mRNAs. However, the response of IGF-I to GH was not affected by the exposure to DTPA nor zinc excess. Furthermore, zinc repletion of primary cultured hepatocytes isolated from zinc-deprived rats did not increase IGF-I nor GHR mRNAs. Therefore, the IGF-I decline induced in vivo by zinc deficiency might be not caused by reduced extracellular zinc availability at the hepatocyte level [Lefebvre, D., 1998].

Alternatively, indirect mechanisms such as hormonal or metabolic alterations secondary to zinc depletion could also contribute to the impaired IGF-I gene expression. Insulin/IGF pathway Mammalian insulin/IGF signaling oversees cellular growth, proliferation, metabolism and survival. The IR and the IGF receptor (IGFR) are receptor tyrosine kinases that become activated upon insulin and IGF binding, respectively [Ullrich, A., 1990]. The multi-site tyrosine auto-phosphorylation of the IR and IGFR subsequently recruits the insulin receptor substrate (IRS) adaptor proteins [Vanhaesebroeck, B., 2001; White, M. F., 1998]. However, the understanding of how the insulin/IGF system regulates, coordinates, and integrates these processes remains at a rudimentary stage.

In our present study, Zn-Met enhanced the level of IGF-I mRNA expression more effectively than $ZnSO_4$ did; these may partly interpret why Zn-Met improved the growth in mice. However, the metabolic pathway of Zn-Met is unclear at present. Furthermore, the mechanism of the two forms of zinc modulating the IGF-I mRNA expression is still unknown.

4.3. Effect of Different Zinc Sources on the Expression of ZnT-1 and ZnT-4 mRNA

As a highly charged, hydrophilic ion, it cannot cross biological membranes by simple diffusion, and specialized mechanisms therefore must exist for its cellular uptake and release. Zinc absorption has been studied extensively in several model systems, particularly perfused intestinal segments and isolated intestinal cells. It has been characterized in many cell types, including fibroblasts, hepatocytes, placental trophoblasts, and endothelial cells. Several characteristics of zinc transport can be deduced from these studies. Zinc transport is a time-, concentration-, pH-, and temperature-dependent process, although there appear to be both saturable and nonsaturable components [Rajinder Kumar, 2000].

In present study on the regulation of ZnT-1 and ZnT-4 in intact animals under varying dietary zinc conditions, the results are important in light of previous ZnT-1 and ZnT-4 studies that were performed in a cell culture model under over-expressing conditions and the paucity of data concerning integrative aspects of ZnT-1 and ZnT-4 expression. ZnT-1 and ZnT-4 mRNAs in the intestine is up-regulated significantly by zinc deficiency in present study. The result of present experiment was consistent with previous study, in which, ZnT-1 showed a significant up-regulation of mRNA expression in colon while ZnT-4 showed up-regulation in both jejunum and colon [Pfaffl, M. W., 2003].

Intestinal ZnT-1 was localized at the basolateral surface of the enterocyte in the upper portion of the villus in the duodenum and jejunum. At the basolateral surface of intestinal enterocytes, efflux of absorbed zinc is thought to be mediated by ZnT-1. Studies suggested that ZnT-1 was a zinc exporter localized at the plasma membrane and was important for eliminating excess, and therefore potentially toxic, levels of zinc [Yamaji, S., 2001]. This places the zinc exporter at an anatomical site and cellular orientation compatible with delivery of dietary zinc to the circulation. Intestinal ZnT-1 is fulfilling a function related to zinc acquisition and/or processing. In this way, ZnT-1 could contribute to overall zinc homeostasis.

Present study demonstrated the relevant physiological regulation of ZnT-1 and ZnT-4 expression by dietary zinc. Although the ZnT-1 gene is zinc-responsive, there are probably compensatory cellular factors that mitigate the magnitude of protein up-regulation. When faced with a deficient or a large excess of intestinal zinc, ZnT-1 is up-regulated. Alternative post-translational processes, such as differences in targeting and protein turnover, may also play a role in modulating the amount of transporter that is functionally able to contribute to zinc export. When the rats were fed diets of various zinc levels, supplementation, but not depletion, could moderately elevate the level of ZnT-1 mRNA in the intestine. The rather modest regulation of ZnT-1 could be explained either because other compensatory factors are limiting the up-regulation of ZnT-1. Taken together, the data are consistent with the notion that the role of ZnT-1 and ZnT-4 is to act as a mechanism for both zinc acquisition and zinc elimination, and thus functions as a component of the zinc homeostatic mechanism [R. J. Mcmahon, 1998].

4.4. Effect of Different Zinc Sources on the Expression of DCT1 mRNA

The regulation of zinc uptake, accumulation and general intracellular homeostasis are necessary to assure an adequate metal supply and to avoid toxicity due to overexposure [Urani, C., 2003].

DCT1 is a metal transporter with affinity to iron, zinc and other cations, that function as a cellular importer for metal uptake and is located at the basolateral membrane in many organs, e.g. duodenum, jejunum, kidney and bone marrow. DCT1 is mainly regulated by the tissue iron concentration. Despite the solid work describing the kinetics and characteristics of zinc transporter, no protein directly associated with the zinc transport was described until recently [Pfaffl, M. W., 2003].

In present experiment, the expression of DCT-1 mRNA was increased by zinc deficiency. Some other studies showed that, the expression of DCT-1 mRNA in jejunum was enhanced by zinc deficiency too [Pfaffl, M. W., 2003]. DCT-1 has been shown to have a key role in the intestinal absorption of zinc; the increment of DCT-1 by zinc deficiency could improve the absorption of zinc from intestine. DCT-1 mediates active transport that is proton coupled and depends on the cell membrane potential. However, some evidences suggested that zinc was not a major substrate for DCT1, and thus the apical membrane transport system for zinc remains elusive [Yamaji, S., 2001].

4.5. Effect of Different Zinc Sources on the Expression of MT-1 mRNA

Zinc homeostasis regulates zinc concentration in cells and tissues quite efficient and prevents the organism from excessive accumulation over a wide range of dietary zinc intake. Therefore, zinc is virtually non-toxic to the living organisms. MT has a high zinc binding capacity, it is one of the strongest biological binding ligands for zinc and regulates the intracellular levels of free zinc through intracellular zinc n concentration and the close correlation between zinc and MT in tissues such as liver and pancreas is well documented [Pfaffl, M. W., 2003].

In present experiment, both intestine and liver MT mRNA was increased by zinc supplementation. It was reported that MT was down-regulated by zinc deficiency in all tissues, massively in liver and in colon and in tendency also in the jejunum and kidney. In parallel with intracellular zinc status it is a potent candidate gene for zinc deficiency [Pfaffl, M. W., 2003].

The molecular mechanism which increases MT is through the binding of the metal transcription factor (MTF-1) to the metal responsive elements (MREs) in the MT promoter region. The activation of MTF-1 by zinc was recently emphasized [Andrews, G. K., 2000]. Thus, among the proposed functions of MT (e.g. free radical scavenger, immune response, transport and storage of metals) [Nordberg, M., 1998], their role in homeostasis and protection against metal toxicity seems predominant [Klaassen, C. D., 1999]. MTF-1 was suggested as a zinc sensor, and to directly bind to zinc with its zinc finger domain, and to bind to MREs in the promoter of zinc homeostasis gene including MT and ZnT [Giedroc, D. P., 2001; Koizumi, S., 1999]. The DNA binding activity of MTF-1 is activated by zinc [Smirnova, I. V., 2000]. Metal-induced phosphorylation of MTF-1 was suggested as the mechanism for increasing MTF-1 activity [LaRochelle, O., 2001]. In addition to regulation of MT gene, Langmade et al. reported that MTF-1 is required for regulation of the mouse ZnT-1 gene [Langsmade, S. J., 2000].

A recent study on zinc uptake into the BBMV prepared from rat renal cortex has revealed the presence of extravesicular as well as intravesicular zinc binding sites. A 40 kDa major zinc binding protein has been purified from renal BBM and physicochemically characterized. Immuno-fluorescence staining localized the protein mainly in proximal tubules indicating its role in the zinc transport. However, the functional characteristics of this protein were yet to be investigated [Rajinder Kumar, 2000].

4.6. Transport and Regulation of Different Forms of Zinc

In present experiment, Zn-Met decreased the level of ZnT-1 and DCT1 mRNAs more efficiently than $ZnSO_4$. The expression of MT-1 mRNA in both intestine and liver of mice treated with Zn-Met was higher than those treated with $ZnSO_4$. We deduced that, the mice could get more zinc from Zn-Met than $ZnSO_4$. Studies showed that uptake of zinc from zinc chelated with citrate was as rapid as from free zinc ions; however, the cells did not take up zinc chelated with EDTA. The cellular uptake of zinc is not dependent upon an available pool of free Zn ions. Instead, the mechanism of transport appears to involve the transport of zinc from low molecular weight ligands that exist in circulation as relatively loosely bound complexes with zinc [Franklin, R. B., 2003]. Based on the effects of the two forms used in present experiment on the expression of ZnTs, DCT1 and MT-1 genes, there might be different transport and regulation ways in $ZnSO_4$ and Zn-Met.

References

Andrews, G. K. Regulation of metallothionein gene expression by oxidative stress and metal ions. *Biochemic al Pharmacology.* 2000, 59: 95–104.

Bhatnagar, S., Taneja, S. Zinc and cognitive development. *Br. J. Nutr.* 2001, 85 (Suppl. 2): S139–45.

Browning, J. D., MacDonal, R. S, Thornton, W. H. Jr, et al. Reduced food intake in zinc deficient rats is normalized by megestrol acetate but not by insulin-like growth factor-1. *J.Nutr.* 1998; 128:136-42.

Campbell, G. L., and Tomlinson, A. Transcriptional regulation of the hedgehog effector C1 by the zinc-finger gene combgap. *Development.* 2000; 127: 4095-103.

Cao, J., Henry, P. R., Guo, R., et al. Chemical characteristics and relative bioavailability of supplemental organic zinc sources for poultry and ruminants. *J. Anim. Sci.* 2000; 78:2039-54.

Chester, J. K., and Quaterman, J. Effects of zinc deficiency on food intake and feeding pattern of rats. *Br. J. Nutr.* 1970; 24:1061-9.

Chesters, J. K. Zinc. In: O'Dell, B. S., and Sunde, R. A. (Eds.), Handbook of Nutritionally Essential Mineral Elements. Marcel Dekker, New York, 1997. pp. 185-230.

Choi, D.W., and Koh, J.Y. Zinc and brain injury. *Annu. Rev. Neurosci.* 1998, 21: 347–75.

Clifford, K. S., and MacDonald, M. J. Survey of mRNAs encoding zinc transporters and other metal complexing proteins in pancreatic islets of rats from birth to adulthood: similar patterns in the Sprague–Dawley and Wistar BB strains. *Diabetes Research and Clinical Practice.* 2000, 49: 77–85.

Cohick, W, and Clemmons, D. The insulin-like growth factors. *Annu Rev Physiol.* 1993; 55:131–53.

Cordanoa, P., Hammona, H. M., Morela, C., et al. mRNA of insulin-like growth factor (IGF) quantification and presence of IGF binding proteins, and receptors for growth hormone, IGF-I and insulin, determined by reverse transcribed polymerase chain reaction, in the liver of growing and mature male cattle. *Domestic Animal Endocrinology.* 2000; 19: 191–208.

Cousins, R. J., and McMahon, R. J. Integrative aspects of zinc transporters. *J. Nutr.* 2000, 130: 1384s–7s.

Coyle, P., Philcox, J. C., Carey, L. C., et al. Metallothionein: the multipurpose protein. *Cellular and Molecular Life Sciences.* 2002, 59: 627–47.

D. Eide. Molecular biology of iron and zinc uptake in eukaryotes. *Curr. Opin. Cell Biol.* 1997, 9: 573–7.

Davis, S. R., and Cousins, R. J. Metallothionein expression in animals: a physiological perspective on function. *Journal of Nutrition.* 2000, 130: 1085–8.

Dunn, M. A., Blalock, T. L., and Cousins, R. J. Metallothionein. *Proc. Soc. Exp. Biol. Med.* 1987; 185, 107–19.

Efstratiadis, A. Genetics of mouse growth. *Int. J. Dev. Biol.* 1998; 42: 955–76.

Florini, JR, Ewton, DZ, and Roof, SL. Insulin-like growth factor-I stimulates terminal myogenic differentiation by induction of myogenin gene expression. *Mol Endocrinol.* 1991; 5:718–24.

Franklin, R.B., Ma, J., Zou, J., et al. Human ZIP1 is a major zinc uptake transporter for the accumulation of zinc in prostate cells. *Journal of Inorganic Biochemistry.* 2003, 96: 435–42.

Froesch, E. R., Schmid, C. H., Schwander, J., and Zapf, J. Actions of insulin-like growth factors. *Ann. Rev. Physiol.* 1990; 47, 443–67.

Froesch, E. R., Schmid, C., Schwander, J., Zapf, J. Actions of insulin-like growth factors. *Annu Rev Physiol.* 1985; 47:443–67.

Giedroc, D. P., Chen, X., and Apuy, J. L. Metal response element (MRE)-binding transcription factor-1 (MTF-1): structure, function, and regulation. *Antioxid. Redox. Signal.* 2001, 3: 597–609.

Gunshin, H., Mackenzie, B., Berger, U. V., et al. Cloning and characterization of a mammalian proton coupled metal ion transporter. *Nature.* 1997, 388: 482–8.

Hambidge, K. M., Casey, C. E., and Krebs, N. F. Zinc, in: Mertz, W. (Ed.), Trace Elements in Human and Animal Nutrition, Academic Press, Orlando, FL, 1986, pp. 1–137.

Hammermueller, J. D., Bray, T. M., and Bettger, W. J. Effect of zinc and copper deficiency on microsomal NADPH-dependent active oxygen generation in rat lung and liver. *J. Nutr.* 1987; 117: 894–901.

Herington AC. Insulin-like growth factors: biochemistry and physiology. In: Robertson DM, Herington AC, editors. Growth factors in endocrinology, Baillie`re's clinical endocrinology and metabolism. *Philadelphia: Baillie`re Tindall.* 1991. pp. 531–51.

Jones, J. I., and Clemmons, D. R. Insulin-like growth factors and their binding proteins: Biological actions. *Endocr. Rev.* 1995; 16: 3–34.

Kincaid, R. L., Chew, B. P., and Cronrath, J. D. Zinc oxide and amino acids as sources of dietary zinc for calves: effects on uptake and immunity. *J. Dairy Sci.* 1997; 80: 1381–8.

Kincaid, R. L., Miller, W. J., Gentry, R. P., et al. Intracellular distribution of zinc and zinc-65 in calves receiving high but non-toxic amounts of zinc. *J. Dairy Sci.* 1976; 59: 552–5.

Klaassen, C. D., Liu, J., and Choudhuri, S. Metallothionein: an intracellular protein to protect against cadmium toxicity. *Annual Review of Pharmacology and Toxicology.* 1999, 39: 267–94.

Koizumi, S., Suzuki, K., Ogura, Y., et al. Transcriptional activity and regulatory protein binding of human metallothionein-IIA gene. *Eur. J. Biochem.* 1999, 259: 635–42.

Kumar, R., and Prasad, R. Functional characterization of purified zinc transporter from renal brush border membrane of rat. *Biochimica et Biophysica Acta.* 2000, 1509: 429-39.

Lackey, B. R., Gray, S. L. and Henricks, D. M. The insulin-like growth factor (IGF) system and gonadotropin regulation: actions and interactions. *Cytokine and Growth Factor Reviews.* 1999; 10: 201–17.

Langmade, S. J., Ravindra, R., Daniels, P. J., et al. The transcription factor MTF-1 mediates metal regulation of the mouse ZnT1 gene. *Journal of Biological Chemistry.* 2000, 275: 34803–9.

LaRochelle, O., Gagne, V., Charron, J., et al. Phosphorylation is involved in the activation of metalregulatory transcription factor 1 in response to metal ions. *J. Biol. Chem.* 2001, 276: 41879–88.

Lefebvre, D., Beckers, F., Ketelslegers, J. M., et al. Zinc regulation of insulin-like growth factor-I (IGF-I), growth hormone receptor (GHR) and binding protein (GHBP) gene expression in rat cultured hepatocytes. *Molecular and Cellular Endocrinology.* 1998, 138: 127–36.

Lipscomb, W. L., and Strater, N. Recent advances in zinc enzymology. *Chem. Rev.* 1996; 96: 2237–42.

Lopantsev, V., Wenzel, H. J., Cole, T. B., et al. Lack of vesicular zinc in mossy fibers does not affect synaptic excitability of CA3 pyramidal cells in zinc transporters 3 knockout mice. *Neuroscience.* 2003, 116: 237–48.

MacDonald, R. S. The role of zinc in growth and cell proliferation. *J. Nutr.* 2000; 130: 1500s–8s.

MacDonald, R. S., Wollard-Biddle, L. C. Browning, J. D., et al. Zinc deprivation of murine 3T3 cells by use of diethylenetrinitrilopentaacetate impairs DNA synthesis upon stimulation with insulin-like growth factor-I (IGF-I). *J. Nutr.* 1998; 128: 1600–5.

Mathews, L. S., Norstedt, G., and Palmiter, R. D. Regulation of IGF-I gene expression by growth hormone. *Proc. Natl. Acad. Sci.* 1986; 83, 9343–7.

Mcmahon, R. J., and Cousins, R. J. Regulation of the zinc transporter ZnT-1 by dietary zinc. *Proc. Natl. Acad. Sci.* 1998, 95:4841–6.

Nakae, J. Distinct and overlapping functions of insulin and IGF-I receptors. *Endocr. Rev.* 2001; 22: 818–35.

Ninh, N. X., Maiter, D., Lause, P., et al. Continuous administration of growth hormone (GH) does not prevent the decrease of IGF-I gene expression in zinc-deprived rats despite normalization of liver GH-binding. *Growth Regul.* 1998; 7, 1–8.

Ninh, N. X., Thissen, J. P., Maiter, D., et al. Reduced liver Insulin-like growth factor-I gene expression in young zinc-deprived rats is associated with a decrease in liver growth hormone (GH) receptors and serum GH-binding protein. *J. Endocrinol.* 1995; 144, 449–56.

Nordberg, M. Metallothioneins: historical review and state of knowledge. *Talanta.* 1998, 46: 243–254

Palmiter, R. D., and Findley, S. D. Cloning and functional characterization of a mammalian zinc transporter that confers resistance to zinc. *EMBO J.* 1995, 14: 639–49.

Palmiter, R. D., Cole, T. B. Quaife, C. J., et al. ZNT-3, a putative transporter of zinc into synaptic vesicles. *Proc. Natl. Acad. Sci.* 1996, 93: 14934–9.

Paski, S. C., and Xu; Z. Labile intracellular zinc is associated with 3T3 cell growth. *Journal of Nutritional Biochemistry.* 2001; 12: 655–61.

Pfaffl, M. W., Windisch, W. Influence of zinc deficiency on the mRNA expression of zinc transporters in adult rats. *J. Trace Elem. Med. Biol.* 2003, 17(2): 97-106.

Reyes, J. G. Zinc transport in mammalian cells. *Am. J. Physiol.* 1996, 270: C401–10.

Saltiel, A. R., and Kahn, C. R. Insulin signalling and the regulation of glucose and lipid metabolism. *Nature.* 2001; 414: 799–806.

Sara, V., and Hall, K. Insulin-like growth factors and their binding proteins. *Physiol Rev.* 1990; 70: 591–614.

Sciaudone, M. P., Chattopadhyay, S., and Freake, H. C. Cheleation of zinc amplifies induction of growth hormone mRNA levels in cultured rat pituitary tumor cells. *J. Nutr.* 2000, 130:158–63.

Smirnova, I. V., Bittel, D. C., Ravindra, R., et al. Zinc and cadmium can promote rapid nuclear translocation of metal response element-binding transcription factor-1. *J. Biol. Chem.* 2000, 275: 9377–84.

Spears, J. W. Zinc methionine for ruminants: relative bioavailability of zinc in lambs and effects of growth and performance of growing heifers. *J. Anim. Sci.* 1989; 67:835–43.

Taylor, C. G., Bettger, W. J., and Bray, T. M. The effect of dietary zinc or copper deficiency on the primary free radical defense system in rats. *J. Nutr.* 1988; 118: 613–21.

Thissen, J. P., Ketelslegers, J. M., and Underwood, L. E. Nutritional regulation of the IGFs. *Endocr. Rev.* 1994; 15, 80–101.

Ullrich, A., and Schlessinger, J. Signal transduction by receptors with tyrosine kinase activity. *Cell.* 1990; 61: 203–12.

Urani, C., Calini, V., Melchioretto, P., et al. Different induction of metallothioneins and Hsp70 and presence of the membrane transporter ZnT-1 in HepG2 cells exposed to copper and zinc. *Toxicology in Vitro.* 2003, 17: 553–9.

Vanhaesebroeck, B. Synthesis and function of 3-phosphorylated inositol lipids. *Annu. Rev. Biochem.* 2001; 70: 535–602.

Wang HS, and Chard T. The role of insulin-like growth factor-I and insulin-like growth factor-binding protein-1 in the control human fetal growth. *J Endocrinology.* 1999; 132:11–9.

Wang, Z. Y., Danscher, G., Ma, A. D., et al. Zinc transporter 3 and zinc ions in the rodent superior cervical ganglion neurons. *Neuroscience.* 2003, 120: 605–16.

Wedekind, K. J., Horton, A. E., and Baker, D. E. Methodology for assessing zinc bioavailability: efficacy estimates for zinc methionine, zinc sulfate and zinc oxide. *J. Anim. Sci.* 1992; 70: 178–97.

White, M. F., and Yenush, L. The IRS-signaling system: a network of docking proteins that mediate insulin and cytokine action. *Curr. Topics in Micro. and Immun.* 1998; 228: 179–208.

Yamaji, S., Tennant, J., Tandy, S., et al. Zinc regulates the function and expression of the iron transporters DMT1 and IREG1 in human intestinal Caco-2 cells. *FEBS Letters.* 2001, 507: 137–41.

In: Focus on Nutrition Research
Editor: Tony P. Starks, pp. 187-205

ISBN 1-59454-768-8
© 2006 Nova Science Publishers, Inc.

Chapter VIII

In Vivo and in Vitro Immunomodulatory Effects of Peptidoglycan Derived from *Lactobacillus*

Jin Sun[1], Guowei Le[1,2], Yonghui Shi[1,1,2] *,
Xiyi Ma[1] and Guanhong Li[1]

[1] Institute of Food Nutrition and Safety, School of Food Science and Technology, Southern Yangtze University, 170 Huihe Road, Wuxi, Jiangsu 214036, P. R. China
[2] Key Laboratory of Industrial Biotechnology, Ministry of Education, Southern Yangtze University, 170 Huihe Road, Wuxi, Jiangsu 214036, P. R. China

Abstract

Aim: The functioning of host immune system, at the systemic as well as local (gastraintestinal tract) level, can be influenced by signals provided by commensal-associated molecular patterns (CAMPs) of probiotics (such as Lactobacilli). Peptidoglycan (PG) is an important CAMP present on the cell surface of *Lactobacillus*. The purpose of this study was to evaluate the immunomodulatory activity of PG. derived from *Lactobacillus*.

Methods: Five- to six-week old KM and BALB/c mice were used to investigate the immunomodulatory activity of PG derived from *Lactobacillus*. Mice were intraperitoneally injected (i.p.) with physiologic saline as control and different dose of PG in physiologic saline. Mice were killed, and the spleens, peritoneal macrophages and blood were collected to assess the effects of PG on a range of immune responses (phagocytic activity, natural killer (NK) cell activity, cytokine and nitric oxide (NO) production, 50% complent hemolysis, serum lysozyme activity). Peritoneal macrophage

---

[1] To whom correspondence should be sent: Tel.: +86-510-5869236; Fax: +86-510-5869236. *E-mail address*: yhshi@sytu.edu.cn

(PMΦ) and splenocyte mRNA were extracted to assess the gene expression profile using high-density oligonucleotide microarrays. The activity of PG was also studied in vitro and in vivo using colon tumor cell CT26 (CT26) and mice inoculated with CT26, respectively.

Results: PG has broad immunomodultory effects on host immune system including both natural and acquired immune response. Phagocytic activity of macrophages from mice treated with Pg was significantly dose-dependently improved. Administration of PG was also found to significantly increase NK activity of splenocytes and cytotoxic T lymphocytes (CTL) activity. Similarly, PG enhanced significantly the production of both NO ($P<0.01$) and tumor necrosis factor-alpha (TNF-α) ($P<0.01$) by macrophages. IL-1 production was increased in high PG dose-treated mice, while no significant difference ($P>0.05$) in IL-2 production was observed in all PG-treated groups with comparison to control group. A significant increase in serum lysozyme ($P<0.01$) and 50% complement hemolytic (CH50) activity ($P<0.01$) was also observed in PG-treated mice as compared with control mice. PG exhibited potent antitumor activity against CT26 in vivo but not in vitro. The gene expression profile revealed that the PG activated macrophages to release molecules that invoke pro-T helper 1-type immune (Th1)/cell-mediated immune response.

Conclusions: The present study has demonstrated that PG derived from *Lactobacillus* possesses immunostimulating activity on healthy and tumor-inoculated mice. PG is responsible for certain immune responses induced by *Lactobacillus*. Antitumor effect of *Lactobacillus* is likely attributable to activation of MΦ by PG expressed on the bacterial cell surface.

Key Words: Peptidoglycan, *Lactobacillus,* mice, immunomodulatory activity, gene expression

Introduction

Lactobacilli are normal components of the healthy human intestinal microflora [1]. It has been shown that Lactobacillus affect selected aspects of immune function that may involve one or several components of the humoral, cellular or nonspecific immunity [2], suggesting the potential use of *Lactobacillus* as natural food products with immunoenhancing properties or immunomodulatory medicines to prevent infection of pathogenic bacteria [3,4] and induction of cancer [5,6,7]. It is not known entirely, however, how *Lactobacillus* affects the immune system and exerts these immunostimulative effects. It is suggested that Lactobacillus activate innate immunity response and mediate a protective inflammatory response in the gut [8]. The first defense mechanism in inflammation is innate immunity and involves epithelium barrier, phagocyte and release of cell derived inflammatory mediators (i.e. cytokines). A characteristic feature of innate immunity is an ability of distinguishing between potentially pathogenic microbial components and harmless antigens by "pattern recognition receptors (PRRs)". Toll like receptors (TLRs) are important PRRs involved in the activation of pro-inflammatory reactions [9]. It has been found that pathogenic microbes express highly conserved molecular structures called pathogen associated molecular patterns (PAMP) [10]. PAMPs include microbial cell wall components such as lipopolysaccharide (LPS), lipoteichoic acid (LTA) and peptidoglycan (PG) [11]. Active innate immune cells expressed

TLRs are capable of recognizing common features of PAMPs [12]. TLR2 is an important TLRs member that recognizes PG. It was demonstrated that recognition of microbes activates Nf-κB signalling pathway and in this way it triggers cytokine production, up-regulation of co-stimulatory molecules on antigen presenting cells leading to activation of T cells [13]. Recent studies indicate that in addition to pathogenic microbes and their products, immune responses can be primed or activated by non-pathogenic commensal bacteria, including the probiotic such as *Lactobacillus* and *Bifidobacteria* species [2]. Probiotics share distinct commensal-associated molecular patterns (CAMPs) [14], which enhance epithelial barrier function in the gut, activate NF-κB and cytokine production in monocyte/macrophages and natural killer (NK) cells and induce phagocytic activity in neutrophils [15].

Seth (2004) demonstrated that the beneficial effects of commensal bacteria or probiotics were due to recognition of their surface molecules by TLRs[16]. This recognition triggers TLRs to regulate genes that foster homeostasis of the intestinal epithelium. It also confers a protective effect on these cells and induces tissue repair. Elucidating the interaction between host and probiotic cell surface molecules will be the key to this protective effect. However, there were few reports of systematic investigation of host cell responses to CAMPs from various probiotic strains. In recent years, we have studied the immunemodulatory effects of *Lactobacillus*-derived PG. It has been found that *Lactobacillus*-derived PG, a kind of CAMP, enhanced immune surveillance of mice. To delineate this response in a more comprehensive way, a genome-wide analysis of the immunity response to PG has been undertaken. The results demonstrated that most genes participating in the immune response were transcriptionally modulated after PG treatment. Many of the genes regulated by PG were concerned with activation of macrophage, and PG-activated macrophage release molecules that invoke pro-T helper 1-type immune (Th1)/cell-mediated immune (CMI) responses. Due to this induced response, anti colon tumor effect of Lactobacillus PG was also studied and the results suggested that *Lactobacillus*-derived PG could be used as potential functional food additive in cancer prevention.

Material and Methods

Preparation of Lactobacillus-Derived Peptidoglycan

Peptidoglycan of *Lactobacillus sp.* derived from livestock feces was prepared by method as described by Sarka [17] with some modification. Briefly, *lactobacillus sp.* was grown in MRS liquid medium for 48 hr at 37°C without shaking. The culture was quickly chilled in ice bath and the bacteria were harvested by centrifugation (2,000×g, 10min, 4°C) and washed several times with sterile water. The cells were inactivated in boiling water bath for 20 min. The bacteria suspension was sonicated for 20 min to break the bacteria and then centrifuged at 1,000×g for 15min to sediment unbroken bacteria, the supernatant containing the cell walls was decanted and were pelleted by centrifugation at 10,000×g for 10 min. The crude cell walls were incubated in 2% sodium dodecyl sulfate for 30 min at 60°C to remove noncovalently bound material. After washing four times with sterile water and twice with dehydrated alcohol, respectively, covalently bound proteins were removed by digestion with

0.02% trypsin in 0.1 M Tris-HCl buffer (pH 7.5) for 20 hr at 37°C. The walls were washed several times with sterile water and lyophilized. The walls were resuspended in 10% trichloroacetic acid and stirred for 20 min at 60°C. The peptidoglycan was concentrated by centrifugation and washed extensively with sterile water. All reagents used were sterile, and disposable plastic ware or glassware baked at 180°C was used to avoid contamination with endotoxin.

Animals

KM and BALB/c conventional mice weighing 18-20 g, 5–6 wk of age, were obtained from Shanghai slac Co. The animals were housed in individual cages at appropriate temperature and offered feed and water *ad libitum* and received humane care in accordance with the animal care provisions.

Experimental Design

Sixteen BALB/c mice were randomly allocated to two groups of 8 mice each. After acclimatization for 1 week, mice were intraperitoneally injected (i.p.) with 0.5 ml/day of physiologic saline as control or PG in physiologic saline (1mg/ml) for two consecutive days. PMΦ was obtained on the third day for phagocytic activity assay.

Sixteen KM mice were randomly allocated to two groups of 8 mice each. After acclimatization for 1 week, mice were orally administered i.p. with 0.5 ml/day of physiologic saline or PG in physiologic saline (1mg/ml) for consecutive seven days. Mice were immunized i.p. with 2% sheep erythrocyte (10 mg in physiologic saline) on the 9th days. Blood and PMΦ were obtained on 14th day for the determination of 50% complement hemolysis (CH50) and nitric oxide (NO) production by PMΦ, respectively.

Eighteen KM mice were randomly allocated to three groups of 6 mice each. After acclimatization, mice were administered i.p. with 0.5ml PBS as control, 0.025 mg or0.05mg PG in 0.5ml PBS for five consecutive days. Spleens were removed from mice on the 6th day and a spleen cell suspension was prepared for the determination of NK activity, IL-2 and IFN-γ. Meanwhile, peritoneal macrophages were collected for the measurement of IL-1 and TNF-α.

KM mice (n=6) was injected i.p. with 0.5ml physiologic saline (control) or PG suspended in 0.5ml of physiologic saline (1mg/ml) for two days (once a day) and blood was sampled on the third day to study effect of PG on serum lysozyme activity.

In vivo and in vitro anti-tumor activities of PG were studied using colon tumor cell CT26 (CT26) and mice inoculated with CT26. CT26 were incubated in complete RPMI1640 medium supplemented with 10% fetal calf serum at 37°C in 5% CO2. Log phase cells were collected, treated by 0.25% trypsinase, washed twice by RPMI1640, resuspended in RPMI1640 to a density of 5×10^6 cells/ml. Thirty BALB/C mice were inoculated with 0.2ml cells in the left hind limb and were randomly allocated to three groups of 10 mice each. Mice were then administered i.p. with 0.5 ml physiologic saline as control, 0.1mg or 0.5mg PG in

0.5 ml physiologic saline every two days for 16 days, staring 24 h after inoculation of the tumor. Mice were sacrificed on the 17th day, solid tumor and spleens were removed from mice and weighed. The inhibition rate was calculated by comparing the weights of the tumor of the treated group with those of the control. For in vitro study, CT26 (5×104 cells/ml) was incubated with or without 100µg/ml or 2000µg/ml PG (0.1ml/well) in 40-well flat-bottomed plates at 37°C in 5% CO_2 for 48 hr, the supernatant was discarded and 20µl of 5g/L MTT was added to each well. After Incubation for another 4-6 hr, suspension was centrifuged at 1500r/min, 4°C for 5min, supernatant was discarded and 100µl of dimethyl sulfoxide was added and then the absorbance at 492 nm (OD492) was measured.

Three groups of three male BALB/c mice each were injected i.p. with phosphate-buffered saline (PBS) as control or PG (25mg/kg wt in PBS) once a day. At 4 hr after treating either once (acute treatment) or once for three consecutive days (chronic treatment), mice were killed. Peritoneal macrophage and splenic lymphocyte were isolated and 1×107 of each two type cells were mix together in each treatment and stored at −70°C in 2 ml Trizol reagent for future use.

Blood

After eyeball was removed, blood was sampled in a centrifuge tube, stayed for 3 hr at 4°C, and centrifuged at $1000 \times g$ for 10 min to yield serum.

Peritoneal Macrophages

Resident peritoneal macrophages were collected by washing the peritoneal cavity of each mouse with D-Hanks. The eluate was centrifuge at $600 \times g$ for 10 min. The cells were washed twice with RPMI-1640 medium containing fetal calf serum (100 ml/l), 100 IU/ml penicillin and 100 mg/ml streptomycin to a density of 2×106 cells/ml. Suspension of 2×106 cells/ml were plated in 24-well tissue culture plates with 1 ml in each well. After a 48-h incubation at 37°C in 5% CO_2, the supernatants were collected and stored at -20°C for further determination of IL-1 and tumor necrosis factor-alpha (TNF-α).

Spleen-Cell Suspensions

Spleens were removed aseptically from mice and placed individually into 2 ml complete RPMI-1640 medium. Single-cell suspensions were prepared by chopping the spleens into small pieces with sterile scissors and then forcing the spleen tissue through a silk mesh with a pore size of 200 µm in diameter. The resulting suspension was then transferred to a tube containing 5ml complete RPMI-1640 and centrifuged at $600 \times g$ for 10 min. The cell pellet was resuspended in ACK lysis buffer (Tris-NH4Cl) and incubated for 5 min with occasional mixing to lyse the erythrocytes. After washing twice in complete RPMI-1640, the cells were adjusted to a final concentration of 2×106 cells/ml in complete RPMI-1640. Splenic lymphocytes (2×106 cells/well) were added to the 24-well flat-bottomed plate and were cultured at 37°C in 5% CO2 for 48h. The supernants were collected and stored at -20°C for further determination of IL-2 and interferon (INF)-γ.

Cytokines and Nitric Oxide (NO)

IL-1 in culture supernatants was determined according to the method as described by Zhu et al. [18]. Briefly, thymus cell suspensions (100μl; 4×107cells/ml in complete RPMI-1046) were added to each well of a 96-well plate and cultured in the presence of concanavalin A (ConA) (0.5-0.7μg /ml; Sigma) and culture supernatant of macrophage (5μL). After removing of the supernatant, methyl thiazolyl tetrazolium (MTT) (5mg/ml) was added at 20μl/well. After a further cultivation for 4-6 h, supernatant was removed, and dimethyl sulphoxide (DMSO) was added at 100μl/well. OD492 was then measured.

For the determination of IL-2, spleen cells of naïve mice were cultured in the presence of ConA (5μg /ml; Sigma) for 48 h. After removing supernatants, cells were resuspended in RMOI1640 containing fetal calf serum and further cultured for 30-60h at 37°C in 5% CO2. Test samples (100μl) were added to cell suspensions (2×106cells/well in complete RPMI-1046) in 96-well flat-bottomed plates and culture for 32-40 h at 37°C in 5% CO2. After removing of the supernatant, methyl thiazolyl tetrazolium (MTT) (5mg/ml) was added at 20μl/well. After a further cultivation for 4-6 h, supernatant was removed, and dimethyl sulphoxide (DMSO) was added at 100μl/well. OD492 was then measured.

The amounts of TNF-α in culture supernatants were quantified by the method as described by Zhang [19]. Briefly, L929 cells (90μl, $2-3 \times 105$ cells/ml) were added to each well of a 96-well flat-bottomed plate and cultured for 18h at 37°C in 5% CO2. Actinomycin-D (10μl, 800ng/ml) and culture supernatant of macrophage (100μl) were added and cultured further for 20 h. For negative control, RPMI-1046 was added only. After removing of the supernatant, methyl thiazolyl tetrazolium (MTT) (5mg/ml) was added at 20μl/well. After a further cultivation for 4-6 h, supernatant was removed, and dimethyl sulphoxide (DMSO) was added at 100μl/well. OD492 was then measured.

IFN-γ was determined by the method as described by Zhang [19]. Briefly, macrophage cell suspensions (200μl, 1×106 cells/ml) of naïve mice were added to 96-well flat-bottomed plates and cultured for 2h at 37°C in 5% CO2. Unadherent cells were washed away, culture supernatant of spleen cell (100μl) was added and cultured in the presence of ConA (10μg /ml; Sigma) for 48h at 37°C in 5% CO2. NO in suspension was then determined as follows:

Determination of NO was conducted with NO assay kit according to manufacturer's instruction. In aqueous solutions, NO is metabolized rapidly into nitrite. NO production was measured as nitrite (NO2-), accumulated in the culture medium, by Griess reagent (1% sulfanilamine, 0.1% naphtyletylene diamine dihydrochoride and 2,5% phosphoric acid). Nitrite reacts with Griess and forms purple azo dye, which can be detected spectrophotometrically. Standard curve was made using serial dilution of natrium nitrosum. For sample, 0.3 ml of cultured macrophage supernatant was used.

Phagocytosis

Assessment of the phagocytic capacity of peritoneal macrophages was based on the method by Zhu et al [18]. Briefly, two or three drops of peritoneal macrophages eluate was added on a glass slide and incubated at 37°C for 1 h, and then washed twice with physiologic saline to remove the unadherent cells. Two drops of yeast suspension was added on the glass slide, and then followed by a incubation for 30-40 min at 37°C. After incubation, the cover slips were removed, washed with physiologic saline, fixed with 1% glutaraldehyde for 2-3 min, air-dried, and stained with methylene blue for 1-2 min. The cover slips were then mounted onto glass slides and the percentage of phagocytic cells with ingested yeasts was determined by counting at 100 cells under oil immersion.

Natural Killer Cell Activity

Mouse lymphadenoma cell YAC-1 (target cell) suspension (100μl, 2×105 cells/ml) and spleen cell suspension (100μl, 2×105 cells/ml) were added to 50-well plate and incubated for 20 h at 37°C in 5% $CO2$. After removing of the supernatant, methyl thiazolyl tetrazolium (MTT) (5mg/ml) was added at 20μl/well. After a further cultivation for 4-6 h, supernatant was removed, and dimethyl sulphoxide (DMSO) was added at 100μl/well. OD492 was then measured. The natural killer cell activity was calculated as follows:

Natural killer cell activity (%) = [OD target cell-(ODsample-ODeffec control)]/ODtarget control

Cytotoxic T Lymphocytes (CTL) Activity

After different PG treatment, spleen cells from mice inoculated with CT26 were used to determine CTL activity. CT26 (target cell) suspension (100μl, 2×105/mL) and spleen cell suspension (100μl, 2×105/mL) were added to 50-well plate and incubated for 20 h at 37°C in 5% $CO2$. After removing of the supernatant, methyl thiazolyl tetrazolium (MTT) (5mg/ml) was added at 20μl/well. After a further cultivation for 4-6 h, supernatant was removed, and dimethyl sulphoxide (DMSO) was added at 100μl/well. OD492 was then measured. The CTL activity was calculated as follows:

CTL activity (%) = [ODtarget cell-(ODsample-ODeffec control)]/ODtarget control

Serum Lysozyme (LSZ) and 50% Complement Hemolytic (CH50) Activity

For determination of serum LSZ activity, Peptidoglycan was suspended in 1/15 mol/L PBS (pH6.2) (OD450 is about 0.6). Three milliliter of the suspension was mixed with 100ul

PBS-diluted serum on rice. OD450 was determined. After incubated at 37°C for 30 min with agitating (120rpm), reaction was ended in ice bath for 10min. Absorbance was determined at 450nm. One unit of the enzyme was defined as that one milliliter of the enzyme solution that decreases the OD492 of PG suspension by 0.1.

CH50 activity was measured after serum was diluted with physiologic saline for 100 folds. One milliliter of diluted serum which was stored at 0°C was mixed with 0.5ml 10% sheep erythrocyte cell (SRBC) and 1ml 10% serum of guinea pig. They were incubated at 37°C for 30 min before the reaction was ended in ice bath. The mixture was centrifuge at 1000×g for 10min and 1ml supernatant was mixed with Du reagent (NaCl 1.0 g/L potassuim cyanide 0.05 g/L ferri- potassuim cyanide 0.2 g/L). Absorbance at 540 nm was measured (ODsample). In another assay, 0.25ml SRBC was diluted with Du reagent to 4ml, and incubated for 10min. After centrifugation, OD540 of supernatant was measured. CH50 was calculated as follows:

CH50 activity = (ODsample/ODSRBC) × dilution fold

High-Density Oligonucleotide Arrays

Gene expression analysis was performed by using the Affymetrix MOE430A GeneChip. GenenChip were made according to laboratory methods in the Affymetrix GeneChip expression manual (see Protocol for Eukaryotic Sample and Array Processing in http://www.Affymetrix.com).

The level of gene expression was normalized for all conditions using a computational technique in which the output of the experimental array is multiplied by a factor (normalization factor) to make the average intensity equivalent to the average intensity of all the other arrays. The data were further processed using GeneChip analysis Microarray Suite 5.0 (Affymetrix) and Data Mining Tool Version 2. The first software performs statistical analysis of array data and generates both signal intensity values representing the relative expression level of each gene on the array and associated. A comparison analysis was performed, which directly compares probe pairs from one GeneChip to another. This type of analysis has been shown to significantly reduce array variability relative to comparisons of expression signals alone. The signal log ratio (SLR) was used to estimate the change in expression level for a transcript between a baseline and an experiment array. This change was expressed as the log2 ratio. Fold Change from log ratios could be calculated as Corrected formula: FoldChange=2single log ratio (single log ratio≥0) or (-1)×2–single log ratio (single log ratio<0). So, a log2 ratio of 1 was the same a change of 2 fold.

Functional Cluster Analysis

Before applying the cut-off filtering criterion, the gene expression values were subjected to functional cluster analysis using MAPPFinder [21], a software that creates a global gene expression profile from microarray data by integrating the annotations of the Gene Ontology (GO) Project (http://www.geneontology.org.; accessed February, 2003) with the free software package GenMAPP (http://www.GenMAPP.org.; accessed February, 2003). Using the GenMAPP Expression Dataset Manager tool, we converted the gene expression values (.xls) into an expression data set file (.gex) and defined the criteria for meaningful gene changes in expression. Having created the expression Dataset file, we obtained functional cluster results using the MAPPFinder program. MAPPFinder builds a local copy of the GO hierarchy using the three Ontology files (process, component, and function) available from GO. For each term, MAPPFinder calculates (1) a first set of percentages for the genes specifically associated with that term of the GO hierarchy, (2) a second set of percentages for the total number of genes associated with that term and all its ''children'', and (3) a z score (i.e. the level of confidence that a term has more or less genes meeting the criterion than would be expected by chance). The cut-off filtering criterion used is at least 30% of genes changed and changed gene is more than 5 and absolute Z is mare than 3.

Statistical Analysis

Significant differences between the experimental and control groups were determined using ANOVA (SPSS ver. 10.0). Difference was considered significant when $P<0.05$.

Result

Natural Killer-Cell Activity and Phagocytic Function of Peritoneal Macrophages

The phagocytic activities of peritoneal macrophages are shown in Fig.1. Peritoneal macrophages from mice administrated i.p. with Lactobacillus PG for five days showed significantly greater phagocytic activity than those from control mice and the effect was dose-dependent.

The activity was increase with the increase of dose. Injection with PG also had a stimulatory effect on NK-cell activity of splenocytes. Spleen cells from mice administrated with different dose of PG exhibited higher NK-cell cytotoxic activity (31.8–50.6%) against the target cells, YAC-1 compared to those from control ones ($P<0.01$).

Twenty four hours after inoculation of the colon tumor cell CT26, BALB/c mice were injected with 0.1mg or 0.5mg PG in 0.5 ml physiologic saline every two days in 16 days, CTL activity was enhanced in a dose-dependent pattern. Forty percent of tumor cells were killed in the high PG dose treatment group.

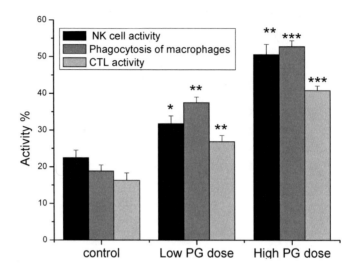

Figure 1. The effect of PG on the activities of CTL, NK and PMφ in mice. Values are means ± SD. **
difference between values of control and low PG dose group is significant (P<0.01); ***: difference between
values of control and low PG dose group is significant (P<0.01) and difference is significant between low PG
dose group and high PG dose group (P<0.05).

Cytokine Production

As is shown in table 1, after co-incubation with supernatant of cultured macrophage,
conA-induced proliferation of thymus cell, an index for IL-1 production in macrophage, was
increased only in high PG dose treated mice (p<0.05). ConA-induced L929 cells
proliferation, which indicate the TNF-α production, was enhanced both in low PG dose
(P<0.05) and high PG dose (P<0.01) treatment groups. Spleen cells culture supernatant of
both treatment did not affect the proliferation of spleen cell of naïve mice, which suggested
that PG treatment did not induce IL-2 production in spleen. Culture supernatant of spleen
cells from PG-treated mice, however, significantly induced the production of NO by
macrophage of naïve mice, indicating the increased production of IFN-γ (P<0.01). It is shown
in Fig. 2 that NO production by macrophage of PG-treated mice was also enhanced (P<0.01).

Table 1. The effect of PG on the activities of Cytokines.

Group	IL-1	IL-2	TNF-α	IFN-γ
Control	0.286±0.032a	0.176±0.018	1.118±0.073a	132.3±3.31A
Low PG dose	0.342±0.025ab	0.186±0.009	0.843±0.062b	104.5±2.0B
High PG dose	0.445±0.057b	0.223±0.019	0.667±0.083C	92.6±2.7C

Notes: TNF-α activity have inverse ratio to optical density; IFN-γ activity have inverse ratio to
fluorescence intensity. Values are means ± SD. Values in the same column with same superscript
are not different. Values in the same column with different superscripts in capital letters are very
significantly different at P< 0.01 level. Values in the same column with different small superscripts
are significantly different at P< 0.05 level.

Effects of PG on Serum LSZ and CH50 Activity

After two days of PG treatment, the blood was sampled to determine serum lysozyme (LSZ) activity. The result revealed that injecting with 0.5mg of PG for two day significantly increased serum LSZ activity (P<0.01). The CH50 activity was used in the study to reflect effect of PG on adoptive immune response. After treated with PG for 1 week, mice were immunized with sheep erythrocyte. The effects of injecting Lactobacillus PG on 50% complement hemolytic activity (CH50) are shown in Fig2. A significant increase was found after PG treatment (P<0.01).

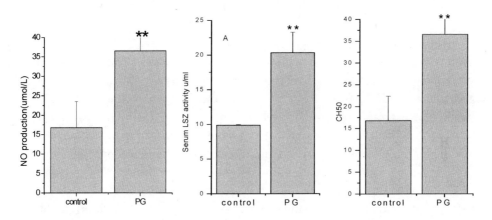

Figure 2. Serum LSZ, CH50 level and macrophage NO production after PG treatment. Values are means ± SD, ** P<0.01.

Weight of Colon Tumor and Spleen

Result indicated that there was a dose-dependent in vitro inhibition on CT26 colon cancer development in mice treated with PG (P<0.01) (Table 2). The inhibition ratio of high PG dose treatment group was 54.2%. Spleen weight, however, was increase after administration of different dose of PG (Table 2). On the other hand, PG did not inhibit the in vitro growth of tumor cell line (Table 3).

Table 2. Inhibitory effect of PG on the growth of CT26 in mice.

Group	CT26 tumor		Spleen	
	Weight (g)	Inhibition (%)	Weight (g)	Relativity (%)
Control	1.786±0.276c	-	0.199±0.041b	100.0
Low dose PG	1.364±0.236B	23.7	0.261±0.091ab	130.9
High dose PG	0.818±0.305A	54.2	0.273±0.078a	137.2

Notes: Values are means ± SD. Values in the same column with same superscript are not different. Values in the same column with different superscripts in capital letters are significantly different at P< 0.01 level. Values in the same column with different superscripts are significantly different at P< 0.05 level.

Table 3. Effect of PG on the CT26 cell proliferation in vitro.

Group	OD192	Inhibition
Control	0.414±0.031*	-
Low PG dose	0.435±0.034	-5.1%
High PG dose	0.412±0.037	0.5%

- Values are means ± SD.

Gene Expression Profile of PMΦ and Splenetic Cell

MAPPFinder was used to assign the differentially expressed genes (n = 5,085 for acute PG treatment and n=3,995 after chronic PG treatment) to non-mutually exclusive categories regarding biological processes, molecular functions, and/or cellular components. These categories contain 11,239 functional gene groups (GO terms) into which genes, differentially expressed in the array, can be clustered on the basis of their known biological roles. Moreover, MAPPFinder calculates the percentage of genes meeting the defined criterion, for each GO term. The criterion used was that at least 30% of genes changed and changed gene is more than 5 and absolute Z is mare than 3. MAPP Finder connects 2861 genes in its dataset of the 4277 detected genes after acute PG treatment and 2264 genes in its dataset of the 3464 detected genes (chronic PG treatment) to a GO term. The GO terms highlighted by MAPPFinder as being "notable" are summarized in Table 4 and Table 5. For both treatments, the functional groups identified are related to response to stimulus, defense response and immune response. After chronic treatment, more biological process was affected including cell-cell adhesion; alcohol metabolism and fatty acid biosynthesis.

Discussion

Probiotic could optimally modulate host innate (non-specific or natural) and acquired (specific) immune systems. This is essential for host to defense against invading pathogens [22] and spontaneously developing cancers [23]. The results of present studies demonstrate that several indices of natural and acquired immunity were enhanced in healthy mice of CT26-incubated mice injected with Lactobacillus PG. PG induced immune response was similar to that induced by some Lactobacillus.

Macrophages Phagocytic and NK cells are the major effectors of natural immunity. Treating mice with Lactobacillus PG resulted in enhanced phagocyte function of peritoneal macrophages (37.5-52.8 %). Enhanced phagocytic activity of peripheral blood leucocytes or peritoneal macrophages from human subjects [24,25] and animals [26] given dietary lactic acid bacteria (LAB) has been also observed. It has been shown that the level of enhancement depends on the strain, dose and viability of LAB used [27]. In present experiment, the PG was found to enhance the phagocytic activity of macrophages in a dose-dependent way. Considering these results, it could be speculated that PG is essential for immunostimulating function of LAB.

**Table 4. Notable functional categories of genes
highlighted by MAPPFinder after acute PG treatment.**

GO Name	Number in GO	Percent Changed	Z Score
Significantly increased:			
Biological Process			
ribosome biogenesis and assembly	69	97.6	4.117
ribosome biogenesis	68	97.6	4.117
response to stimulus	1521	78.9	4.083
response to external stimulus	1371	79	3.871
response to biotic stimulus	941	79.3	3.508
response to pest/pathogen/parasite	502	83.5	3.177
defense response	912	81.1	3.919
immune response	698	80.2	3.373
Cellular Component			
cytosol	221	82.8	3.168
cytosolic ribosome (sensu Eukarya)	48	100	4.397
ribosome	159	96.4	5.585
cytosolic ribosome (sensu Eukarya)	48	100	4.397
ribonucleoprotein complex	281	91.6	5.585
extracellular	2467	74.1	3.283
Molecular Function			
signal transducer activity	1908	76.3	3.796
receptor activity	1374	77.8	3.644
structural molecule activity	497	87.2	5.22
structural constituent of ribosome	266	94.6	5.552
Significantly decreased:			
Biological Process			
intracellular transport	460	63.4	4.104
protein transport	416	62.8	3.624
intracellular protein transport	399	63.8	3.693
transcription	1359	56	3.551
transcription\, DNA-dependent	1298	55.9	3.435
regulation of transcription	1295	56.1	3.497
regulation of transcription, DNA-dependent	1801	56.2	3.501
Cellular Component			
microtubule associated complex	90	82.4	3.001
Molecular Function			
protein transporter activity	227	70.4	4.15

Criterion: at least 30% of genes changed and changed gene is more than 5 and absolute Z is mare than 3

Table 5. Notable functional categories of genes highlighted by MAPP Finder after chronic PG treatment.

GO Name	Number in GO	Percent Changed	Z Score
Significantly increased:			
Biological Process			
cell-cell adhesion	182	47.2	3.016
alcohol metabolism	152	48.1	3.867
fatty acid biosynthesis	41	66.7	3.282
sterol biosynthesis	18	70	3.237
cholesterol biosynthesis	15	75	3.219
organismal physiological process	1185	42.7	6.12
defense response	912	41.4	5.383
immune response	698	43.1	5.43
innate immune response	105	54.5	4.466
inflammatory response	118	53.5	4.253
regulation of physiological process	32	100	4.193
response to stimulus	1521	36.4	4.401
response to external stimulus	1371	38.2	4.919
response to biotic stimulus	941	41.1	5.515
response to pest/pathogen/parasite	502	43.7	3.97
response to wounding	302	50	4.339
response to pest/pathogen/parasite	502	43.7	3.97
Cellular Component			
extracellular	2467	36.7	6.003
extracellular space	2298	35.5	5.22
Molecular Function			
receptor binding	417	41.8	3.108
cytokine activity	217	56.5	4.879
chemokine activity	35	73.7	4.84
G-protein-coupled receptor binding	40	73.7	4.84
chemokine receptor binding	34	73.7	4.84
serine-type endopeptidase activity	172	52	3.058
trypsin activity	107	60	3.077
serine-type peptidase activity	175	53.8	3.337
serine-type endopeptidase activity	172	52	3.058

Table 5. Continued

GO Name	Number in GO	Percent Changed	Z Score
intramolecular isomerase activity	26	77.8	3.606
significantly decreased:			
Cellular Component			
cell	7894	86.2	3.403
intracellular	4702	88.6	5.036
cytoplasm	2532	89.7	4.196
mitochondrion	582	96.8	3.956
Molecular Function			
protein transporter activity	227	98.5	3.248

Criterion: at least 30% of genes changed and changed gene is more than 5 and absolute Z is mare than 3

Thus, different strain of LAB may stimulate phagocytosis differently just because of their difference in PG content, structure and because of their dissimilarities in the ability to produce PG in the gut. In addition, viability of LAB determins their PG producing ability in gut and affect immunostimulating function.

NK-cell activity was also enhanced in PG treated mice. Increased NK-cell activity in mice injected with *L. casei* [28] and orally administered with LAB [29] was reported. Activated NK cell activity probably attributes to PG released by these bacteria.

T cells are the main effectors and regulators of cell mediated immunity. On activation by antigen or pathogen, T cells synthesize and secrete a variety of cytokines that serve as growth, differentiation and activation factors for other immunocompetent cells. T cells can be subdivided into two functional types, Th1 and Th2, based on their cytokine profile. Th1 cells produce IL-2, IFN-γ and tumour necrosis factor and are vital for cell-mediated immunity. On the other hand, Th2 cells predominantly produce IL-4, IL-5 and IL-10 and are associated with humoral immunity and allergic responses [30]. In the present study, spleen cells from mice injected i.p. with *Lactobacillus* PG produced significantly greater amounts of IFN-γ following stimulation with ConA. The production, however, are not increase with the increase of PG dose. Using genechip analysis, it is found that expression of pro-Th1 cytokine, IL-12, was up regulated in early PG treatment followed by increased expression of IFN-γ in late time period of PG treatment. This clearly shows that PG treatment results in the selective activation of Th1 cells, which was further supported by the result that mice treated with PG had higher CTL activity and IFN-γ production than control mice. Gill (2000) found that the Lactobacillus ability to stimulate IFN-γ production was species-dependent [29]. According to our studies, this may be because of the different cell surface PG of different Lactobacillus.

When MAPPfinder program was used to analysis the effect of PG treatment on biological pathway, it was found that, after both treatments, most influenced pathway was early response of inflammatory response pathway (Fig. 3). Expression pattern of genes involved in this pathway indicate that *Lactobacillus* PG induced macrophages to release cytokines such as IL-1α, IL-1β, IL-6 and IL-12α. After acute PG administration expression of IL-12α and MHC type 2 molecules of macrophages increased significantly.

This revealed the enhanced antigen presentation of macrophage and appearance of pro-Th 1 polarization signal. Stimulated by these cytokines, T cell was activated followed by regulation of B cell by T cell produced costimulatory molecules. Up-regulated expression of activated-T cell specific genes such as proto-oncogene tyrosine-protein kinase LCK and CD28 indicate the activation of T cell. Products of these two genes are critical in early events of T cell activation. After chronic treatment, expression of INF-γ was up regulated. This means the appearance of Th1 immune response. Companied by costimulatory molecules of T cell, IL-6 produced by macrophage plays an essential role in the final differentiation of B-cells into Ig-secreting cells and IL-1 stimulates B-cell maturation and proliferation.

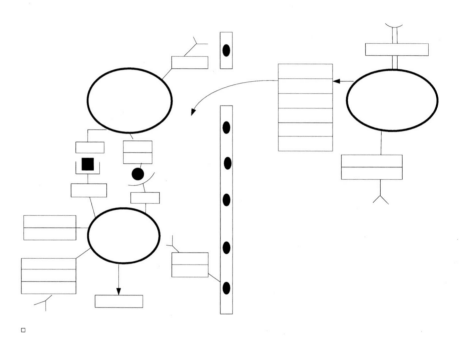

Figure 3. Functional mapping of genes to pathways for early inflammatory response. Pathway is obtained by processing the genechip data by Mappfinder program. The original author of this pathway is Nick Fidelman(E-mail:nsalomonis@Gladstone.ucsf.edu). If gene expression changed, its LSR was followed in parentheses to acute (left) and chronic (right) treatment. Genes whose expression increased in response to PG have plus LSR; those whose expression decreased have negative LSR. NC refers to change in gene expression is not significant. Mice in acute PG treatment were treated with PG for once. Mice in chronic PG treatment were treated with PG for three times.

Furthermore, injection with Lactobacillus PG was found to enhance antibody responses to systemically administered immunogens (sheep erythrocyte) as reflected by increased CH50 activity. The antibody response of PG-treated mice to sheep erythrocyte was significantly higher (91.26) than those of control mice (47.44).

Enhanced phagocytic activity, NK cell activity, T- and B-cell function, and antigen-specific antibody responses are likely to result in an increased resistance to invading pathogens and tumor incidence. When CT26-incubated mice were treated with PG, a dose-dependent inhibition on CT26 development was found. On the other hand, PG did not show direct inhibitory effect in in vitro growth of tumor cell line. This phenomenon demonstrates that the anti-tumor activity of PG against CT26 was probably a consequence of immunostimulation and not a result of direct anti-proliferation activity. Activated NK cell is the major army to inhibit tumor [31]. NK cells are capable of kill cancer cells by antibody-directed cellular cytotoxicity (ADCC) or by direct lysis. These two types of tumoricidal activity require macrophage activation. Interaction between PAMPs and cell surface PRRs induce macrophage activation. Microarry analysis and immunology index indicated the activation of PMø by Lactobacillus PG, which may provide signal for NK cell activation.

The precise mechanisms by which *Lactobacillus spp.* stimulate the immune system are not fully understood. It is possible that oral administration of *Lactobacillus* or their products are able to gain access to the gut-associated lymphoid tissue, especially Peyer's patches and/or to the systemic immune system. It has been found that foreign *Lactobacillus murinus* and cell fragments can penetrate the gut wall by translocation through the epithelial layer or through Peyer's patches [32]. Indigenous intestinal bacteria including *lactobacilli* are also able to cross the intestinal mucous layer and they can survive in the spleen or in other organs for many days where they stimulate phagocytic activity. The interaction between Lactobacillus or Lactobacillus-derived products (CAMPs) and immunocompetent cells (e.g. macrophages, T cells), results in the secretion of cytokines [33] that are known to have a multitude of effects on the functioning of the immune system.

In conclusion, the present study has demonstrated that *Lactobacillus*-derived PG, an important CAMP, possesses immunostimulating activities on healthy or tumor-inoculated mice and PG is responsible for certain immune response induced by *Lactobacillus*. The stimulation of cell-mediated and humoral immunity suggests that PG expressed on surface of *Lactobacillus* may be beneficial for optimizing and/or enhancing immunocompetence in healthy, immunosuppressed or immunocompromised subjects and be functional molecules of *Lactobacillus*. However, it is not known enough how the PG could influence gastrointestinal mucus immune system. Some valid in vitro model should be established for further study.

References

[1] Hans, GH; Heilig, J; Erwin, G; Zoetendal; Elaine, E; Vaughan; Philippe Marteau; Antoon, DL; Akkermans; Willem, M; De Vos.Molecular Diversity of Lactobacillus spp. and Other Lactic Acid Bacteria in the Human Intestine as Determined by Specific Amplification of 16S Ribosomal DNA. *Appl. Environ. Microbiol.* 2002; 68(1):114-123

[2] Kent, L; Erickson; Neil, E; Hubbard. Probiotic immunomodulation in health and disease. *J Nutr* 2000; 130: 403S-409S

[3] Reid, Gregor; Jeremy, Burton.Use of Lactobacillus to prevent infection by pathogenic bacteria. *Microbes and Infection* 2002; 4: 319-324

[4] Van Neil, CW; Feudtner, C; Garrison, MM; Christakis, DA. *Lactobacillus* therapy for acute infectious diarrhea in children: a meta-analysis. *Pediatrics* 2002; 109: 678–84.

[5] Rafter, JJ. The role of lactic acid bacteria in colon cancer prevention. *Scand. J. Gastroenterol.* 1995; 30: 497–502.

[6]   Bolognani, F; Rumney, CJ; Pool-Zobel, BL; Rowland, IR. Effect of lactobacilli, bifidobacteria and inulin on the formation of aberrant crypt foci in rats. *Eur J Nutr* 2001; 40:293–300.

[7]   Wollowski, I; Ji, S; Bakalinsky, AT; Neudecker, C; Pool-Zobel, BL. Bacteria used for the production of yogurt inactivate carcinogens and prevent DNA damage in the colon of rats. *J Nutr* 1999; 129: 77–82.

[8]   Bernard, Dugas; Annick, Mercenier; Irene, Lenoir-Wijnkoop; Cécile Arnaud; Nathalie Dugas; Eric Postaire. Immunity and probiotics. *Immunol. Today* 1999; 20(9):387-390

[9]   Takeda, K; Kaisho, T; Akira, S. Toll-like Receptors. *Annu. Rev. Immunol.* 2003; 21: 335-376

[10]   Poltorak, A; He, X; Smirnova, I; Liu, MY; Huffel, CV; Du, X; Birdwell, D; Alejos, E; Silva, M; Galanos, C; Freudenberg, M; Ricciardi-Castagnoli, P; Layton, B; Beutler, B. Defective LPS signaling in C3H/HeJ and C57BL/10ScCr mice: mutations in Tlr4 gene. *Science* 1998; 282:2085-2088

[11]   Astarie-Dequeker, C; Ndiaye, EN; Le Cavec, V; Rittig, MG; Prandi, J; Maridonnear-Parini, I. The mannose receptor mediates uptake of pathogenic and nonpathogenic mycobacteria and bypasses bactericidal responses in human macrophages. *Infect Immun* 1999; 67: 469-477

[12]   Akira, S; Hemmi, H. Recognition of pathogen-associated molecular patterns by TLR family. *Immunol Lett* 2003; 85:85–98.

[13]   Medzhitov, R; Janeway, Jr; Ch. Innate immune recognition: mechanisms and pathways. *Immunol Rev* 2000; 173:89–97.

[14]   Elke, Cario; Dennis Brown; Mary McKee; Kathryn Lynch-Devaney; Guido Gerken; Daniel, K; Podolsky. Commensal-associated molecular patterns induce selective Toll-Like receptor trafficking from apical membrane to cytoplasmic Compartments in polarized intestinal epithelium. *AJP* 2002, 160 (1): 165-173

[15]   Madsen, K; Cornish, A; Soper, P; Mckaigney, C; Jijon, H; Yachimec, C; Doyle, J; Jewell, L; De Simone, C. Probiotic bacteria enhance murine and human intestinal epithelial barrier function. *Gastroenterology* 2001; 121:580-591

[16]   Seth, Rakoff-Nahoum; Justin Paglino; Fatima Eslami-Varzaneh; Stephen Edberg; Ruslan Medzhitov. Recognition of commensal microflora by Toll-like receptors is required for intestinal homeostasis *Cell* 2004; 118 (7): 229-241

[17]   Sarka, B; Dominic, MD; Michael, J Pabst. Structure of biologically active muramyl peptides from peptidoglycan of Streptococcum Sanguis. *Journal of Mass Spectrometry* 1998; 33:1182-1191

[18]   Lipin Zhu; Xueqin Chen. Methods of immunology. BeingJin: publishing house of the people's surgeon. 2000, 219-220

[19]   Juntian Zhang. Methods in modern pharmacology. BeingJin: *associated publishing company of Beijing medical collage and Xiehe medical collage of China*, 1998: 728-729

[20]   Ruoyu Ni. Detection of IFN-γ through NO2 released by macrophages. *Journal of Immunology (Shang hai)* 1995; 2: 10-13

[21] Doniger, SW, Salomonis N, Dahlquist KD, Vranizan K, Lawlor SC, Conklin BR. MAPPFinder: using Gene Ontology and GenMAPP to create a global gene-expression profile from microarray data. Genome Biol 2003; 4: R7.

[22] Lori Kopp-Hoolihan.Prophylactic and therapeutic uses of probiotics. *J Am Diet Assoc.* 2001; 101: 229-238, 241

[23] Ingrid Wollowski; Gerhard Rechkemmer; Beatrice, L Pool-Zobel.Protective role of probiotics and prebiotics in colon cancer. *Am J Clin Nutr* 2001; 73(suppl): 451S-5S.

[24] Mikes, Z; Ferenicik, M; Jahnova, E; Ebringer,; Ciznar, I. Hypocholesterolemic and immunostimulatory effects of orally applied Enterococcus faecium M-74 in man. *Folia Microbiologica* 1995; 40, 639–646.

[25] Schiffrin, EJ; Brassart, D; Servin, A; Rochat, F; Donnet-Hughes, A. Immune modulation of blood leukocytes in humans by lactic acid bacteria: criteria for strain selection. *American Journal of Clinical Nutrition* 1997; 66, 515S–520S.

[26] Paubert-Braquet, M; Gan, XH; Gaudichon, C; Hedef, N; Serikoff, A;Bouley, C; Bonavida, B; Braquet, P. Enhancement of host resistance against Salmonella typhimurium in mice fed a diet supplemented with yogurt or milks fermented with various Lactobacillus casei strains. *International Journal of Immunotherapy* 1995 11, 153–161.

[27] Gill, HS. Stimulation of the immune system by lactic cultures. *International Dairy Journal* 1998; 8, 535–544.

[28] Kato, I; Yokokawa, T; Mutai, M. Antitumor activity of Lactobacillus casei in mice. *Japanese Journal of Cancer Research (Gann)* 1981; 72, 517–523.

[29] Gill, HS; Rutherfurd, K; Prasad JJ; Gopal PK. Enhancement of natural and acquired immunity by *Lactobacillus rhamnosus* (HN001), *Lactobacillus acidophilus* (HN017) and *Bifidobacterium lactis* (HN019). *British Journal of Nutrition* 2000; 83:167-176

[30] Xin Tong-jing. Basic and clinic of Th genus cell polarization colony. *Military affairs medicinal publishing company, Beijing, China* 2002:25

[31] Takeda, K; Clausen, BE; Kaisho, T; Tsujimura, T; Terada, N; Forster, I; AkiraM, S. Enhanced Th1 activity and development of chronic enterocolitis in mice devoid of Stat3 in macro-phages and neutrophils. *Immunity* 1999; 10: 39-49

[32] Deitch, E; Specian, E; Steffen, E; Berg, R. Translocation of *Lactobacillus murinus* from the gastrointestinal tract. *Curr. Microbiol.* 1990;20, 177–184.

[33] Hamann, L; El-Samalouti, V; Ulmer, AJ; Flad, HD; Rietschel, ET. Components of gut bacteria as immunomodulators. *Int. J. Food Microbiol.* 1998; 41:141-154

In: Focus on Nutrition Research
Editor: Tony P. Starks, pp. 207-222
ISBN 1-59454-768-8
© 2006 Nova Science Publishers, Inc.

Chapter IX

Advances in the Diagnosis and Treatment of Feeding Disorders in Children with Developmental Disabilities

Steven M. Schwarz[1], William McCarthy and Mimi N. Ton
State University of New York Downstate College of Medicine
Department of Pediatrics,Long Island College Hospital
Brooklyn, New York, USA

Abstract

Feeding difficulties, secondary nutritional deficiencies and growth failure frequently complicate management and heighten morbidity for infants, children and adults with developmental disabilities. Oral-motor dysfunction, poor coordination of swallowing, esophageal motility disorders and aversive feeding behaviors represent common problems that comprise significant obstacles to growth, hinder the achievement of developmental potential and increase dependency upon both acute and chronic healthcare resources. The association between feeding disorders and significant malnutrition has been reported in up to 90% of non-ambulatory children with cerebral palsy. Failure to assess and treat these problems in a timely fashion results in malnutrition and growth failure, maximizes the risk of feeding-related complications, increases hospitalization rates and contributes to impaired quality of life. In the present monograph, we consider the background and significance of feeding disorders in children with disabilities, and review our proposed diagnostic and therapeutic algorithm for managing these problems.

[1] Corresponding author: Steven M. Schwarz, MD, FAAP, FACN, Professor of Pediatrics, State University of New York Downstate College of Medicine,Chairman, Department of Pediatrics,Long Island College Hospital,339 Hicks Street,Brooklyn, New York, USA 11201,Tel:718-780-1146,Fax:718-780-2569, E-mail: sschwarz@chpnet.org

The influences of diagnosis-specific management strategies on patient growth and clinical outcomes are evaluated, and newer methods for calculating energy requirements are discussed. Utilizing a diagnosis-specific approach, we recently reported our clinical experiences in a group of 79 children with moderate to severe motor and/or cognitive disabilities, who were referred for feeding problems. Our initial two-year follow-up data demonstrated that interventions directed at increasing energy intake significantly improved overall nutritional status and reduced clinical morbidity. Further clinical, nutritional and growth data were collected over a 5-year period, in 21 developmentally disabled children who required percutaneous endoscopic gastrostomy (PEG) feedings to achieve nutritional rehabilitation. At the conclusion of the monitoring period, 21 patients had undergone 109.3 patient-years of PEG feedings (mean 5.2 years, range 1-11 years). Gastrostomy feedings resulted in significant weight gain and were associated with marked improvements in body mass index (BMI) and BMI Z-scores. The data herein also confirm our earlier observations, suggesting that reductions in feeding-associated morbidity and acute care hospitalization rates occurred as a consequence of aggressive nutritional management. The significance of these findings for subsequent treatment of feeding disorders in developmentally disabled children is discussed.

Introduction

The increasing prevalence of major motor and cognitive disabilities in childhood, a consequence in part of improved survival rates for very low birth weight infants, has resulted in significant home and institution-based healthcare burdens. Although exact frequency data regarding co-morbid conditions occurring in special needs populations are not available, published reports suggest that major gastrointestinal problems occur in 80-90% of developmentally challenged children and adults. [1] Disabled children are at particularly increased risk for developing feeding difficulties leading to suboptimal energy intake and secondary nutrient deficiencies. In children with a diagnosis of cerebral palsy, for example, clinical evidence of malnutrition has been reported in up to 90% of non-ambulatory subjects. [2] Feeding problems often arise as a consequence of poor oral motor coordination, swallowing dysfunction and esophageal dysmotility. [3-6] Complications (e.g. aspiration pneumonia, esophagitis) limit growth, reduce developmental potential and negatively impact life quality for both patients and families. As a consequence, these disorders demand significant consumption of healthcare and allied specialty resources.

Gastroesophageal reflux (GER), oral motor dysfunction and aversive feeding behaviors have been observed with high frequency in patients with major motor and cognitive disabilities. [7-10] Together, these functional disorders comprise the major feeding abnormalities observed in disabled subjects. As indicated above, failure to assess and treat these feeding problems in a timely fashion will hasten the onset of significant nutrient deficits, heighten the incidence of feeding disorder-related complications, increase hospitalization rates and costs of care. [11,12] The data reviewed herein will discuss current approaches to both evaluating and managing feeding disorders in children with neurodevelopmental disabilities, and the importance of effective medical/surgical interventions on growth and clinical outcomes will be discussed.

Definitions and Clinical Presentation

Feeding disorders in children with developmental disabilities have been described using a variety of terminologies. For descriptive purposes, commonly encountered problems may be subdivided into three major diagnostic categories, shown in Table I:

1. *Oropharyngeal dysphagia*. This descriptive term comprises problems related to oral motor function and swallowing efficiency and includes abnormalities of deglutition, such as poor liquid and/or solid oral bolus formation, ineffective propulsion and poor swallowing coordination. [13] Oropharyngeal dysphagia encompasses oral motor functional disorders (abnormalities in sucking, chewing and lingual movement), swallowing discoordination (with or without laryngeal penetration) and pharyngoesophageal dyskinesia.

2. *Gastroesophageal reflux (GER)*. GER is a common problem encountered in developmentally normal infants and children. However, it occurs with markedly increased frequency and severity in disabled patients, persisting well into later childhood in this population. In fact, recently published data demonstrated that GER was the most prevalent condition associated with food refusal and suboptimal nutrient consumption in a group of 349 children with neurodevelopmental abnormalities, including patients with primary diagnoses of cerebral palsy, trisomy 21 and autism. [14] GER involves the retrograde propulsion of gastric contents into the esophagus, and it is often associated with delayed esophageal acid clearance, both in normal and in neurologically impaired children. In developmentally disabled subjects (often with diminished gag reflex responses), GER may also be associated with laryngeal penetration, nasopharyngeal and tracheal aspiration of the acid refluxate.

3. *Aversive feeding behaviors*. Encountered commonly in children with primary diagnoses of autism or pervasive developmental delay, aversive feeding problems include behavioral disorders that are neither structurally nor solely neurologically founded, as well as sensory-based feeding problems. These neurobehavioral disorders involve food refusal unrelated to oropharyngeal dysphagia and/or GER.

Two broad neurodevelopmental diagnostic groups generally typify children with disabilities and nutritional problems. The first group includes patients who demonstrate significant motor impairment, often accompanied by cognitive deficits. The largest number of these children is assigned the diagnosis of idiopathic cerebral palsy-mental retardation. Here, nutritional deficiencies are commonly associated with poor oral motor coordination and swallowing disorders. Accordingly, oropharyngeal dysphagia and GER represent the most prevalent feeding-related problems. [15] Typical symptoms in affected individuals include excessive drooling leading to ineffective oral feedings (oropharyngeal dysphagia), post-prandial emesis (GER) and feeding-associated irritability (both diagnostic categories). Caregivers report problems such as prolonged meal times, coughing or gagging during meals and feeding refusal (secondary to dyspepsia with or without esophagitis). The most frequently encountered nutritional complications in affected patients are consequences of inadequate energy intake and micronutrient deficiencies. [16] Problems directly related to swallowing abnormalities and/or dysmotility include laryngotracheal aspiration, esophagitis and esophageal stricture formation. GER-related reactive airway disease may develop secondary to microaspiration of gastric contents. In an experimental cat model, altered pulmonary function may also result from a reflexive increase in airway resistance, secondary to acid reflux into the mid-esophagus without tracheal aspiration. [17] The second major diagnostic group of disabled children with associated feeding problems includes patients with autism and pervasive developmental delay. Typically, gross motor deficits associated with these diagnoses are minor, if present at all. While GER-related problems must also be considered in this population [14], feeding and nutritional problems commonly occur secondary to behavioral food refusal or sensory-based textural aversions. In both patient groups described above, macro- and micronutrient deficiencies have been reported, although significant clinical evidence of malnutrition is more common in children with severe motor impairments. [2]

Evaluation and Treatment

The importance of feeding and nutritional problems in developmentally disabled children has been established in large population studies. For example, prospective data collected from 14,000 births enrolled in the Avon (UK) Longitudinal Study of Parents and Children identified 33 infants diagnosed with cerebral palsy. [18] In these infants, a weak suck was reported at four weeks of age in nearly 50%, and feeding problems at four weeks were highly predictive for subsequent swallowing dysfunction and undernutrition by four to eight years of age. In a review of the Oxford (UK) Register of Early Childhood Impairments, 93% of children with disabilities carried a diagnosis of cerebral palsy and nearly 50% were non-ambulatory. [9] Children with moderate to severe neurodevelopmental disabilities commonly manifested feeding problems, with persistent vomiting described in 22%, choking with feeds in 56% and prolonged feeding times in 28% of affected children. In this review, parents and other caregivers used adjectives such as stressful and unenjoyable to describe mealtimes.

Recent clinical data from the UK demonstrate that only 20% of neurologically impaired children achieved 100% of the estimated average requirement for energy intake. [16] These results also confirmed the direct relationship between the severity of motor impairment and degree of nutritional and growth deficits. Clearly, feeding disorders that commence during infancy are associated with subsequent growth failure and long-term difficulties with self-feeding; and these are problems are predictive for adverse developmental outcomes. [18,19] However, when feeding disorders are recognized early in life, prompt diagnostic evaluation and nutritional intervention may avoid feeding-associated complications and maximize the potential for growth. Thus, in one study of 51 children with cerebral palsy, supplemental tube feedings led to maximum linear growth only when nutritional intervention commenced within six months of the primary neurological insult. [20] In children for whom nutritional rehabilitation began after eight years of age, linear growth did not approach catch-up levels, despite the achievement of significant weight gain.

Since malnutrition in infants and children with neurodevelopmental disabilities often arises insidiously and is progressive over time, recording of energy intake and assessment of nutritional status in at-risk patients should be should be carried out monthly during the first year of life and at least yearly thereafter. Feeding patterns and problems of deglutition and/or emesis should also be addressed during each routine healthcare visit. Interval histories should include information regarding the duration of mealtimes, presence of the feeding-related symptoms and, in toddlers and in older children, occurrence of any specific food preferences or aversions. Once a feeding disorder is suspected, previous studies have shown that an aggressive diagnostic and therapeutic approach to these problems will offer the greatest likelihood to prevent significant malnutrition and to effect successful nutritional rehabilitation. [15,21-23] A multidisciplinary team approach should involve physicians, nurses, behavioral specialists, speech-language pathologists, feeding therapists and parents as caregivers, in order to increase the potential for improved clinical outcomes.

Nutritional Assessment

We have previously reported our experiences in evaluating and treating feeding problems in a group of 79 children with moderate to severe developmental disabilities. [15] Similar to earlier investigations discussed above, the severity of malnutrition in these children correlated with their degree of neurodevelopmental impairment. The most severely compromised, non-ambulatory patients exhibited varying degrees of spasticity associated with either diplegia or quadriplegia. Nutritional assessments of these children, including anthropometric measurements, indicated poor subcutaneous tissue stores as evidence of chronic malnutrition. Specifically, overall nutritional status was evaluated by calculating Z-scores for weight and height. The Z-scores for height and weight are defined as:

$$Z = (x - X) \div \sigma,$$

where x equals the patient's weight or height measurement, X equals the age-specific population mean value derived from United States National Center for Health Statistics (NCHS) data, and σ represents the standard deviation for the particular measurement and cohort. This Z-score equation may be employed when evaluating growth variables that follow a normal or near-normal distribution pattern in selected populations. Because of the prevalence of genetic disorders associated with impaired linear growth in severely disabled patients, these Z-score values may not be normally distributed in our study population. Accordingly, in our recent long-term follow-up study, described below, body mass index (BMI) Z-scores were measured. [24] Age-specific median values for BMI, however, may also be skewed in healthy populations. As a result, published NCHS normative data for BMI Z-scores employ a Box-Cox transformation to remove skewness and transform these values to a nearly normal distribution. [25] This is known as the LMS technique [26] and is defined by the equation:

$$Z = (x \div M)^L - (1 \div LS)$$

where x = patient BMI, M = age-specific population median value, L = Box-Cox transformation, and S = coefficient of variation.

While Z-scores indicate relative nutritional status compared to age-matched population norms, triceps and subscapular skin-fold thickness measurements are utilized to determine fat and lean body mass, in order to estimate body composition and gauge the short-term effects of nutritional management. Additional screening studies include determinations of micronutrient levels in plasma, especially calcium, phosphorous and vitamin D. Recent studies have shown that intake of micronutrients are inadequate and may contribute to osteopenia and pathological fractures in non-ambulatory children. [27] The combined anthropometric and biochemical assessment information is then used to estimate specific energy requirements (see below) and plan the course of nutritional rehabilitation.

Diagnostic and Therapeutic Approaches

In our published series of disabled children referred for feeding and nutritional assessments, [15] GER was the most prevalent feeding disorder and affected 56% of subjects (Table II).

This finding is consistent with previously published data in disabled children and adults, where rates of pathologic GER as high as 70% have been reported. [28,29] Videofluoroscopic swallowing studies demonstrated abnormal swallowing kinetics (i.e. oropharyngeal dysphagia) in 26% of our patients. All children in this series who exhibited these functional feeding disorders also manifested significant motor disabilities. Finally, 18% of children in this patient cohort presented for evaluation and management of aversive feeding behaviors. No patient in this diagnostic group (pervasive developmental delay was the most common primary diagnosis) suffered disabling motor abnormalities, and all children demonstrated normal swallowing and gastroesophageal function. Based upon these data, an algorithmic model for evaluating and managing feeding disorders in developmentally disabled children has been proposed (Figure 1). This approach will be discussed below, in the context of describing specific therapeutic alternatives.

Feeding and Swallowing Evaluation

Following completion of the initial history and dietary assessment, a trained speech-language pathologist evaluates children with suspected aversive feeding behaviors. Observation of feeding patterns and identification of any behavioral and sensory-based solid/liquid or textural preferences will identify problems with swallowing function that might indicate the need for additional diagnostic studies. If swallowing problems are suspected during the initial speech-language evaluation, a videofluoroscopic swallowing study (VFSS, also referred to as the modified barium swallow) may be used to identify mechanisms of solid and liquid bolus formation and retrograde bolus propulsion. We perform this study in most children with moderate to severe disabilities who are referred for feeding evaluations. The VFSS will determine the occurrence of aspiration and/or laryngeal penetration (a precursor to aspiration), identify problems related to swallowing thin vs. thickened liquids and assess difficulties with solid food intake. This study is especially important for patients who are non-ambulatory or who manifest signs of progressive supranuclear palsy, since "silent" aspiration of thin and/or thickened liquids is a common finding in these patients. [8,30] The VFSS may also provides some information regarding esophageal peristalsis, although dysmotility syndromes (Table I) and delayed esophageal clearance (except as a consequence of GER) have not been reported with great frequency in neurodevelopmentally impaired children.

Table 1. Classification of common feeding disorders in children with developmental disabilities

Oropharyngeal dysphagia

Poor bolus formation
- thin liquids
- thickened liquids
- solids

Impaired retrograde propulsion
- thin liquids
- thickened liquids
- solids

Laryngeal penetration (± aspiration)
- thin liquids
- thickened liquids

Pharyngoesophageal dyskinesia (± aspiration)
- Gastroesophageal reflux
- With aspiration
- Without aspiration

Aversive feeding behaviors
- Behavioral
- Neurological-behavioral
- Sensory-based

Table II. Feeding disorders in 79 children with developmental disabilities.

Feeding Disorder	Number (%)
Gastroesophageal reflux	44 (56)
Oropharyngeal dysphagia	21 (26)
Aversive feeding behaviors	14 (18)

(modified from Schwarz SM, et al. *Pediatrics* 2001, 108; 671-676.)

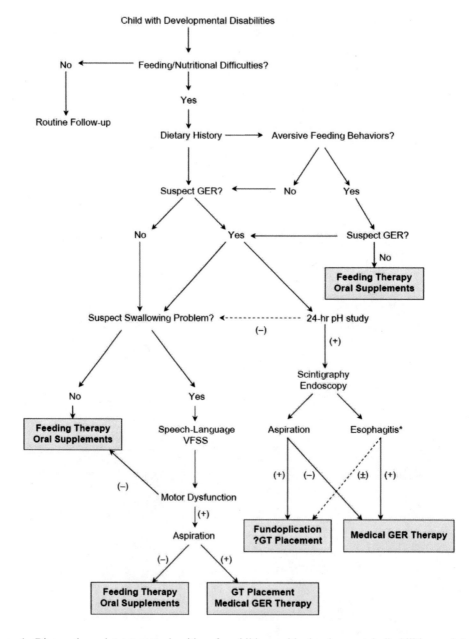

Figure 1. Diagnostic and treatment algorithm for children with developmental disabilities and feeding problems (modified from Schwarz SM et al. Pediatrics 2001; 108: 671-676).

A recently described procedure that employs fiberoptic endoscopy to evaluate swallowing function in pediatric patients may contribute to our diagnostic capabilities without requiring x-ray exposure. [31] Should the swallowing study demonstrate oropharyngeal aspiration, primary endoscopic placement of a gastrostomy tube is generally indicated. Exceptions to this treatment plan include laryngeal aspiration for thin liquids only with normal thickened liquid swallowing kinetics, as well as evidence of laryngeal penetration that is dependent upon feeding position. Here, appropriate guidance with respect to diet and feeding technique, together with feeding therapy (usually conducted on a weekly or twice per week basis) will significantly reduce the risk for aspiration. In those cases with oropharyngeal dysphagia where *PO* feedings are maintained, close follow-up is required in order to screen for any subsequent deterioration in oral motor coordination, heralding the need for gastrostomy placement. On the other hand, for some malnourished patients whose oral intake is initially limited to thickened formula, we have observed that improved nutritional status and ongoing feeding therapy may result in improved swallowing function for thin liquids.

Evaluation and Treatment of GER

Our data and the findings of other groups have confirmed the high incidence of GER in this patient cohort. In patients with suspected GER, routine evaluation includes 24-hr intraesophageal pH monitoring, esophagogastroduodenoscopy, and ^{99}Technetium-sulfur colloid milk scintigraphy to detect aspiration. Fundoplication will be absolutely required as first-line therapy only for those patients who demonstrate GER-associated aspiration, and surgery may be recommended for children manifesting moderate to severe esophagitis. Even for the patient with esophagitis, however, intensive nutritional support and a pharmacologic trial of acid blockade (either H_2-receptor antagonists or proton pump inhibitors) are warranted prior to referring patients for fundoplication. In fact, one study demonstrated a significant, objective improvement in GER, evaluated by pH monitoring, following nutritional rehabilitation of disabled children. [32] Medical management of GER includes, as its cornerstone, the use of acid blocking medications. Both H_2-receptor antagonists and proton pump inhibitors may effect some increase in lower esophageal sphincter tone, mediated via the trophic effects of increased circulating gastrin levels following inhibition of the acid-regulated gastrin negative feedback loop. However, the primary pharmacological effects of these agents involve reduced gastric hydrochloric acid secretion, and their major therapeutic role is to ameliorate dyspepsia, prevent acid-induced esophageal injury and accelerate healing of esophagitis. The use of prokinetic agents remains a controversial therapeutic alternative. Before the introduction of cisapride (Propulsid™), urecholine (Bethanacol™) and metoclopramide (Reglan™) were the most commonly prescribed prokinetics. Although the latter two agents appear to reduce the frequency and duration of GER episodes during pH monitoring, no clear evidence has supported their clinical superiority to conservative management and gastric acid reduction. After its introduction and prior to its market withdrawal because of potential cardiac side effects, cisapride was the most widely prescribed prokinetic agent used for management of GER associated disease n the United States. This agent exerts gastrointestinal motility changes that are mediated via 5-HT_4 receptors and/or enhanced release of acetylcholine. In 1999, a position paper by the European Society of Pediatric Gastroenterology, Hepatology and Nutrition reviewed available safety and efficacy data and concluded that cisapride was the most effective prokinetic studied to date, with a wide safety profile across all age groups. [33] Conversely, a recent, systematic review of the drug challenged the validity of these clinical trials. [34] Thus, while cisapride does appear to reduce the reflux index (i.e. the percent time of pH less than 4) during pH monitoring, convincing evidence that supports its clinical effectiveness is lacking. In any case, because of concerns regarding its potential cardiotoxicity (limited, to date, to identifiable at-risk patients), the drug is largely unavailable in this country, except on a compassionate use basis. The macrolide antibiotic erythromycin may present another alternative for GER management, particularly when reflux is associated with prolonged gastric emptying times. Erythromycin acts as a motilin receptor agonist in the gastrointestinal tract, when used in sub-antimicrobial doses; and, both animal and human studies have demonstrated a prokinetic effect. In the pediatric population, studies in pre-term infants have shown beneficial effects of erythromycin in promoting tolerance to enteral feedings or enhancing motility. [35]

When considering gastrostomy alone (i.e. without fundoplication) as primary therapy for feeding disorders in disabled children, earlier reports have suggested that gastrostomy placement, *per se*, may be associated with development or exacerbation of GER. [36,37] However, recent studies have refuted this argument; [38,39] and, in our prospective series, no patient who received a gastrostomy alone (without fundoplication) required anti-reflux surgery during a two-year follow-up period. [15]

Other Therapies

For children without a clinical history suggesting GER and without evidence of aspiration during the VFSS, oral nutritional supplements, using defined formula diets, may be sufficient intervention to improve nutritional status. Management of aversive feeding behaviors will also require feeding therapy directed at overcoming food refusal, treating sensory-based eating disorders and assuring adequate nutrient intake. Because of its significance in neurodevelopmentally disabled children, GER should be considered with a high index of suspicion, particularly in patients with oral motor problems and without complaints of vomiting, as well as for children with aversive feeding behaviors that may result from subclinical reflux with secondary esophagitis.

Nutritional Requirements

Feeding disorders continue to represent significant barriers to improving positive, long-term clinical outcomes for disabled children, despite the fact that well-established diagnostic and therapeutic methods are available to evaluate and treat both behavioral and neurological-structural problems. The diagnostic-treatment algorithm shown in Figure 1 indicates diagnosis-specific interventions that limit the occurrence of feeding-associated complications and improve the likelihood for achieving nutritional rehabilitation. After developing strategies for addressing functional and behavioral feeding disorders, optimal management of children with disabilities depends upon accurately determining nutritional requirements, aimed at achieving appropriate body mass and maximizing growth potential. However, conventional mathematical formulas for estimating steady-state energy expenditure, including the Harris-Benedict and World Health Organization equations, may be inaccurate in this clinical setting. These equations are based upon the age, gender, weight and height of developmentally normal subjects; and, they often overestimate energy expenditure in disabled patients, particularly those who are non-ambulatory. [5,40] For example, in children and adolescents with spastic quadriplegia, prior studies have shown that the mean ratio between total energy expenditure and resting energy expenditure (TEE:REE) is significantly lower than the mean ratio in normal controls. The TEE:REE ratio is also lower in adequately nourished quadriplegic children than the average value in poorly nourished subjects manifesting similar neurodevelopmental disabilities. [5] Furthermore, TEE may be reduced as a consequence of physical immobility, particularly in quadriplegic patients. [41,42] These problems may be even more complex in nutritionally growth stunted children, where evidence suggests that endogenous fat oxidation is impaired. Therefore, after instituting effective management strategies to treat feeding disorders, reduced steady-state energy expenditure of growth impaired, non-ambulatory children may actually increase the likelihood of excessive weight gain and subsequent obesity. [42]

To account for these unique problems related to estimating nutritional requirements in non-ambulatory subjects, prior studies have proposed modified calculations of energy requirements. Corrected estimates of basal metabolic rates or the recommended daily allowance (RDA) for energy intake provided by the United States National Research Council (for patients without disabling motor impairments) consider factors such as muscle tone, movement and activity to determine requirements for non-ambulatory patients. [43-45] Newer equations for predicting energy expenditure, based upon estimates of fat-free body mass (FFM) derived from skin-fold thickness measurements, have recently been proposed for non-ambulatory, adult patients by Dickerson et al. [40] For these institutionalized, quadriplegic subjects, REE may be accurately expressed by the equation:

$$REE \text{ (kcal/d)} = [22.3 \times FFM \text{ (kg)}] - [9.4 \times Age \text{ (y)}] + 557$$

For patients who retained spontaneous upper extremity movement, a more "classical" estimate of energy expenditure (i.e. Harris-Benedict equation) was found to be an appropriate tool for establishing energy requirments. [40]

Outcomes and Conclusion

Few available studies have examined long-term clinical outcomes of nutritional intervention for children with neurodevelopmental disabilities. Investigations in disabled adult patients have shown that management strategies aimed at reducing complications from swallowing disorders may be life-sustaining. Thus, in one report, unadjusted Kaplan-Meier curves indicated that institutionalized patients with feeding tubes were significantly (p<0.001) less likely to die than were subjects without feeding tubes, when followed for two years. [46] For children with neurodevelopmental disabilities, goals of nutritional management should include improving nutritional status, reducing feeding related complications, decreasing costs of care and, where feasible, maximizing overall level of functioning. Previous work has demonstrated that motor and cognitively impaired children who receive comprehensive, multidisciplinary nutritional services are adequately nourished and achieve nutritional intakes that meet estimated requirements. [17] In severely disabled children with cerebral palsy and oropharyngeal dysphagia, tube feedings improve quality of life indicators, both for the child and for the caregiver. [47] Gastrostomy tube (GT) feedings have been associated with late complications, including extruded or "buried" tubes, gastric metaplasia adjacent to the GT site, and gastric mucosal ulceration. [48] While these problems must be considered when contemplating GT insertion, our experience indicates that the benefits gained from assuring adequate nutriture via GT far outweigh the inherent risks from long-term, indwelling feeding tubes.

Gastrostomy tube feedings have been shown to be associated with a decrease in the severity of GER symptoms in neurologically impaired children, and they may also reduce the need for anti-reflux surgery. In our earlier report, the efficacy of GT feedings alone for nutritional management in disabled children with swallowing dysfunction, with or without GER, was confirmed. [15] Recently, we reviewed long-term nutritional outcomes following percutaneous endoscopic gastrostomy (PEG) placement (without fundoplication) for the management of disability-related feeding disorders. At the conclusion of a mean 5-year post-PEG monitoring period, comprising 109.3 patient-years, BMI and BMI Z-scores improved significantly, demonstrating the efficacy of this method of nutrition support (Table III).

As an important corollary to observed effects on nutritional status, examining the influences of therapy on co-morbidities related to feeding disorders must also be used to assess the clinical consequences of these diagnosis-specific interventions. Problems such as aspiration pneumonia, feeding-associated hypoxemia, reactive airway disease and bedsores secondary to immobility and nutritional deficiencies significantly increase acute-care hospitalizations and the costs of care. In our recent follow-up study, the acute-care hospitalization rate decreased from 0.4 hospital admissions per patient-year in the two years prior to nutritional intervention, to 0.15 admissions per patient-year over the two years following commencement of diagnosis-specific therapy (p<0.01). [15] Based upon an average length of stay of approximately five days for children admitted to our hospital (frequently longer for children with developmental disabilities), at least 180 hospital days were saved over a two-year period, for this group of 79 children.

Table III. Body Mass Index (BMI) measurements 5.2 ± 2.5 years following percutaneous endoscopic gastrostomy placement in 21 children with developmental disabilities

Measurement	N	Initial (m±sd)	Final (m±sd)	p-value
BMI	21	12.6±2.7	16.2±2.4	<0.05
Z-score (BMI)	21	-3.7±1.8	-0.7±1.6	<0.05

At a time when costs of care are a major concern for practitioners, clinical departments and healthcare administrators in the U.S., management strategies are judged not only by their effects on immediate clinical status and long-term morbidity, but also by the impact of diagnostic and treatment protocols on the utilization of limited and diminishing financial resources. Prompt diagnosis and appropriate management of feeding disorders certainly enhance long-term clinical outcomes and improve quality of life measures for children with neurodevelopmental disabilities. Importantly (and, not surprisingly), effective management strategies may also obviate repeated and prolonged hospitalizations that have characterized this challenging patient population. As a consequence, appropriate diagnostic and therapeutic approaches, directed at ameliorating feeding disorder-related complications, will reduce the financial burdens on families, healthcare providers and institutions providing long-term care for children with major motor and cognitive impairments.

References

[1]   Chong SK. Gastrointestinal problems in the handicapped child. *Curr Opin Pediatr 2001*; 13:441-446

[2]   Dahl M, Thommessen M, Rasmussen M, Selberg T. Feeding and nutritional characteristics in children with moderate or severe cerebral palsy. *Acta Paediatr 1996*; 6: 697-701

[3]   Reilly S, Skuse D, Poblete X. Prevalence of feeding problems and oral motor dysfunction in children with cerebral palsy: a community survey, *J Pediatr 1996*; 6: 877-882

[4]   Gisel EG, Birnbaum R, Schwartz S. Feeding impairments in children: diagnosis and effective intervention. *Int J Orofacial Myology 1998*; 24: 27-33

[5]   Stallings VA, Zemel BS, Davies JC, Cronk CE, Charney EB. Energy expenditure of children and adolescents with severe disabilities: a cerebral palsy model. *Am J Clin Nutr 1996*; 4: 627-34

[6]   Rempel GR, Colwell SO, Nelson RP. Growth in children with cerebral palsy fed via gastrostomy. *Pediatrics 1988*; 82: 857-862

[7]   Waterman ET, Koltai PJ, Downey JC, Cacace AT. Swallowing disorders in a population of children with cerebral palsy. *Int J Pediatr Otolaryngol 1992*; 24: 63-71

[8]   Rogers B, Arvedson J, Buck G, Smart P, Msall M. Charactersitics of dysphagia in children with cerebral palsy. *Dysphagia 1994*; 9: 69-73

[9]   Sullivan PB, Lambert B, Rose M, Ford-Adams M, Johnson A, Griffiths P. Prevalence and severity of feeding and nutritional problems in children with neurological impairments: Oxford Feeding Study. *Dev Med Child Neurol 2000*; 42: 674-680

[10]   Burklow KA, Phelps AN, Schultz JR, McConnell K, Rudolph C. Classifying complex pediatric feeding disorders. *J Pediatr Gastroeneterol Nutr 1998*; 27: 143-147

[11]   Morton RE, Wheatley R, Minford J. Respiratory tract infections due to direct and reflux aspiration in children with severe neurodisability. *Dev Med Child Neurol 1999*; 41: 329-334

[12]   Toder DS. Respiratory problems in the adolescent with developmental delay. *Adolesc Med 2000*; 11: 617-631

[13]   Lefton-Greif MA, Crawford TO, Winkelstein JA, Loughlin GM, Koerner CB, Zaburak M, Lederman HM. Oropharyngeal dysphagia and aspiration in patients with ataxia-telangiectasia. *J Pediatr 2000*; 136: 225-231

[14]   Field D, Garland M, Williams K. Correlates of specific childhood feeding problems. *J Paediatr Child Health 2003*; 39:299-304

[15]   Schwarz SM, Corredor J, Fisher-Medina J, Cohen J,Rabinowitz S. Diagnosis and treatment of feeding disorders in children with developmental disabilities. *Pediatrics 2001*; 108: 671-676

[16]   Sullivan PB, Juszczak E, Lambert BR, Rose M, Ford-Adams ME, Johnson A. Impact of feeding problems on nutritional intake and growth: Oxford feeding study II. *Dev Med Child Neurol 2002*; 44:461-467

[17]   Boyle JT, Tuchman DN, Altschuler SM, Nixon TE, Pack AI, Cohen S. Mechanisms for the association of gastroesophageal reflux and bronchospasm. *Am Rev Respir Dis 1985*; 31: S16-20

[18]   Motion S, Northstone K, Edmond A, Stucke S, Golding J. Early feeding problems in children with cerebral palsy: weight and neurodevelopmental outcomes. *Dev Med Child Neurol 2002*; 44: 40-43

[19]   Stallings VA, Charney EB, Davies JC, Cronk CE. Nutritional status and growth of children with diplegic or hemiplegic cerebral palsy. *Dev Med Child Neurol 1993*; 35: 997-1006

[20]   Sanders KD, Cox K, Cannon R, Blanchard D, Pitcher J, Papathakis P, et al. Growth response to enteral feeding by children with cerebral palsy. *J Parenter Enteral Nutr 1990*; 14: 23-26

[21]   Pesce KA, Wodarski LA, Wang M. Nutritional status of institutionalized children and adolescents with developmental disabilities. *Res Dev Disabil 1989*; 10: 33-52

[22]   Rogers B, Stratton P, Msall M, Andres M, Champlain MK, Koerner P, Piazza J. Long-term morbidity and management strategies of tracheal aspiration in adults with severe developmental disabilities. *Am J Ment Retard 1994*; 98: 490-498

[23]   Brant CQ, Stanich P, Ferrari AP Jr. Improvement in children's nutritional status after enteral feeding by PEG: and interim report. *Gastrointest Endosc 1999*; 50: 183-188

[24]   Schwarz SM, McCarthy W, Ton M. Long-term nutritional effects following percutaneous endoscopic gastrostomy in children with developmental disabilities. *Pediatr Res 2005*. in press (abstract)

[25] Box GE, Cox DR. An analysis of transformations. *Journal of the Royal Statistical Society* 1964; 26:211–252

[26] Cole TJ. The LMS method for constructing normalized growth standards. *European Journal of Clinical Nutrition 1990*; 44:45–60

[27] Duncan B, Barton LL, Lloyd J, Marks-Katz M. Dietary considerations in osteopenia in tube-fed nonambulatory children with cerebral palsy. *Clin Pediatr 1999*; 38: 133-137

[28] Bohmer CJ, Niezen-de Boer MC, Klinkenberg-Knol EC, Deville WL, Nadorp JH, Meuwissen SG. The prevalence of gastroesophageal reflux in institutionalized intellectually disabled individuals. *Am J Gastroenterol 1999*; 94: 804-810

[29] Puntis JW, Thwaites R, Abel G, Stringer MD. Children with neurological disorders do not always need fundoplication concomitant with percutaneous endoscopic gastrostomy. *Dev Med Child Neurol 2000*; 42: 97-99

[30] Litvan I, Sastry N, Sonies BC. Characterizing swallowing abnormalities in progressive supranuclear palsy. *Neurology 1997*; 48: 1654-62

[31] Hartnick CJ, Hartley BE, Miller C, Willging JP. Pediatric fiberoptic endoscopic evaluation of swallowing. *Ann Otol Rhinol Laryngol 2000*; 109: 996-999

[32] Lewis D, Khoshoo V, Pencharz PB, Golladay ES. Impact of nutritional rehabilitation on gastroesophageal reflux in neurologically impaired children. *J Pediatr Surg 1994*; 29: 167-169

[33] Vandenplas Y, Belli DC, Benatar A, Cadranel S, Cucchiara S, Dupont C, Gottrand F, et al. The role of Cisapride in the treatment of pediatric gastroesophageal reflux. *J Pediatr Gatroenterol Nutr 1999*; 28: 518-528

[34] Bourke B, Drumm B. Cochrane's epitaph for cisapride in childhood gastro-esophageal reflux. *Arch Dis Child 2002*; 86: 71-72

[35] Ng PC, So KW, Fung KSC, Lee CH, Fok TF, Wong E. Randomised controlled study of oral erythromycin for treatment of gastrointestinal dysmotility in preterm infants *Arch Dis Child Fetal Neonatal Ed 2001*; 84:F177-F182

[36] Mollitt DL, Golladay ES, Seibert JJ. Symptomatic gastroesophageal reflux following gastrostomy in neurologically impaired patients. *Pediatrics 1985*; 75: 1124-1126

[37] Berezin S, Schwarz SM, Newman LJ, Halata M. Gastroesophageal reflux secondary to gastrostomy tube placement. *Am J Dis Child 1986*; 140: 699-701

[38] Borowitz SM, Sutphen JL, Hutcheson RL. Percutaneous endoscopic gastrostomy without an antireflux procedure in neurologically disabled children, *Clin Pediatr 1997*; 36: 25-29

[39] Puntis JW, Thwaites R, Abel G, Stringer MD. Children with neurological disorders do not always need fundoplication concomitant with percutaneous endoscopic gastrostomy. *Dev Med Child Neurol 2000*; 42: 97-99

[40] Dickerson RN, Brown RO, Gervasio JG, Hak EB, Hak LJ, Williams JE. Measured energy expenditure of tube-fed patients with severe neurodevelopmental disabilities. *J Am Coll Nutr 1999*; 18: 61-68

[41] Chad KE, McKay HA, Zello GA, Bailey DA, Failkener RA, Snyder RE. Body composition in nutritionally adequate ambulatory and non-ambulatory children with cerebral palsy and a healthy reference group. *Dev Med Child Neurol 2000*; 42: 334-339

[42] Hoffman DJ, Sawaya AL, Verreschi I, Tucker KL, Roberts SB. Whay are nutritionally stunted children at increased risk of obesity? Studies of metabolic rate and fat oxidation in shantytown children from Sao Paulo, Brazil. *Am J Clin Nutr 2000*; 72: 702-707

[43] National Research Council, Food and Nutrition Board. Recommended dietary allowances. 10th ed. Washington, DC: National Academy Press, 1989

[44] Cully WJ, Middleton TO. Caloric requirements of mentally retarded children with and without motor dysfunction. *J Pediatr 1969*; 75: 380-386

[45] Krick J, Murphy PE, Markham JF, Shapiro BK. A proposed formula for calculating energy needs of children with cerebral palsy. *Dev Med Child Neurol 1992*; 34: 81-487

[46] Rudberg MA, Egleston, BL, Grant MD, Brody JA. Effectiveness of feeding tubes in nursing home residents with swallowing disorders. *J Parenter Enteral Nutr 2000*; 24: 97-102

[47] Smith SW, Camfield C, Camfield P. Living with cerebral palsy and tube feeding: A population-based follow-up study. *J Pediatr 1999*; 135: 307-310

[48] Mathus-Vliegen, Koning H, Taminiau JAJ, Moorman-Voestermans CGM. Percutaneous endoscopic gastrostomy and gastrojejunostomy in psychomotor retarded subjects: a follow-up covering 106 patient years. *J Pediatr Gastroenterol Nutr 2001*; 33: 488-494

Index

A

access, 90, 116, 169, 203
acclimatization, 190
accumulation, 39, 47, 63, 124, 156, 167, 180, 181, 183
acetylcholine, 12, 216
achievement, x, 207, 211
acid, viii, 11, 15, 18, 19, 24, 29, 30, 33, 35, 36, 39, 42, 43, 44, 45, 48, 49, 50, 51, 52, 53, 54, 55, 56, 57, 58, 59, 60, 61, 63, 65, 66, 67, 68, 69, 70, 112, 131, 148, 167, 169, 170, 177, 178, 188, 190, 192, 198, 200, 209, 210, 215
acquired immunity, 198, 205
activation, x, 43, 125, 129, 130, 131, 133, 134, 138, 181, 184, 188, 189, 201, 202, 203
active oxygen, 183
active site, 168
active transport, 181
activity level, ix, 71, 132
adenine, 142
adenosine, 36
adenosine triphosphate, 36
adhesion, 18, 198, 200
adipocyte, ix, 121, 122, 123, 127
adiponectin, 127
adipose, 17, 22, 61, 69, 122, 124, 125, 126, 127, 158, 167
adipose tissue, 17, 22, 61, 69, 125, 126, 158
adiposity, ix, 121, 122, 124, 125, 126, 127, 128, 129, 137, 138, 144
adjustment, 142
administrators, 219
adolescence, 90, 116

adolescents, ix, 71, 72, 73, 90, 91, 92, 95, 97, 116, 117, 118, 120, 217, 219, 220
adult population, ix, 8, 71, 120
adulthood, 116, 182
adults, x, 5, 27, 72, 90, 94, 100, 116, 120, 156, 160, 207, 208, 212, 220
adverse event, 24
advertising, 96
affect, vii, 1, 2, 12, 21, 28, 46, 50, 53, 89, 96, 97, 117, 129, 131, 134, 151, 168, 178, 184, 188, 196, 201
Africa, 56, 63, 68
age, viii, 9, 33, 34, 35, 36, 37, 38, 42, 44, 46, 50, 65, 67, 74, 75, 76, 77, 92, 96, 145, 151, 153, 154, 156, 158, 159, 162, 190, 210, 211, 212, 216, 217
agent, 23, 25, 31, 32, 215
aggregation, viii, 25, 26, 33, 37
aging, 31, 36, 37, 45, 46, 48, 66, 67
aging process, 46
agonist, 14, 129, 132, 136, 142, 147, 148, 216
air pollutants, viii, 33
alanine, 68
albumin, 35, 38, 153
alcohol, 19, 189, 198, 200
alcohols, 23, 31
aldolase, 66
algorithm, x, 207, 214, 216
alternative, 14, 19, 94, 124, 178, 215
alternatives, 212
alters, 25, 32, 67, 68
Alzheimer's disease, 46, 47, 48
amines, 130
amino acids, 35, 50, 52, 54, 56, 57, 58, 65, 66, 67, 68, 69, 70, 145, 183
amphetamines, 129
amygdala, 143

anabolism, 166

angina, vii, 1, 2, 13, 19, 21, 22, 23

angiotensin converting enzyme, 24

animals, viii, 12, 26, 49, 50, 51, 52, 53, 54, 55, 56, 58, 59, 60, 62, 63, 64, 65, 66, 129, 130, 131, 132, 133, 166, 168, 169, 177, 178, 180, 183, 190, 198

anorexia, 126, 127, 130, 131, 134, 135, 136, 146, 147, 148, 177

ANOVA, 171, 195

antibiotic, 216

antibody, 170, 202

antigen, 189, 201, 202

antioxidant, viii, 6, 7, 9, 13, 14, 15, 19, 22, 23, 25, 27, 31, 32, 34, 35, 42, 43, 44, 45, 47

antioxidative activity, 14

antisense oligonucleotides, 125

antitumor, 188

anxiety, 90

appetite, ix, 121, 137, 140, 142, 146

aqueous solutions, 192

ARC, 124, 127, 128, 130

Argentina, v, 149, 152, 160, 161, 162

arginine, viii, 33, 42, 136, 141

argument, 216

arteries, 6, 12

artery, 6, 12, 13, 22, 28

ascorbic acid, 34, 35, 39

aspiration, 208, 209, 210, 213, 215, 216, 218, 220

aspiration pneumonia, 208, 218

assessment, 47, 157, 211, 212

association, x, 5, 7, 8, 9, 28, 35, 73, 78, 88, 89, 90, 91, 98, 151, 158, 207, 220

assumptions, 75

astrocytes, 35

ataxia, 22, 31, 220

atherogenesis, 7, 17, 18, 22

atherosclerosis, 7, 13, 14, 15, 18, 22, 23, 27, 28, 29, 31

atherosclerotic plaque, 13, 18, 23

atoms, 58

ATP, 21, 36, 56, 129

atrophy, 53, 69

attention, vii, 96

attitudes, 76, 78, 83, 97, 118

Australia, ix, 8, 69, 71, 72, 94, 95, 117, 120

autism, 209, 210

automobiles, 152

autooxidation, 39, 40

availability, 58, 96, 179

B

bacteria, 188, 189, 198, 201, 203, 204, 205

Bangladesh, 159

barium, 213

barriers, 216

behavior, 117, 118, 119, 130, 137, 141, 142, 143, 146, 147

behavioral disorders, 209

behavioral variation, 137

Beijing, 170, 204, 205

Belgium, 120

beneficial effect, 1, 6, 7, 9, 12, 13, 16, 18, 19, 21, 24, 26, 189, 216

beta-carotene, 22

beverages, ix, 2, 71

bile, 11

binding, 11, 13, 38, 44, 47, 124, 125, 128, 134, 138, 146, 151, 160, 166, 167, 168, 178, 179, 181, 183, 184, 185, 200

binding globulin, 11, 160

bioavailability, 6, 168, 177, 182, 185

biological activity, 11

biological processes, 166, 198

biological systems, viii, 34, 178

biomarkers, 37, 46

biosynthesis, 24, 26, 34, 137, 198, 200

biotic, 199, 200

birth, 182, 208

birth weight, 208

black tea, 3, 5, 6, 7, 8, 9, 27, 28

blame, 74, 75, 80, 82, 83, 98, 106

bleeding, 25

blood, 3, 6, 8, 9, 11, 12, 14, 15, 16, 18, 19, 21, 22, 25, 28, 29, 30, 34, 35, 44, 47, 51, 54, 58, 63, 66, 70, 125, 128, 137, 168, 169, 187, 190, 191, 197, 205

blood flow, 12

blood plasma, 22

blood pressure, 8, 14, 18, 19, 22, 29, 30

blood stream, 58

blood vessels, 25, 44, 47

blood-brain barrier, 137

bloodstream, vii, 7

BMI, x, 77, 78, 80, 82, 83, 85, 88, 89, 97, 98, 145, 208, 211, 212, 218, 219

body, vii, viii, ix, x, 2, 6, 15, 19, 22, 27, 33, 34, 36, 37, 45, 49, 50, 53, 54, 59, 60, 61, 66, 67, 70, 71, 72, 74, 75, 76, 77, 78, 80, 81, 82, 83, 85, 86, 87, 88, 89, 90, 94, 96, 97, 98, 100, 101, 105, 106,

112, 116, 117, 118, 120, 122, 124, 125, 126, 127, 128, 129, 130, 136, 137, 138, 142, 143, 144, 145, 146, 148, 157, 158, 166, 178, 179, 208, 211, 212, 217
body composition, 70, 212
body fat, 126, 127
body image, ix, 71, 74, 75, 77, 78, 96, 97, 117
body mass index, x, 77, 78, 97, 116, 120, 158, 208, 211
body shape, 72, 94, 97
body size, 80, 81, 82, 86, 87, 166
body weight, 36, 53, 54, 59, 60, 61, 76, 78, 83, 90, 122, 130, 136, 137, 138, 142, 143, 144, 145, 146, 148
bone marrow, 69, 180
boredom, 73, 78, 83, 88, 90
boys, 72, 74, 76, 77, 78, 79, 80, 83, 88, 89, 90, 91, 99, 116
brain, viii, 33, 34, 35, 36, 37, 38, 39, 42, 43, 45, 46, 47, 48, 122, 123, 125, 126, 128, 130, 131, 134, 136, 137, 138, 139, 140, 141, 142, 143, 144, 145, 146, 147, 148, 167, 168, 182
brainstem, 134
Brazil, 50, 66, 121, 222
breakdown, 6, 53
breakfast, 73, 103, 104
breast cancer, 67
Britain, 158
buffer, 39, 42, 56, 171, 190, 191
buildings, ix, 149, 151, 156

C

cabbage, 101
cadmium, 184, 185
caffeine, 3
calcium, 18, 25, 39, 47, 93, 151, 152, 154, 155, 158, 159, 162, 212
caloric restriction, 67
calorie, 105
campaigns, 26
cancer, 17, 19, 22, 27, 31, 35, 118, 188, 189, 203, 205
cancer cells, 203
capillary, 24
carbohydrate, 130, 141, 148, 166
carbon, 24, 34, 65
carbonyl groups, 42
carcinogenesis, 22
cardiac muscle, 53

cardiac surgery, 21, 22
cardiomyopathy, 21, 30
cardiovascular disease, vii, 1, 2, 6, 16, 17, 19, 21, 22, 23, 24, 25, 26, 27, 28, 35
cardiovascular risk, 13, 17, 18, 29
cardiovascular system, vii, 1, 2, 9
caregivers, 210, 211
Caribbean, 23
carotid arteries, 17
casein, 11, 13
cast, 6, 13, 14
catabolism, 52, 53, 56, 58, 65, 69
catecholamines, 34, 38
Catholic school, 97
cation, 165, 166, 167, 168, 177
cDNA, 171, 172
cell, viii, x, 6, 7, 13, 34, 35, 38, 39, 42, 43, 46, 48, 125, 129, 131, 166, 167, 177, 179, 180, 181, 184, 185, 187, 188, 189, 190, 191, 192, 193, 194, 195, 196, 197, 198, 200, 201, 202, 203, 205
cell culture, 180
cell death, 39, 46
cell line, 48, 197, 202
cell membranes, 35, 167
cell surface, x, 187, 188, 189, 201, 203
central nervous system, 48, 122, 136, 137, 140, 141, 143
central obesity, 132
cerebellum, 42
cerebral palsy, x, 207, 208, 209, 210, 218, 219, 220, 221, 222
cerebrospinal fluid, 127
Chad, 221
channels, 43, 46
chemiluminescence, 42
chemokine receptor, 200
chicken, 53, 102, 113, 114, 152
childhood, 208, 209, 220, 221
children, x, 24, 100, 120, 156, 203, 207, 208, 209, 210, 211, 212, 213, 214, 215, 216, 217, 218, 219, 220, 221, 222
China, 5, 165, 187, 204, 205
cholecalciferol, 150, 156, 160
cholesterol, vii, 2, 3, 5, 6, 7, 9, 10, 11, 12, 15, 16, 17, 18, 19, 22, 23, 24, 25, 26, 27, 28, 29, 44, 45, 47, 48, 200
chopping, 191
chromatography, 42, 67
chronic venous insufficiency, 25
cigarette smoking, viii, 25, 33

circadian rhythm, 132
circulation, 16, 124, 161, 180, 182
classes, 3, 38, 166
classification, 21
Classification and Regression Tree (CART), 74, 80, 85
cleavage, viii, 33, 128
clinical trials, 1, 3, 8, 10, 11, 12, 23, 24, 25, 26, 28, 216
cloning, 124, 147, 148, 168
cluster analysis, 194
CNS, 124, 125, 126, 127
CO2, 190, 191, 192, 193
coagulation, 18
coagulation factors, 18
cocaine, ix, 121, 122, 123, 127, 145
coding, 167
coefficient of variation, 212
coenzyme, vii, 1, 2, 19, 20, 23, 30, 31
cognition, 34, 95
cognitive deficit, 209
cognitive development, 182
cognitive dissonance, 94
cognitive function, 48
cognitive impairment, 35, 36, 219
cognitive performance, 34
cohort, 9, 211, 212, 215
collagen, 34, 35, 44, 47
colon, 180, 181, 188, 189, 190, 195, 197, 203, 204, 205
colon cancer, 197, 203
communication, 22, 140
community, 35, 93, 96, 97, 162, 219
competition, 11
complement, 127, 188, 190, 197
complementary DNA, 147
complexity, 136, 177
compliance, 12, 30
complications, x, 15, 21, 22, 207, 208, 210, 217, 219
components, 15, 17, 23, 25, 38, 92, 96, 180, 188, 198
composition, 3, 23, 25, 36, 59, 67, 68, 69, 70, 131, 221
compounds, vii, viii, 1, 2, 3, 10, 11, 19, 33, 35, 37
concentration, 5, 8, 17, 18, 19, 26, 35, 36, 37, 38, 40, 41, 51, 53, 58, 59, 61, 66, 124, 160, 165, 166, 168, 170, 172, 177, 178, 179, 180, 181, 191
concordance, 45, 94
conditioning, 50
confidence, 76, 77, 98, 195
confidence interval, 76, 77, 98

confounders, 99
confusion, 8, 14
congestive heart failure, 21, 30
conservation, 63
consumers, 19, 26
consumption, 2, 3, 5, 6, 7, 8, 9, 10, 11, 12, 13, 14, 15, 17, 26, 27, 28, 30, 40, 91, 92, 94, 95, 118, 130, 152, 155, 158, 208, 209
contamination, 190
control, ix, 9, 25, 37, 42, 43, 50, 51, 52, 53, 54, 56, 58, 61, 62, 63, 64, 65, 93, 106, 121, 122, 123, 124, 125, 129, 134, 138, 142, 145, 146, 148, 165, 166, 169, 171, 173, 174, 175, 177, 185, 187, 188, 190, 191, 192, 193, 195, 196, 201, 202
control group, 58, 63
controlled trials, 18
conversion, 17, 19, 34, 150, 156
cooking, 96
coping, 117
copper, 38, 39, 42, 47, 183, 185
corn, 15, 101, 178
coronary arteries, 7, 13
coronary artery disease, 6
coronary heart disease, vii, 2, 15, 17, 18, 22, 23, 27, 28, 29, 30, 31
correlation, 8, 12, 14, 18, 129, 158, 181
cortex, 44, 47, 124, 181
corticotropin, ix, 121, 122
Costa Rica, 17
costimulatory molecules, 202
costs, 208, 218, 219
coughing, 210
coupling, 131
covering, 222
craving, 148
creatine, 37, 38
creatinine, 151, 152
cross-sectional study, 117
CSF, 40
CTA, 170
Cuba, 23
cultivation, 192, 193
culture, 94, 95, 96, 119, 178, 189, 191, 192, 196
CVD, vii, 1, 2, 3, 6, 8, 10, 13, 14, 19, 120
cyanide, 194
cycles, 61, 171, 172
cycling, 171
cytokines, 145, 201, 203
cytoplasm, 201
cytotoxicity, 203

D

daily living, 162
damage, viii, 21, 22, 33, 36, 37, 38, 39, 42, 43, 44, 45, 46, 47, 48
data analysis, 74
data set, 74, 78, 89, 90, 98, 195
death, 8, 17, 18, 38, 39, 44, 46, 167
defects, 167, 178
defense, 48, 185, 188, 198, 199, 200
defense mechanisms, 48
deficiency, ix, 15, 22, 31, 34, 43, 44, 46, 47, 52, 65, 67, 70, 124, 125, 134, 144, 149, 150, 151, 152, 156, 160, 161, 162, 166, 167, 171, 177, 178, 179, 180, 181, 182, 183, 185
deficit, 157
deformation, 16
degenerate, 44
degradation, 23, 36, 53, 55, 58, 61, 63, 65, 69, 124
degradation rate, 53
delivery, 125, 137, 180
demand, 208
dementia, 44, 46
demographics, 96
denaturation, 171
dengue, 117
density, 11, 28, 38, 39, 47, 127, 160, 188, 190, 191
depolarization, 130, 135
deposition, 38, 132
depression, 34, 78, 83, 88, 90, 117, 139, 148
deprivation, 50, 53, 65, 68, 70, 146, 162, 177, 184
destruction, viii, 33, 132
detection, 51, 117, 170
diabetes, 100, 101, 138, 143
diarrhea, 203
diastolic blood pressure, 14
diet, vii, 1, 2, 7, 8, 9, 12, 13, 14, 15, 17, 18, 19, 26, 27, 48, 50, 59, 69, 93, 104, 105, 109, 110, 120, 124, 125, 127, 129, 141, 142, 144, 161, 165, 168, 169, 176, 177, 179, 205, 215
dietary fat, 96, 119
dietary habits, vii, 2
dietary intake, ix, 15, 71, 72, 151, 157
dietary supplementation, 12
dieting, 116, 118
differentiation, 166, 178, 183, 201, 202
diffusion, 167, 179
digestion, 189
dilation, 6, 12

disabilities, x, 207, 208, 209, 210, 211, 212, 213, 214, 217, 218, 219, 220, 221
disability, 159, 162, 218
discomfort, 90, 94
disorder, 44, 147, 156, 208, 211, 212, 219
dissatisfaction, 83
distribution, 120, 161, 184, 212
diversity, 120, 143
DNA, 29, 39, 44, 46, 47, 48, 166, 171, 177, 181, 184, 199, 203, 204
DNA damage, 29, 44, 46, 48, 204
DNA polymerase, 171, 177
docosahexaenoic acid, 15, 30
dogs, 102, 137, 142
domain, 125, 181
donors, 136
dopamine, 34, 35, 129, 137, 141, 143, 144, 145, 146
dosage, 2, 21, 25, 27
drought, 61
drug therapy, 24
drugs, ix, 23, 24, 31, 121, 129, 130, 131, 135, 136, 168
drying, 3
duodenum, 180
duration, 3, 12, 21, 65, 153, 211, 215
dyspepsia, 210
dysphagia, 209, 215, 219, 220

E

eating, ix, 19, 45, 71, 72, 73, 78, 80, 83, 85, 86, 87, 88, 89, 90, 91, 92, 93, 94, 95, 96, 97, 115, 117, 119, 128, 130, 133, 139, 142, 216
eating disorders, ix, 71, 72, 90, 216
economic problem, viii, 71, 72
economic status, 97
edema, 25
egg, 114
eicosapentaenoic acid, 15, 30
elastin, 44, 47
elderly, ix, 48, 150, 151, 153, 156, 158, 159, 160, 161, 162, 163
elderly population, ix, 150, 151, 153, 156, 159, 160, 161
elders, 34
electrons, 35, 37
electrophoresis, 171, 173, 174, 175, 176
emotion, 78
emotions, 73, 74, 75, 89, 90
encoding, 124, 182

endocrine, 137, 166

endocrinology, 183

endoscopy, 215

endothelial cells, 6, 13, 125, 179

endothelium, 6

energy, viii, ix, x, 21, 35, 36, 49, 50, 53, 56, 59, 60, 61, 62, 63, 65, 67, 71, 73, 75, 78, 121, 122, 123, 124, 125, 126, 127, 129, 130, 132, 134, 136, 138, 139, 140, 141, 148, 167, 208, 210, 211, 212, 217, 221, 222

England, 8, 66

environment, 19, 36, 94, 95, 96, 97, 124

environmental factors, 93, 96, 122, 158, 159

enzymes, 3, 8, 21, 31, 34, 35, 37, 38, 166, 168, 177

EPA, 15, 17, 18

epidemic, 140

epidemiology, vii, 2, 3, 8

epilepsy, 147

epinephrine, 142

epithelia, 167

epithelium, 167, 188, 189, 204

erythrocytes, 191

esophagitis, 210

esophagus, 210

essential fatty acids, vii, 1, 2, 15

ester, 141

estimating, 217

ethanol, 28, 48

ethnicity, 145

Europe, vii, 1, 2, 94, 160

evidence, vii, 1, 2, 5, 7, 8, 9, 12, 13, 14, 17, 18, 19, 21, 23, 25, 26, 27, 28, 34, 35, 38, 39, 43, 45, 122, 124, 130, 131, 136, 138, 140, 159, 177, 208, 210, 211, 215, 216, 217

evolution, 124

excitability, 184

excretion, 5, 14, 58, 66, 69, 142

exercise, 9, 21, 72, 73, 78, 80, 82, 85, 86, 87, 89, 91, 93, 94, 95, 96, 97, 98, 104, 106, 119

exposure, viii, ix, 33, 150, 151, 152, 153, 154, 155, 156, 157, 158, 159, 161, 162, 179, 215

expression, x, 43, 44, 46, 47, 124, 127, 128, 129, 132, 134, 136, 138, 142, 147, 165, 166, 167, 168, 169, 174, 175, 176, 178, 179, 180, 181, 182, 183, 185, 186, 194, 201, 202, 205

extracellular matrix, 43, 47

extraction, 23, 61

F

failure, x, 21, 151, 207, 208, 210

family, 9, 96, 109, 111, 124, 168, 204

family members, 96, 109, 111

fasting, 30, 50, 51, 52, 53, 60, 66, 67, 68, 69, 126, 133, 134, 135, 144, 145

fat, vii, viii, 2, 5, 15, 19, 49, 61, 68, 72, 73, 74, 75, 76, 77, 78, 80, 81, 82, 83, 85, 86, 87, 88, 89, 90, 91, 92, 93, 96, 98, 102, 104, 105, 106, 113, 118, 119, 120, 122, 124, 129, 130, 132, 141, 142, 147, 162, 212, 217, 222

fat reduction, 119

fatigue, 21

fatty acids, viii, 15, 17, 18, 19, 29, 30, 36, 40, 49, 50, 59, 60, 61, 62, 63, 64, 65, 68, 69

feces, 189

feedback, 124, 215

feelings, 90

females, 72, 73, 77, 89, 91

fermentation, 3

fetal growth, 185

fibers, 184

fibrinogen, 17

fibroblasts, 179

filtration, 159

financial resources, 219

financing, 65

Finland, 22, 116

fish, 15, 17, 18, 19, 102, 105, 114, 152, 157

fish oil, 15, 18, 19

fitness, 73, 96, 100, 101

flavonoids, vii, 1, 2, 3, 7, 9, 25, 27

fluctuations, 8, 90

fluid, 70, 114

fluorescence, 181, 196

fluoxetine, 141

food, vii, viii, ix, 49, 50, 51, 52, 53, 59, 63, 65, 69, 70, 71, 72, 73, 75, 89, 90, 91, 92, 93, 94, 95, 96, 99, 102, 103, 104, 105, 106, 112, 114, 115, 116, 117, 118, 119, 120, 122, 123, 124, 125, 126, 127, 128, 129, 130, 131, 132, 133, 134, 135, 136, 137, 140, 143, 144, 146, 148, 150, 152, 154, 155, 156, 169, 171, 177, 182, 188, 189, 209, 210, 211, 213, 216

food intake, 72, 73, 90, 92, 117, 122, 123, 125, 126, 127, 128, 129, 130, 131, 132, 134, 135, 136, 137, 143, 144, 146, 148, 150, 152, 154, 155, 171, 177, 182, 213

food products, 156, 188

Ford, 220
fractures, ix, 149, 150, 151, 212
France, 94, 120, 156, 162
free radicals, viii, 14, 33, 35, 36, 37, 38, 45
friends, 74, 75, 77, 82, 98, 103, 106, 109, 111
frontal cortex, 134, 138
fruits, 22, 34, 35, 45
fuel, vii
functional changes, 36
furniture, 152

G

ganglion, 185
gastric mucosa, 218
gastrin, 215
gastrocnemius, 61
gastroesophageal reflux, 220, 221
gastrointestinal tract, 122, 205, 216
gastrojejunostomy, 222
gel, 40, 42
gender, 72, 73, 77, 99, 150, 153, 154, 158, 217
gender differences, 72, 73
gene, x, 123, 124, 125, 126, 128, 130, 131, 134, 137,
    138, 142, 145, 146, 148, 166, 167, 168, 172, 178,
    179, 180, 181, 182, 183, 184, 188, 194, 198, 199,
    201, 202, 204, 205
gene expression, 125, 131, 142, 146, 167, 168, 172,
    178, 179, 182, 183, 184, 188, 194, 202
generation, 30, 36, 183
genes, x, 124, 128, 165, 167, 168, 170, 182, 189,
    195, 198, 199, 200, 201, 202
genetic disorders, 167, 211
genome, 189
genotype, 145
girls, 72, 75, 77, 78, 84, 85, 88, 89, 90, 91, 99, 116
gland, 35
glasses, 102, 114
glia, 42, 44
glial cells, 47, 48
glucocorticoid receptor, 131
gluconeogenesis, 68
glucose, 58, 60, 68, 69, 127, 131, 147, 148, 167, 185
glutamate, 140, 142, 143, 144, 145, 147
glutathione, 46
goals, 218
government, 26, 76, 97
grades, 99, 100
grass, 56
gray matter, 141

grazing, 66
groups, 38, 50, 51, 54, 55, 56, 58, 59, 61, 63, 74, 75,
    78, 79, 82, 83, 84, 88, 89, 90, 93, 94, 117, 159,
    162, 188, 190, 191, 195, 196, 198, 209, 215
growth, x, 44, 47, 70, 125, 126, 165, 166, 168, 171,
    172, 176, 177, 178, 179, 182, 183, 184, 185, 197,
    201, 202, 207, 208, 209, 210, 211, 217, 220, 221
growth factor, 44, 47, 125, 165, 166, 177, 178, 182,
    183, 184, 185
growth hormone, 126, 165, 166, 178, 183, 184, 185
guidance, 215
guilt, 73, 78, 83, 88, 90
guilty, 74, 75, 77, 78, 80, 85, 86, 87, 88, 89, 98, 105,
    106
Guinea, 43
gut, 137, 188, 201, 203, 205

H

hands, 111
hazards, 117
HE, 47
healing, 215
health, vii, viii, 1, 2, 3, 8, 10, 14, 15, 26, 27, 29, 34,
    71, 72, 73, 76, 78, 90, 91, 92, 93, 96, 98, 104,
    117, 118, 119, 120, 159, 203
health effects, vii, 2
health status, 96
heart attack, 18, 22
heart disease, 17, 18, 23, 28, 30, 31, 100, 101, 104
heart failure, vii, 1, 2, 19, 21
heart rate, 18, 30
height, 97, 211, 217
hepatocytes, 178, 179, 184
high blood pressure, 18, 100, 101
high density lipoprotein, 23
high fat, 73, 91, 118, 125
high school, 76, 97, 116
hip, 151, 156, 159
hip fractures, 151, 159
hippocampus, 37, 42, 139, 142, 143
histidine, 42, 53, 168
histology, 66
homeostasis, ix, 6, 43, 121, 122, 125, 126, 127, 129,
    136, 138, 148, 151, 167, 168, 180, 181, 189, 204
hormone, ix, 11, 66, 121, 122, 123, 125, 126, 127,
    128, 129, 131, 134, 137, 139, 143, 146, 150, 152,
    159, 160, 165, 166, 178
hospitalization, x, xi, 207, 208, 218
host, x, 187, 188, 189, 198, 205

House, 153, 155
housing, ix, 96, 149, 150, 151, 153, 156
HTLV, 44, 47
human brain, 35, 46, 48
human subjects, 198
humoral immunity, 201, 203
hydrogen, 39
hydrogen peroxide, 39
hydrolysis, 42, 61, 62, 64, 65
hydroxyl, 11, 37
hydroxyl groups, 11
hypercholesterolemia, 23, 31
hyperinsulinemia, 125
hyperparathyroidism, 151, 161, 162
hypertension, 2, 8, 9, 14, 15, 19, 22, 25, 26, 27, 29,
    30
hypotensive, 8, 15
hypothalamus, 122, 124, 125, 126, 127, 128, 129,
    130, 131, 132, 133, 134, 135, 136, 138, 139, 140,
    143, 144, 145, 146, 147
hypothermia, 144
hypothesis, viii, 7, 9, 11, 12, 14, 34, 36, 44, 77, 96
hypoxemia, 218

I

identification, 61, 83, 88, 89, 117, 124, 138, 212
idiopathic, 209
IFN, 190, 192, 196, 201, 204
IL-6, 17, 18, 123, 126, 201, 202
immersion, 193
immobilization, 159
immune function, 188
immune response, x, 181, 187, 188, 189, 197, 198,
    199, 200, 202, 203
immune system, x, 22, 168, 187, 188, 198, 203, 205
immunity, 34, 188, 189
immunocompetent cells, 201, 203
immunocompromised, 203
immunoglobulin, 44, 47
immunomodulation, 203
immunomodulatory, x, 187, 188
immunoreactivity, 128, 140, 141
immunostimulatory, 205
in situ hybridization, 143
in vitro, 1, 5, 7, 13, 26, 37, 38, 39, 40, 45, 134, 140,
    188, 190, 197, 198, 202, 203
incidence, 3, 7, 9, 36, 94, 202, 208, 215
inclusion, 65
income, ix, 150, 151, 152, 154, 158, 159, 160

indication, 147
indicators, 218
indices, 162, 198
inducer, 133
induction, 132, 183, 185, 188
industrial chemicals, viii, 33
infancy, 210
infants, x, 207, 208, 209, 210, 211, 216
infection, 142, 188, 203
inflammation, 17, 188
inflammatory disease, 24
inflammatory mediators, 168, 188
influence, ix, 12, 17, 28, 50, 59, 60, 65, 95, 121, 122,
    136, 145, 168, 177, 203
informed consent, 152
infrastructure, 94, 96
ingestion, 3, 5, 6, 7, 9, 10, 11, 13, 14, 15, 26, 28,
    126, 131
inhibition, ix, 8, 13, 14, 18, 22, 23, 24, 25, 26, 46,
    121, 125, 128, 130, 133, 135, 136, 138, 139, 142,
    191, 197, 202, 215
inhibitor, 25, 144, 146, 147, 148
initiation, 36
injections, 134, 143
injury, 13, 26, 32, 39, 44, 48, 182, 215
innate immunity, 188
inoculation, 191, 195
inositol, 185
input, 56
insertion, 218
insight, 74
institutions, 219
insulin, 68, 122, 123, 125, 126, 127, 128, 129, 131,
    137, 138, 139, 140, 142, 143, 145, 146, 147, 148,
    167, 178, 179, 184, 186
insulin resistance, 123, 145
insulin sensitivity, 124, 127
insulin signaling, 125, 137, 138, 147
integration, 122
intensity, 194, 196
interaction, 117, 132, 136, 145, 147, 163, 189, 203
interactions, ix, 23, 24, 25, 75, 78, 122, 138, 140
interest, vii, 2
interferon, 192
interleukins, 126
intervention, 11, 12, 64, 83, 88, 93, 95, 119, 210,
    216, 217, 218, 219
intervention strategies, 83, 88
intestine, x, 126, 165, 166, 167, 168, 169, 170, 175,
    176, 177, 180, 181, 182

intima, 17, 22
intoxication, 160
iodine, 170
ion transport, 168, 183
ions, 40, 41, 182, 184, 185
iron, 36, 43, 46, 168, 180, 183, 186
iron transport, 168, 186
irritability, 210
ischaemic heart disease, 44
isoflavonoid, 14, 15, 27
isoflavonoids, 12, 15
isolation, 67
Israel, 161

J

Japan, 3, 7, 8, 120
jejunum, 180, 181
Jordan, 68

K

kidney, 19, 167, 180
kinase activity, 37, 124, 125, 145, 185
kinetic studies, 45
kinetics, 35, 180, 212, 215
knowledge, vii, ix, 2, 10, 26, 71, 73, 89, 91, 92, 93,
    94, 95, 96, 97, 118, 168, 185

L

lactation, 51
lactic acid, 198, 203, 205
lactobacillus, 189
language, 211, 212
laxatives, 72, 110
LDL, 3, 5, 7, 11, 13, 14, 17, 18, 22, 23, 24, 25, 26,
    27, 30, 39, 40, 41, 43
lead, 6, 12, 13, 19, 22, 23, 50, 51, 52, 104
lean body mass, 212
learning, 118
leisure, ix, 71, 159
leisure time, 159
leptin, ix, 121, 122, 123, 124, 125, 126, 127, 128,
    129, 130, 133, 134, 135, 136, 137, 138, 139, 140,
    141, 144, 145, 146, 147
lesions, 37, 38
leucine, 58
life quality, 208

lifestyle, ix, 8, 19, 26, 94, 150, 151, 156, 157, 161
ligands, 147, 181, 182
likelihood, 211, 217
lipid metabolism, 18, 30, 127, 166, 185
lipid peroxidation, 39, 40, 43, 44, 45, 47
lipids, 7, 17, 27, 28, 38, 39, 45, 47, 48, 50, 59, 66,
    67, 70, 185
lipolysis, 32
lipoproteins, 15, 28, 30, 40, 45
liquid chromatography, 42
liquids, 213, 215
liver, 5, 11, 19, 66, 69, 165, 166, 167, 168, 169, 170,
    171, 175, 176, 178, 181, 182, 183, 184
liver cells, 5
livestock, 60, 189
living conditions, 156
locus, 123, 128
longevity, viii, 33, 167
low fat diet, 93
low-density lipoprotein, 3, 7, 45
lower esophageal sphincter, 215
LTA, 188
lung cancer, 68
lycopene, vii, 1, 2, 19, 20, 22, 23, 25, 31
lymphocytes, 191
lymphoid, 47, 203
lymphoid tissue, 203
lysis, 191, 203
lysozyme, 187, 188, 190, 197

M

macromolecules, 38
macrophages, 23, 187, 188, 189, 190, 191, 193, 195,
    198, 201, 203, 204
magazines, 103
males, 72, 73, 77, 91
malignancy, 151
malnutrition, x, 68, 207, 208, 210, 211
management, x, 50, 66, 207, 212, 215, 217, 218,
    219, 220
manipulation, 92
mapping, 202
marital partners, 118
market, 157, 215
mass, 42, 66, 74, 75, 124, 125, 126, 127, 147, 217
mass spectrometry, 42
matrix, 58
maturation, 202
meals, 73, 91, 92, 94, 96, 104, 110, 210

measurement, 190, 211

measures, ix, 71, 72, 77, 143, 219

meat, 17, 68, 73, 91, 94, 102, 104, 105, 113, 114, 157

media, 17, 22, 96

median, 98, 211, 212

mediation, 125

medication, 151

Mediterranean, 29

melanin, ix, 121, 122, 123, 128, 139, 146

melanocyte stimulating hormone, 127

melanoma, 117

melatonin, 19, 20, 26, 32, 48

membranes, 15, 167, 177, 179

memory, 35

memory performance, 35

men, 11, 18, 22, 29, 45, 48, 74, 75, 86, 94, 98, 106, 116, 120, 132, 150, 152, 157, 158, 160, 162

mental health, 116

mental retardation, 37, 209

mercury, 18, 19

meta analysis, 17

metabolism, 11, 31, 36, 43, 50, 51, 66, 67, 69, 124, 131, 132, 134, 136, 139, 141, 145, 146, 148, 151, 155, 166, 167, 168, 179, 183, 198, 200

metabolites, 14

metals, 168, 181

methodology, 96

MHC, 201

mice, x, 123, 124, 125, 126, 127, 128, 129, 130, 132, 134, 136, 137, 138, 139, 140, 141, 142, 144, 145, 147, 148, 165, 167, 169, 171, 172, 175, 176, 177, 178, 179, 182, 184, 187, 188, 189, 190, 191, 192, 193, 195, 196, 197, 198, 201, 202, 203, 204, 205

microcirculation, 12, 24

micrograms, 171

micronutrients, 44, 212

microstructure, 147

migration, 14

milk, 11, 12, 14, 29, 66, 73, 102, 114, 118, 130, 157, 158, 167, 168, 215

Ministry of Education, 187

mitochondria, 19

mitogen, 125

mixing, 191

mobility, 40, 42, 163

model system, 179

models, ix, 34, 37, 75, 89, 92, 93, 94, 96, 99, 117, 122, 123, 124, 132

molecular oxygen, 35, 36, 38

molecular structure, 188

molecular weight, 36, 44, 47, 168, 182

molecules, 18, 36, 38, 39, 188, 189, 201, 202, 203

monitoring, x, 2, 27, 208, 215, 218

monograph, 207

monosodium glutamate, 132, 139, 143, 144

mood, 34, 90, 96

mood disorder, 34

morbidity, x, 155, 207, 219, 220

mortality, vii, 1, 2, 9, 15, 16, 17, 18, 19, 22, 27, 28, 29, 68

mothers, 161, 167

movement, 209, 217

mRNA, x, 67, 129, 135, 136, 138, 139, 142, 143, 144, 165, 166, 167, 168, 171, 172, 173, 174, 175, 176, 178, 179, 180, 181, 182, 183, 185, 188

MRS, 189

mucus, 203

multiple factors, ix, 121

multiplication, 90

muscle atrophy, 66

muscle mass, 53

muscles, 53, 54, 61

Muslims, 157

mutant, 138, 167

mutation, 123, 128, 147

mycobacteria, 204

myocardial infarction, vii, 1, 2, 17, 18, 19, 22, 23, 28, 29, 30, 31, 32

myocardium, 19, 53

myosin, 53, 66

N

NaCl, 169, 194

NAD, 35

NADH, 21

National Research Council, 217, 222

natural killer cell, 193

necrosis, 18, 201

needs, 24, 25, 52, 53, 63, 91, 97, 105, 114, 129, 208, 222

negative attitudes, 83, 89, 92

negative emotions, 77, 89, 90

nerve, 32

nervous system, 146

network, ix, 121, 122, 186

neural network, 138

neural networks, 138

neuroblastoma, 43, 46

neurodegeneration, 34
neurodegenerative disorders, 37
neurofibrillary tangles, 38, 42, 44
neurological disease, 36, 43
neurons, 38, 42, 44, 127, 128, 129, 131, 132, 134, 135, 139, 140, 141, 144, 146, 147, 185
neuropeptides, 122, 127
neurotoxicity, 38
neurotransmitter, 36, 130, 132, 140
neurotransmitters, 34, 35, 122, 127, 129
neutrophils, 189, 205
New South Wales, 69
New Zealand, 116
nicotinamide, 142
nitric oxide, 6, 8, 25, 37, 42, 43, 46, 136, 138, 141, 144, 146, 147, 148, 187, 190
nitric oxide synthase, 43, 144, 146, 147, 148
nitrogen, 53, 58, 170
NK cells, 198, 203
non-institutionalized, ix, 150, 151, 159
non-insulin dependent diabetes, 24
nonsense mutation, 167
norepinephrine, 34, 35, 129, 137, 139, 141, 142, 144, 146
normal aging, 48
normal distribution, 211
North America, vii, 1, 2
Norway, 8
nuclei, 124, 126, 127, 128, 130, 131, 134, 137, 139, 145
nucleic acid, 38, 166
nucleus, 37, 126, 127, 131, 132, 133, 135, 139, 141, 142, 143, 145, 146, 178
nucleus tractus solitarius, 131, 139, 141
nurses, 211
nursing, 161, 162, 167, 222
nursing home, 161, 162, 222
nutraceutical, vii, 1, 2, 22, 24, 26
nutrients, vii, 2, 75, 93, 150, 166
nutritional assessment, 212
nutritional deficiencies, x, 207, 209, 218

O

obesity, viii, ix, 25, 71, 72, 94, 116, 117, 119, 120, 121, 122, 123, 124, 125, 126, 127, 128, 129, 130, 132, 136, 138, 139, 140, 141, 142, 144, 145, 146, 147, 148, 217, 222
observations, x, 54, 61, 119, 179, 208
occlusion, 26
oil, 15, 19, 30, 169, 193
oils, 15, 29, 67, 68
older adults, 30, 158
optical density, 196
organ, viii, 33, 122, 151, 168
organism, 181
orientation, 180
osteomalacia, 156
osteoporosis, 160
output, 56, 128, 194
overload, 18
overweight, viii, 71, 72, 74, 75, 78, 80, 81, 82, 83, 85, 86, 87, 88, 89, 90, 91, 92, 94, 98, 106, 108, 116, 119
oxalate, 39
oxidation, viii, 3, 7, 13, 14, 22, 25, 33, 37, 38, 39, 40, 42, 43, 44, 45, 46, 47, 48, 61, 217, 222
oxidation products, 45, 48
oxidative damage, 22, 35, 36, 38, 39, 42, 43, 44, 45, 46, 47
oxidative stress, 6, 8, 14, 15, 35, 37, 38, 39, 43, 44, 46, 182
oxygen, 21, 22, 25, 36, 37, 42, 44, 47
oxygen consumption, 21, 36
ozone, viii, 33

P

pain, 21
pancreas, 124, 126, 181
parameter, 122
parasite, 199, 200
parathyroid, 151, 155, 159, 161, 162, 163
parathyroid hormone, 151, 155, 161, 162, 163
parents, 91, 97, 103, 109, 111, 210, 211
parietal lobe, 44
Parkinson's disease, viii, 25, 34
particles, 23
passive, 167
pasta, 104, 112, 114
pastures, 50, 66
pathogenesis, ix, 13, 22, 39, 40, 43, 44, 46, 121, 136
pathogens, 198, 202
pathologist, 212
pathways, 22, 55, 58, 125, 129, 136, 138, 139, 141, 179, 202, 204
pattern recognition, 188
PCR, 165, 170, 171, 172, 173, 174, 175, 176
peers, 96
penicillin, 191

peptidase, 200

peptide chain, viii, 33

peptides, 131, 139, 143, 145, 204

perceived control, 93

perceived norms, 118

perceptions, 76

perinatal, 68

peripheral blood, 198

peristalsis, 213

peritoneal cavity, 191

peroxidation, 26, 43, 48

peroxide, 43, 46

peroxynitrite, 42, 48

perspective, 141, 161, 183

pH, 168, 180, 190, 215

phagocyte, 188, 198

phagocytosis, 201

pharmacology, 31, 204

pharmacotherapy, 140

phenotype, 140

Philippines, 50, 66

phosphorous, 212

phosphorylation, 124, 125, 126, 179, 181

physical activity, 116, 119

physiology, 144, 183

pigs, 34, 43, 44, 46, 47, 60, 67, 70

pilot study, 29

pine, 25, 31, 32

placebo, 3, 12, 29, 30

placenta, 126

plaques, 17, 38

plasma, 2, 3, 7, 10, 11, 12, 17, 18, 23, 25, 26, 27, 28, 29, 32, 34, 35, 39, 40, 44, 47, 48, 50, 51, 52, 53, 59, 60, 61, 62, 63, 64, 65, 66, 67, 68, 69, 70, 124, 126, 127, 129, 137, 161, 165, 166, 167, 168, 169, 172, 178, 179, 180, 212

plasma levels, 2, 27, 35, 126, 127

plasma membrane, 167, 168, 180

platelet aggregation, 13, 16, 17, 18, 25, 26

plexus, 124

PM, 27, 118

polarization, 202, 205

pollution, 151, 156, 157

polymerase, 165, 183

polymerase chain reaction, 165, 183

polymers, 3, 44

polypeptide, 123, 126

polyunsaturated fatty acids, 15, 29, 30

polyuria, 24

poor, ix, x, 9, 50, 71, 72, 150, 157, 159, 207, 208, 209, 211

population, ix, 9, 34, 71, 73, 76, 90, 91, 92, 93, 97, 117, 150, 151, 153, 154, 156, 157, 158, 159, 160, 161, 162, 209, 210, 211, 212, 216, 219, 222

Portugal, 49, 54, 56, 61

positive correlation, 9

potassium, 134

potato, 73, 114

poultry, 177, 182

precipitation, 152

predictors, 74, 75, 76, 77, 78, 80, 82, 83, 85, 89, 90, 92, 98, 99, 119, 150, 154

preference, 15, 96

pregnancy, 24

preparation, 98

pressure, ix, 8, 15, 16, 18, 21, 47, 71, 72, 106

preterm infants, 221

prevention, vii, 1, 2, 13, 23, 27, 31, 34, 116, 118, 119, 189, 203

preventive programs, 151

primary hyperparathyroidism, 151

probability, 98

probe, 194

probiotic, 189

problem behavior, 119

problem behaviors, 119

production, viii, 3, 6, 17, 18, 21, 25, 38, 49, 50, 51, 66, 67, 69, 70, 123, 126, 128, 129, 166, 168, 178, 187, 188, 189, 190, 192, 196, 197, 201, 204

productivity, 66

prognosis, 117

program, 26, 119, 151, 195, 201, 202

proliferation, 14, 43, 47, 166, 177, 179, 184, 196, 198, 202, 203

promoter, 181

propagation, 40

proposition, 132

prostate, 17, 19, 29, 183

prostate cancer, 17, 19, 29

protein oxidation, viii, 34, 36, 37, 38, 41, 42, 43, 44, 45, 46, 48

protein synthesis, 53, 65, 68, 69, 177

proteins, viii, 11, 25, 34, 37, 38, 39, 40, 42, 43, 44, 45, 46, 47, 48, 51, 53, 54, 57, 58, 65, 66, 67, 125, 128, 141, 166, 167, 168, 177, 179, 182, 183, 185, 186, 189

protocol, 42, 152

proton pump inhibitors, 215

proto-oncogene, 202

psychology, 117
psychosocial factors, 92, 95, 96, 97
public awareness, 26
public health, 150
pulse, 12, 18
purchasing power, 159
purification, 67
P-value, 82
pyramidal cells, 184

Q

quality of life, viii, x, 21, 33, 207, 218, 219
quartile, 74, 75, 98

R

radiation, 154, 156, 157, 161
range, vii, x, 2, 6, 7, 9, 13, 15, 19, 74, 75, 76, 78, 98,
    133, 158, 160, 168, 181, 187, 208
reactive airway disease, 210, 218
reactive oxygen, viii, 6, 8, 33, 36, 37, 38, 46
reagents, 190
receptors, 5, 11, 13, 14, 24, 125, 126, 127, 128, 129,
    131, 132, 134, 135, 137, 139, 140, 141, 143, 145,
    146, 147, 167, 177, 183, 184, 185, 188, 204, 216
recognition, 189, 204
recovery, 21, 22, 66, 68
reduction, vii, 1, 2, 5, 6, 7, 10, 11, 12, 14, 16, 17, 18,
    19, 21, 22, 23, 25, 53, 59, 67, 130, 132, 215
regression, 74, 76, 77, 89, 90, 98, 99, 117, 150, 153,
    154, 158
regression analysis, 74, 76, 89, 99, 153, 158
regression line, 150, 154
regulation, x, 43, 48, 66, 122, 128, 130, 134, 137,
    138, 139, 141, 143, 144, 165, 166, 169, 179, 180,
    181, 182, 183, 184, 185, 189, 199, 200, 202
regulators, 123, 125, 178, 201
rehabilitation, x, 208, 211, 212, 215, 217, 221
relationship, 3, 16, 17, 73, 74, 89, 91, 92, 131, 145,
    162, 168, 210
relationships, ix, 73, 92, 98, 121
relatives, 151
relaxation, 8, 25, 94
relevance, viii, ix, 36, 47, 49, 121, 127, 136
religion, 96
repair, 45
replacement, 11, 12
reproduction, 138, 142, 167, 168

residues, viii, 33, 42, 44
resistance, 8, 12, 18, 24, 45, 48, 124, 125, 144, 147,
    178, 185, 202, 205, 210
resources, x, 60, 69, 207, 208
respiratory, 35
responsiveness, 144
retardation, 166
retention, 63, 178
reverse transcriptase, 171
ribonucleic acid, 144
ribosome, 199
rice, 104, 112, 114, 194
rickets, 156, 161
risk, vii, ix, x, 1, 2, 3, 6, 7, 8, 9, 10, 13, 14, 15, 16,
    17, 18, 19, 22, 23, 25, 26, 27, 28, 29, 30, 31, 35,
    38, 45, 73, 74, 75, 83, 88, 89, 150, 151, 156, 157,
    158, 207, 208, 211, 215, 216, 222
risk factors, vii, 1, 2, 8, 9, 18, 19, 22, 23, 25, 26, 28,
    31, 89
RNA, 168, 170, 171
rodents, 5, 58, 60, 124, 126
room temperature, 3
rural areas, 157

S

safety, 24, 25, 140, 216
sample, 76, 78, 79, 80, 81, 82, 83, 84, 85, 86, 87, 88,
    89, 97, 98, 119, 128, 161, 192
sampling, 51
satisfaction, 72, 116
saturated fat, 7, 15, 17, 19, 67
saturated fatty acids, 67
scarcity, 124
school, 72, 73, 76, 85, 88, 89, 97, 98, 103
scores, x, 35, 208, 211, 212, 218
search, 119, 142
secrete, 201
secretion, 18, 67, 126, 132, 133, 139, 162, 178, 203,
    215
sediment, 189
selecting, 118
selenium, 46
self, 83, 88, 93, 96, 117, 210
self-efficacy, 93, 117
sensitivity, 141, 144
septum, 145
series, 15, 41, 73, 212, 216
serine, 125, 200

serotonin, ix, 121, 122, 126, 130, 131, 132, 133, 134, 135, 136, 137, 138, 139, 140, 141, 142, 143, 144, 145, 146, 147, 148

serum, viii, ix, 3, 5, 6, 9, 12, 15, 17, 21, 22, 23, 24, 27, 28, 45, 48, 49, 50, 54, 56, 58, 67, 132, 150, 151, 153, 154, 160, 165, 169, 171, 177, 178, 185, 187, 188, 190, 191, 192, 193, 194, 197

services, 218

severity, viii, 35, 36, 49, 50, 65, 93, 209, 210, 211, 218, 220

shape, ix, 71, 73, 76, 90, 92, 100, 101, 111, 117

shares, 37

sharing, 172, 174, 175, 176

sheep, 50, 51, 58, 59, 63, 67, 68, 69, 70, 190, 194, 197, 202

shortage, 50

shoulders, 111

sign, 166

signaling pathway, 125, 140

signalling, 185, 189

signals, ix, x, 121, 122, 127, 128, 137, 138, 143, 144, 187, 194

sites, 124, 125, 126, 128, 130, 131, 134, 136, 138, 181

skeletal muscle, 66, 68

skewness, 211

skin, 102, 113, 128, 150, 152, 157, 212, 217

small intestine, 68, 169

smokers, 19

smoking, 9, 93, 94, 116

smooth muscle, 6, 8, 9, 14, 43, 47

smooth muscle cells, 14, 43, 47

social influences, 118

social norms, 96

social psychology, 117

social support, 96

sodium, 169, 189

software, 153, 194

South Africa, 50

soy bean, 10

Spain, 33, 66

spastic, 217

spasticity, 211

species, viii, 6, 8, 19, 22, 33, 34, 36, 37, 38, 42, 44, 45, 46, 49, 50, 51, 53, 54, 56, 60, 65, 167, 189, 201

specificity, 168

spectrophotometric method, 48

spectrophotometry, 152, 165, 169, 170

spectrum, 44, 83, 89

speech, 211, 212

spin, 37

spleen, 167, 190, 191, 192, 193, 196, 201, 203

sports, 104

SPSS, 99, 195

stages, 95, 96, 119

standard deviation, 98, 211

standards, 61, 95, 221

starch, 169

starvation, 66, 68, 69, 70

sterile, 39, 189, 191

stimulus, 130, 198, 199, 200

stomach, 126

storage, 167, 181

strain, 123, 198, 201, 205

strategies, x, 66, 96, 168, 208, 217, 219, 220

stratification, 158

stress, 6, 18, 21, 26, 31, 32, 37, 38, 39, 48, 90, 131, 138

striatum, 136, 145

structural characteristics, 168

structural protein, 37

students, 72, 73, 76, 77, 78, 79, 84, 89, 90, 91, 97, 98, 116

subcortical nuclei, 138

subcutaneous tissue, 211

substitution, 19, 139

substrates, 125

sugar, 72, 73, 91, 92, 105, 119, 169

sulfur, 215

summer, 150, 152, 153, 154, 156, 157, 158, 159

Sun, vi, 48, 147

superiority, 215

supply, viii, 9, 15, 42, 49, 180

suppression, 140

surgical intervention, 209

surplus, 37

surveillance, 189

survival, 43, 46, 124, 178, 179, 208

survival rate, 208

susceptibility, 44, 47, 93, 139

suspensions, 191, 192

symptom, vii, 1, 2

symptoms, 25, 29, 209, 211, 218

synaptic vesicles, 167, 185

syndrome, 37, 46, 47, 132

synthesis, ix, 6, 8, 23, 24, 25, 34, 35, 53, 58, 69, 131, 132, 133, 138, 139, 150, 157, 158, 167, 168, 177, 178, 184

systems, ix, 43, 50, 69, 70, 122, 126, 131, 132, 134, 138, 167
systolic blood pressure, 8, 14

T

T cell, 189, 201, 202, 203
T lymphocytes, 188
Taiwan, 8
tangles, 38
targets, 122, 128, 138, 139
taxation, 96
teachers, 76, 97, 116
teenagers, 114
telangiectasia, 220
temperature, 96, 180, 190
test statistic, 98
TGA, 59, 60, 62, 64
theory, 6, 8, 15, 36, 118
therapeutic approaches, 219
therapists, 211
therapy, 11, 13, 21, 24, 31, 37, 44, 47, 119, 203, 215, 216, 218
three-way interaction, 99
threshold, 8, 17, 151
threshold level, 8
thrombosis, 17
thymus, 192, 196
thyroid, 11
time, viii, 39, 40, 41, 71, 90, 91, 93, 96, 107, 130, 150, 152, 153, 154, 156, 158, 180, 201, 211, 216, 219
time constraints, viii, 71
tissue, viii, 9, 29, 33, 36, 37, 38, 46, 67, 68, 70, 134, 170, 177, 180, 189, 191
TLR, 204
TLR2, 189
TMC, 93, 94, 95, 96
TNF, 123, 126, 188, 190, 191, 192, 196
TNF-α, 188, 190, 191, 192, 196
toddlers, 211
total cholesterol, 3, 11, 17, 23
total energy, 217
toxic effect, 48
toxicity, 168, 180, 181, 184
training, 113
transcription, 124, 166, 168, 177, 179, 181, 183, 184, 185, 199
transcription factors, 124, 168, 177
transducer, 124, 199

transduction, 134, 168, 179, 185
transformation, 211, 212
transformations, 221
transforming growth factor, 28
transition, 8, 38, 40
transition metal, 8, 38, 40
translocation, 124, 167, 185, 203
transport, 35, 96, 125, 137, 142, 167, 168, 180, 181, 182, 185, 199
transportation, x, 165, 166
trees, 117
trend, 63, 159
trial, 5, 7, 11, 12, 13, 14, 15, 19, 21, 22, 23, 24, 25, 27, 30, 54, 58, 63, 215
triceps, 212
triggers, 189
triglycerides, 4, 17, 18, 23
trisomy, 209
trisomy 21, 209
trypsin, 190, 200
tryptophan, 131, 133, 138
tumor, x, 137, 178, 185, 188, 189, 190, 191, 195, 197, 202, 203
tumor cells, 178, 185, 195
tumor necrosis factor, 137, 188, 191
turnover, 36, 66, 131, 132, 134, 136, 138, 139, 147, 159, 160, 161, 162
type 2 diabetes, 145
tyrosine, 14, 42, 43, 124, 125, 145, 179, 185, 202

U

UK, 1, 9, 67, 171, 210
UN, 139
underlying mechanisms, 166
undernutrition, viii, 49, 50, 51, 52, 53, 54, 55, 56, 58, 59, 61, 63, 65, 66, 67, 69, 210
United States, 94, 116, 211, 216, 217
urban population, 150, 151
urea, 58, 67
urine, 53, 70
UV, 156, 157
UV radiation, 156, 157

V

vacuum, 63
validity, 216

values, 14, 52, 53, 82, 97, 98, 99, 156, 157, 194, 196, 211
variability, 194
variable(s), 24, 74, 75, 80, 82, 83, 89, 98, 153, 154, 211
variance, 171
variation, 21, 37, 63, 65, 67, 151
vascular cell adhesion molecule (VCAM), 18
vascular dementia, viii, 34, 46, 47
vasculature, 13
vasoconstriction, 12
vasodilation, 6
vasodilator, 6, 18, 28
vegetable oil, 15, 17
vegetables, 22, 35, 45, 72, 73, 93, 95, 101, 114
velocity, 12
venous insufficiency, 32
ventricle, 128
very low density lipoprotein (VLDL), 18
vessels, 6, 12, 44
villus, 180
vitamin C, viii, 34, 35, 36, 39, 41, 42, 43, 44, 45, 46, 47, 48
vitamin D, 150, 151, 152, 153, 154, 155, 156, 157, 158, 159, 160, 161, 162, 177
vitamin D deficiency, 150, 151, 160, 162
vitamin E, 44, 47
vitamins, 34, 45
vomiting, 210
vulnerability, 38

W

walking, 94
water, 3, 6, 35, 102, 110, 130, 169, 170, 189, 190

weight control, 90, 93, 118
weight gain, x, 138, 165, 166, 208, 211, 217
weight loss, viii, ix, 24, 49, 50, 52, 54, 60, 61, 65, 71, 72, 73, 74, 75, 76, 77, 78, 79, 80, 83, 84, 85, 88, 89, 90, 91, 92, 93, 94, 98, 99, 110, 111, 115, 116
weight reduction, 91
welfare, 96
well-being, 92, 98
wheat, 152
winter, ix, 150, 152, 153, 156, 157, 158, 159, 161
wintertime, 59, 69
withdrawal, 131, 215
women, 11, 12, 13, 14, 27, 28, 29, 74, 75, 86, 94, 98, 106, 116, 118, 120, 150, 151, 153, 157, 158, 159, 160, 161, 162
work, 14, 49, 60, 61, 74, 75, 98, 100, 180, 218
World Health Organization, 217
worry, 105

Y

yang, 148
yeast, 193
yield, 191
yin, 148
young women, 159

Z

zinc, x, 165, 166, 167, 168, 169, 171, 172, 176, 177, 178, 179, 180, 181, 182, 183, 184, 185
zinc oxide, 178, 185
zinc sulfate, x, 165, 166, 169, 177, 185